Brain Disorders
SOURCEBOOK

Fourth Edition

Fourth Edition

Brain Disorders
SOURCEBOOK

Basic Consumer Health Information about Acquired and Traumatic Brain Injuries, Brain Tumors, Cerebral Palsy and Other Genetic and Congenital Brain Disorders, Infections of the Brain, Epilepsy and Other Seizure Disorders, and Degenerative Neurological Disorders Such as Dementia, Huntington Disease, and Amyotrophic Lateral Sclerosis (ALS)

Along with Information on Brain Structure and Function, Current Research, a Glossary of Terms Related to Brain Disorders, and a Directory of Resources for More Information

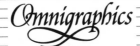

Omnigraphics

Bibliographic Note
Because this page cannot legibly accommodate all the copyright notices, the Bibliographic
Note portion of the Preface constitutes an extension of the copyright notice.

* * *

Omnigraphics, Inc.
Editorial Services provided by Omnigraphics, Inc.,
a division of Relevant Information, Inc.

Keith Jones, *Managing Editor*

* * *

Copyright © 2015 Relevant Information, Inc.
ISBN 978-0-7808-1352-6
E-ISBN 978-0-7808-1397-7

Table of Contents

Part III: Brain Infections

Part IV: Acquired and Traumatic Brain Injuries

Part VIII: Other Brain Disorders

Part IX: Additional Help and Information

Preface

About This Book

Millions of Americans and their families experience the daily challenges of living with physical, mental, or emotional difficulties that result from brain disorders caused by heredity, infection, injury, tumors, or degeneration. For example, an estimated four million people are currently living with the effects of stroke, which is the leading cause of serious, long-term disability in adults. Another 5 million individuals live with Alzheimer disease, and each year 1.7 million Americans suffer a traumatic brain injury. Although damage to the brain may result in permanent disability, with appropriate treatment and follow-up care, many affected individuals are able to participate fully in life's activities.

Brain Disorders Sourcebook, Fourth Edition provides readers with updated information about basic brain function and the development and changes our brains experience as we age. It describes degenerative neurological disorders, such as Alzheimer's disease and other dementias, Parkinson disease, and amyotrophic lateral sclerosis (ALS). It also discusses brain injuries, infections, tumors, and congenital and seizure, disorders. Information on current research, a glossary of related terms and a directory of organizations about brain disorders is also included.

How to Use This Book

This book is divided into parts and chapters. Parts focus on broad areas of interest. Chapters are devoted to single topics within a part.

Part I: An Overview of the Brain describes the architecture of the human brain and the biology of thought. It details brain development through the aging process, including the effects of maltreatment on early brain development. The impact of drug addiction on the brain is discussed, and the dangers of exposure to environmental toxins are described. The wide range of tests used to diagnose neurological disorders is described.

Part II: Degenerative Brain Disorders offers an overview of dementia and details on specific forms, including frontotemporal, progressive supranuclear, lewy body, and multi-infarct dementias. Degenerative diseases including Alzheimer's, ALS, cerebral palsy, Huntington's, and Parkinson's disease are also described, as are less-known diseases such as Binswanger, Creutzfeldt-Jakob, and Batten diseases.

Part III: Brain Infections discusses different infections that can lead to neurological damage or disorders, including infection from the tapeworm parasite and, complications of AIDS. Other viral and bacterial infections with neurological complications resulting from inflammation of veins, arteries and capillaries are also covered.

Part IV: Acquired and Traumatic Brain Injuries includes detailed coverage of mild and traumatic brain injury types, signs and symptoms, diagnosis, and treatment options.. It also provides an overview of stroke, types of strokes, risks, treatment options, and the research that is currently being done.

Part V: Congenital Brain Disorders highlights the complications of arteriovenous malformations, which are defects of the circulatory system that are generally believed to arise during embryonic or fetal development or soon after birth. It also covers the conditions that may damage or cause the abnormal or incomplete development of the nervous system in a child.

Part VI: Brain Tumors discusses the conditions that can occur due to high pressure within the spaces that surround the brain and spinal cord, and the excessive accumulation of fluid in the brain. Specific types of brain tumors are described, as well as their classification, treatment and managment.

Part VII: Seizures includes a detailed discussion of epilepsy and nonepileptic seizures, including information about their diagnosis, treatment, and management. Information on specific seizure disorders affecting or beginning in infants and children, including febrile seizures, infantile spasms, and Lennox-Gastaut syndrome is also included.

Part VIII: Other Brain Disorders includes information on neurological conditions, such as agnosia, Chiari malformation, encephalocele, multiple sclerosis, narcolepsy, peripheral neuropathy, restless leg syndrome and Wernicke-Korsakoff syndrome. Information about headache and memory loss is also included.

Part IX: Additional Help and Information provides information on current brain disorder-related research, a glossary of terms and a directory of organizations that are resources for additional information and offer help and support for patients and families dealing with brain disorders.

Bibliographic Note

This volume contains documents and excerpts from publications issued by the following U.S. government agencies: Agency for Toxic Substances and Disease Registry (ATSDR); Centers for Disease Control and Prevention (CDC); Child Welfare Information Gateway; Genetic and Rare Diseases Information Center (GARD); National Institute on Aging (NIA); National Institute on Drug Abuse (NIDA); National Eye Institute (NEI); National Institutes of Health (NIH); and National Institute of Neurological Disorders and Stroke (NINDS).

About the Health Reference Series

The *Health Reference Series* is designed to provide basic medical information for patients, families, caregivers, and the general public. Each volume takes a particular topic and provides comprehensive coverage. This is especially important for people who may be dealing with a newly diagnosed disease or a chronic disorder in themselves or in a family member. People looking for preventive guidance, information about disease warning signs, medical statistics, and risk factors for health problems will also find answers to their questions in the *Health Reference Series*. The *Series*, however, is not intended to serve as a tool for diagnosing illness, in prescribing treatments, or as a substitute for the physician/patient relationship. All people concerned about medical symptoms or the possibility of disease are encouraged to seek professional care from an appropriate health care provider.

A Note about Spelling and Style

Health Reference Series editors use *Stedman's Medical Dictionary* as an authority for questions related to the spelling of medical terms and the *Chicago Manual of Style* for questions related to grammatical structures, punctuation, and other editorial concerns. Consistent adherence is not always possible, however, because the individual volumes within the *Series* include many documents from a wide variety of different producers, and the editor's primary goal is to present material from each source as accurately as is possible. This sometimes means that information in different chapters or sections may follow other guidelines and alternate spelling authorities.

Our Advisory Board

We would like to thank the following board members for providing guidance to the development of this Series:

Dr. Lynda Baker, Associate Professor of Library and
Information Science, Wayne State University,
Detroit, MI

Nancy Bulgarelli, William Beaumont Hospital Library,
Royal Oak, MI

Karen Imarisio, Bloomfield Township Public Library,
Bloomfield Township, MI

Karen Morgan, Mardigian Library, University of
Michigan-Dearborn, Dearborn, MI

Rosemary Orlando, St. Clair Shores Public Library,
St. Clair Shores, MI

Health Reference Series Update Policy

The inaugural book in the *Health Reference Series* was the first edition of Cancer Sourcebook published in 1989. Since then, the Series has been enthusiastically received by librarians and in the medical community. In order to maintain the standard of providing high-quality health information for the layperson the editorial staff at Omnigraphics felt it was necessary to implement a policy of updating volumes when warranted.

Medical researchers have been making tremendous strides, and it is the purpose of the *Health Reference Series* to stay current with the most recent advances. Each decision to update a volume is made on an individual basis. Some of the considerations include how much new information is available and the feedback we receive from people who use the books. If there is a topic you would like to see added to the update list, or an area of medical concern you feel has not been adequately addressed, please write to:

Editor
Health Reference Series
Omnigraphics, Inc.
155 W. Congress, Suite 200
Detroit, MI 48226

Part One

An Overview of the Brain

Chapter 1

Brain Basics: Know Your Brain

Introduction

The brain is the most complex part of the human body. This three-pound organ is the seat of intelligence, interpreter of the senses, initiator of body movement, and controller of behavior. Lying in its bony shell and washed by protective fluid, the brain is the source of all the qualities that define our humanity. The brain is the crown jewel of the human body.

For centuries, scientists and philosophers have been fascinated by the brain, but until recently they viewed the brain as nearly incomprehensible. Now, however, the brain is beginning to relinquish its secrets. Scientists have learned more about the brain in the last 10 years than in all previous centuries because of the accelerating pace of research in neurological and behavioral science and the development of new research techniques.

This chapter is a basic introduction to the human brain. It may help you understand how the healthy brain works, how to keep it healthy, and what happens when the brain is diseased or dysfunctional.

This chapter includes excerpts from "Brain Basics: Know Your Brain," National Institute of Neurological Disorders and Stroke (NINDS), April 28, 2014; and from "Alzheimer's Disease: Unraveling the Mystery," National Institute of Aging (NIA), January 22, 2015.

3

The Architecture of the Brain

The brain is like a committee of experts. All the parts of the brain work together, but each part has its own special properties. The brain can be divided into three basic units: the forebrain, the midbrain, and the hindbrain.

The hindbrain includes the upper part of the spinal cord, the brain stem, and a wrinkled ball of tissue called the **cerebellum** (1). The hindbrain controls the body's vital functions such as respiration and heart rate. The cerebellum coordinates movement and is involved in learned rote movements. When you play the piano or hit a tennis ball you are activating the cerebellum. The uppermost part of the brainstem is the midbrain, which controls some reflex actions and is part of the circuit involved in the control of eye movements and other voluntary movements. The forebrain is the largest and most highly developed part of the human brain: it consists primarily of the **cerebrum** (2) and the structures hidden beneath it (see "The Inner Brain").

When people see pictures of the brain it is usually the cerebrum that they notice. The cerebrum sits at the topmost part of the brain and is the source of intellectual activities. It holds your memories, allows you to plan, enables you to imagine and think. It allows you to recognize friends, read books, and play games.

The cerebrum is split into two halves (hemispheres) by a deep fissure. Despite the split, the two cerebral hemispheres communicate with each other through a thick tract of nerve fibers that lies at the base of this fissure. Although the two hemispheres seem to be mirror images of each other, they are different. For instance, the ability to form words seems to lie primarily in the left hemisphere, while the right hemisphere seems to control many abstract reasoning skills.

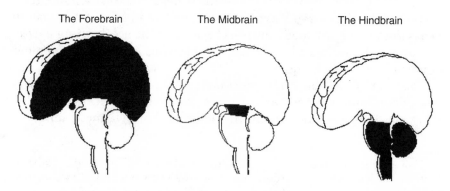

Figure 1.1. *Basic Units of the Brain*

For some as-yet-unknown reason, nearly all of the signals from the brain to the body and vice-versa cross over on their way to and from the brain. This means that the right cerebral hemisphere primarily controls the left side of the body and the left hemisphere primarily controls the right side. When one side of the brain is damaged, the opposite side of the body is affected. For example, a stroke in the right hemisphere of the brain can leave the left arm and leg paralyzed.

The Geography of Thought

Each cerebral hemisphere can be divided into sections, or lobes, each of which specializes in different functions. To understand each lobe and its specialty we will take a tour of the cerebral hemispheres, starting with the two **frontal lobes** (3), which lie directly behind the forehead. When you plan a schedule, imagine the future, or use reasoned arguments, these two lobes do much of the work. One of the ways the frontal lobes seem to do these things is by acting as short-term storage sites, allowing one idea to be kept in mind while other ideas are considered. In the rearmost portion of each frontal lobe is a **motor area** (4), which helps control voluntary movement. A nearby

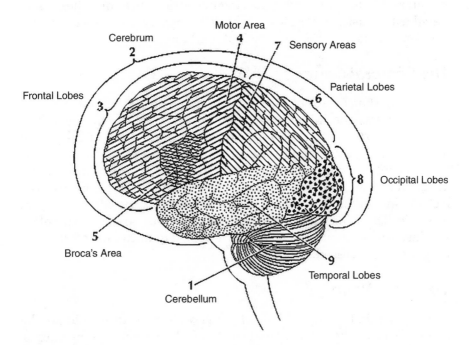

Figure 1.2. *Lobes and Areas of the Brain*

place on the left frontal lobe called **Broca's area** (5) allows thoughts to be transformed into words.

When you enjoy a good meal—the taste, aroma, and texture of the food—two sections behind the frontal lobes called the **parietal lobes** (6) are at work. The forward parts of these lobes, just behind the motor areas, are the primary **sensory areas** (7). These areas receive information about temperature, taste, touch, and movement from the rest of the body. Reading and arithmetic are also functions in the repertoire of each parietal lobe.

As you look at the words and pictures on this page, two areas at the back of the brain are at work. These lobes, called the **occipital lobes** (8), process images from the eyes and link that information with images stored in memory. Damage to the occipital lobes can cause blindness.

The last lobes on our tour of the cerebral hemispheres are the **temporal lobes** (9), which lie in front of the visual areas and nest under the parietal and frontal lobes. Whether you appreciate symphonies or rock music, your brain responds through the activity of these lobes. At the top of each temporal lobe is an area responsible for receiving information from the ears. The underside of each temporal lobe plays a crucial role in forming and retrieving memories, including those associated with music. Other parts of this lobe seem to integrate memories and sensations of taste, sound, sight, and touch.

The Cerebral Cortex

Coating the surface of the cerebrum and the cerebellum is a vital layer of tissue the thickness of a stack of two or three dimes. It is called the cortex, from the Latin word for bark. Most of the actual information processing in the brain takes place in the cerebral cortex. When people talk about "gray matter" in the brain they are talking about this thin rind. The cortex is gray because nerves in this area lack the insulation that makes most other parts of the brain appear to be white. The folds in the brain add to its surface area and therefore increase the amount of gray matter and the quantity of information that can be processed.

The Inner Brain

Deep within the brain, hidden from view, lie structures that are the gatekeepers between the spinal cord and the cerebral hemispheres.

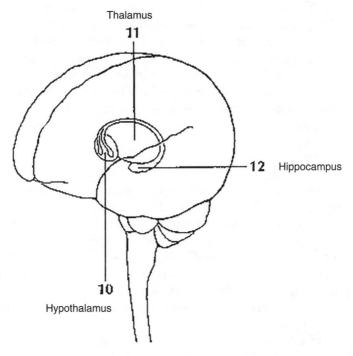

Thalamus

11

12 Hippocampus

10
Hypothalamus

Figure 1.3. *The Inner Brain*

These structures not only determine our emotional state, they also modify our perceptions and responses depending on that state, and allow us to initiate movements that we make without thinking about them. Like the lobes in the cerebral hemispheres, the structures described below come in pairs: each is duplicated in the opposite half of the brain.

The **hypothalamus** (10), about the size of a pearl, directs a multitude of important functions. It wakes you up in the morning, and gets the adrenaline flowing during a test or job interview. The hypothalamus is also an important emotional center, controlling the molecules that make you feel exhilarated, angry, or unhappy. Near the hypothalamus lies the **thalamus** (11), a major clearinghouse for information going to and from the spinal cord and the cerebrum.

An arching tract of nerve cells leads from the hypothalamus and the thalamus to the **hippocampus** (12). This tiny nub acts as a memory indexer—sending memories out to the appropriate part of the cerebral hemisphere for long-term storage and retrieving them when necessary. The **amygdala** (not shown) is an almond-shaped structure involved in processing and remembering strong emotions such as fear. It is located in the temporal lobe just in front of the hippocampus. The **basal ganglia** (not shown) are clusters of nerve cells surrounding the thalamus. They are responsible for initiating and integrating movements. Parkinson's disease, which results in tremors, rigidity, and a stiff, shuffling walk, is a disease of nerve cells that lead into the basal ganglia.

Making Connections

The brain and the rest of the nervous system are composed of many different types of cells, but the primary functional unit is a cell called the neuron. All sensations, movements, thoughts, memories, and feelings are the result of signals that pass through neurons. Neurons consist of three parts. The **cell body** (13) contains the nucleus, where most of the molecules that the neuron needs to survive and function are manufactured. **Dendrites** (14) extend out from the cell body like the branches of a tree and receive messages from other nerve cells. Signals then pass from the dendrites through the cell body and may travel away from the cell body down an **axon** (15) to another neuron, a muscle cell, or cells in some other organ. The neuron is usually surrounded by many support cells. Some types of cells wrap around the axon to form an insulating **sheath** (16). This sheath can include a fatty molecule called myelin, which provides insulation for the axon and helps nerve signals travel faster and farther. Axons may be very short, such as those that carry signals from one cell in the cortex to another cell less than a hair's width away. Or axons may be very long, such as those that carry messages from the brain all the way down the spinal cord.

Scientists have learned a great deal about neurons by studying the synapse—the place where a signal passes from the neuron to another cell. When the signal reaches the end of the axon it stimulates the release of **tiny sacs** (17). These sacs release chemicals known as **neurotransmitters** (18) into the **synapse** (19). The neurotransmitters cross the synapse and attach to **receptors** (20) on the neighboring cell. These receptors can change the properties of the receiving cell. If the receiving cell is also a neuron, the signal can continue the transmission to the next cell.

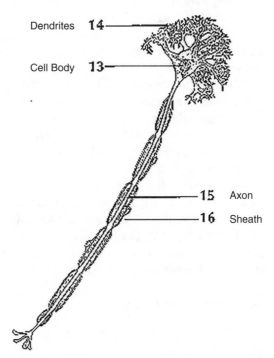

Dendrites **14**

Cell Body **13**

15 Axon

16 Sheath

Figure 1.4. *The Neuron*

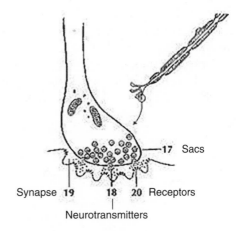

Figure 1.5. *The Synapse*

17 Sacs

Synapse **19** **18** **20** Receptors

Neurotransmitters

Some Key Neurotransmitters at Work

Acetylcholine is called an **excitatory neurotransmitter** because it generally makes cells more excitable. It governs muscle contractions and causes glands to secrete hormones. Alzheimer's disease, which initially affects memory formation, is associated with a shortage of acetylcholine.

GABA (gamma-aminobutyric acid) is called an inhibitory neurotransmitter because it tends to make cells less excitable. It helps control muscle activity and is an important part of the visual system. Drugs that increase GABA levels in the brain are used to treat epileptic seizures and tremors in patients with Huntington's disease.

Serotonin is a neurotransmitter that constricts blood vessels and brings on sleep. It is also involved in temperature regulation. Dopamine is an inhibitory neurotransmitter involved in mood and the control of complex movements. The loss of dopamine activity in some portions of the brain leads to the muscular rigidity of Parkinson's disease. Many medications used to treat behavioral disorders work by modifying the action of dopamine in the brain.

Neurological Disorders

When the brain is healthy it functions quickly and automatically. But when problems occur, the results can be devastating. Some 50 million people in this country—one in five—suffer from damage to the nervous system. Some of the major types of disorders resulting from damage to the nervous system include: neurogenetic diseases (such as Huntington's disease and muscular dystrophy), developmental disorders (such as cerebral palsy), degenerative diseases of adult life (such as Parkinson's disease and Alzheimer's disease), metabolic diseases (such as Gaucher's disease), cerebrovascular diseases (such as stroke and vascular dementia), trauma (such as spinal cord and head injury), convulsive disorders (such as epilepsy), infectious diseases (such as AIDS dementia), and brain tumors.

Chapter 2

Brain Development and Aging

Chapter Contents

Section 2.1

Brain Development in Childhood

Text in this section is excerpted from "Understanding the Effects of
Maltreatment on Brain Development," Child Welfare Information
Gateway, November, 2009.

How the Brain Develops

What we have learned about the process of brain development
has helped us understand more about the roles both genetics and the
environment play in our development. It appears that genetics predisposes us to develop in certain ways. But our experiences, including
our interactions with other people, have a significant impact on how
our predispositions are expressed. In fact, research now shows that
many capacities thought to be fixed at birth are actually dependent
on a sequence of experiences combined with heredity. Both factors are
essential for optimum development of the human brain (Shonkoff and
Phillips, 2000).

The Newborn Brain

The raw material of the brain is the nerve cell, called the *neuron*.
When babies are born, they have almost all of the neurons they will
ever have, more than 100 billion of them. Although research indicates
some neurons are developed after birth and well into adulthood, the
neurons babies have at birth are primarily what they have to work
with as they develop into children, adolescents, and adults.

During fetal development, neurons are created and migrate to form
the various parts of the brain. As neurons migrate, they also differentiate, so they begin to "specialize" in response to chemical signals
(Perry, 2002). This process of development occurs sequentially from
the "bottom up," that is, from the more primitive sections of the brain
to the more sophisticated sections (Perry, 2000a). The first areas of
the brain to fully develop are the brainstem and midbrain; they govern
the bodily functions necessary for life, called the autonomic functions.
At birth, these lower portions of the nervous system are very well

developed, whereas the higher regions (the limbic system and cerebral cortex) are still rather primitive (Zero to Three, 2009).

Newborns' brains allow babies to do many things, including breathe, eat, sleep, see, hear, smell, make noise, feel sensations, and recognize the people close to them. But the majority of brain growth and development takes place after birth, especially in the higher brain regions involved in regulating emotions, language, and abstract thought. Each region manages its assigned functions through complex processes, often using chemical messengers (such as neurotransmitters and hormones) to help transmit information to other parts of the brain and body (Perry, 2000a).

The Growing Baby's Brain

Brain development, or learning, is actually the process of creating, strengthening, and discarding connections among the neurons; these connections are called synapses. Synapses organize the brain by forming pathways that connect the parts of the brain governing everything we do—from breathing and sleeping to thinking and feeling. This is the essence of postnatal brain development, because at birth, very few synapses have been formed. The synapses present at birth are primarily those that govern our bodily functions such as heart rate, breathing, eating, and sleeping.

The development of synapses occurs at an astounding rate during children's early years, in response to the young child's experiences. At its peak, the cerebral cortex of a healthy toddler may create 2 million synapses per second (Zero to Three, 2009). By the time children are 3, their brains have approximately 1,000 trillion synapses, many more than they will ever need. Some of these synapses are strengthened and remain intact, but many are gradually discarded. This process of synapse elimination—or pruning—is a normal part of development (Shonkoff & Phillips, 2000). By the time children reach adolescence, about half of their synapses have been discarded, leaving the number they will have for most of the rest of their lives. Brain development continues throughout the lifespan. This allows us to continue to learn, remember, and adapt to new circumstances (Ackerman, 2007).

Another important process that takes place in the developing brain is myelination. Myelin is the white fatty tissue that insulates mature brain cells by forming a sheath, thus ensuring clear transmission across synapses. Young children process information slowly because their brain cells lack the myelin necessary for fast, clear nerve impulse transmission (Zero to Three, 2009). Like other neuronal growth processes, myelination begins in the primary motor and sensory areas (the brain stem and cortex) and gradually progresses to the higher-order regions that control thought, memories, and feelings. Also, like other neuronal growth processes, a child's experiences affect the rate and growth of myelination, which continues into young adulthood (Shonkoff & Phillips, 2000).

By the age of 3, a baby's brain has reached almost 90 percent of its adult size. The growth in each region of the brain largely depends on receiving stimulation, which spurs activity in that region. This stimulation provides the foundation for learning.

Plasticity—The Influence of Environment

Researchers use the term plasticity to describe the brain's ability to change in response to repeated stimulation. The extent of a brain's plasticity is dependent on the stage of development and the particular brain system or region affected (Perry, 2006). For instance, the lower parts of the brain, which control basic functions such as breathing and heart rate, are less flexible than the higher functioning cortex, which controls thoughts and feelings. While cortex plasticity may lessen as a child gets older, some degree of plasticity remains. In fact, this brain plasticity is what allows us to keep learning into adulthood and throughout our lives.

The developing brain's ongoing adaptations are the result of both genetics and experience. Our brains prepare us to expect certain experiences by forming the pathways needed to respond to those experiences. For example, our brains are "wired" to respond to the sound of speech; when babies hear people speaking, the neural systems in their brains responsible for speech and language receive the necessary stimulation to organize and function (Perry, 2006). The more babies are exposed to people speaking, the stronger their related synapses become. If the appropriate exposure does not happen, the pathways developed in anticipation may be discarded. This is sometimes referred to as the concept of "use it or lose it." It is through these processes of creating, strengthening, and discarding synapses that our brains adapt to our unique environment.

The ability to adapt to our environment is a part of normal development. Children growing up in cold climates, on rural farms, or in large sibling groups learn how to function in those environments. But regardless of the general environment, all children need stimulation and nurturance for healthy development. If these are lacking—if a child's caretakers are indifferent or hostile—the child's brain development may be impaired. Because the brain adapts to its environment, it will adapt to a negative environment just as readily as it will adapt to a positive one.

Sensitive Periods

Researchers believe that there are sensitive periods for development of certain capabilities. These refer to windows of time in the developmental process when certain parts of the brain may be most susceptible to particular experiences. Animal studies have shed light on sensitive periods, showing, for example, that animals that are artificially blinded during the sensitive period for developing vision may never develop the capability to see, even if the blinding mechanism is later removed.

It is more difficult to study human sensitive periods. But we know that, if certain synapses and neuronal pathways are not repeatedly activated, they may be discarded, and the capabilities they promised may be diminished. For example, infants have the genetic predisposition to form strong attachments to their primary caregivers. But if a child's caregivers are unresponsive or threatening, and the attachment process is disrupted, the child's ability to form any healthy relationships during his or her life may be impaired (Perry, 2001a).

While sensitive periods exist for development and learning, we also know that the plasticity of the brain often allows children to recover from missing certain experiences. Both children and adults may be able to make up for missed experiences later in life, but it may be more difficult. This is especially true if a young child was deprived of certain stimulation, which resulted in the pruning of synapses (neuronal connections) relevant to that stimulation and the loss of neuronal pathways. As children progress through each developmental stage, they will learn and master each step more easily if their brains have built an efficient network of pathways.

Memories

The organizing framework for children's development is based on the creation of memories. When repeated experiences strengthen a neuronal pathway, the pathway becomes encoded, and it eventually becomes a memory. Children learn to put one foot in front of the other to walk. They learn words to express themselves. And they learn that a smile usually brings a smile in return. At some point, they no longer have to think much about these processes—their brains manage these experiences with little effort because the memories that have been created allow for a smooth, efficient flow of information.

The creation of memories is part of our adaptation to our environment. Our brains attempt to understand the world around us and fashion our interactions with that world in a way that promotes our survival and, hopefully, our growth. But if the early environment is abusive or neglectful, our brains will create memories of these experiences that may adversely color our view of the world throughout our life.

Babies are born with the capacity for *implicit memory*, which means that they can perceive their environment and recall it in certain unconscious ways (Applegate & Shapiro, 2005). For instance, they recognize their mother's voice from an unconscious memory. These early implicit memories may have a significant impact on a child's subsequent attachment relationships.

In contrast, *explicit memory*, which develops around age 2, refers to conscious memories and is tied to language development. Explicit memory allows children to talk about themselves in the past and future or in different places or circumstances through the process of conscious recollection (Applegate & Shapiro, 2005).

Sometimes, children who have been abused or suffered other trauma may not retain or be able to access explicit memories for their experiences. However, they may retain implicit memories of the physical or emotional sensations, and these implicit memories may produce flashbacks, nightmares, or other uncontrollable reactions (Applegate & Shapiro, 2005). This may be the case with very young children or infants who suffer abuse or neglect.

Section 2.2

The Adolescent Brain

Text in this section is excerpted from "The Teen Brain: Still Under Construction," National Institute of Mental Health (NIMH), 2011.

Introduction

One of the ways that scientists have searched for the causes of mental illness is by studying the development of the brain from birth to adulthood. Powerful new technologies have enabled them to track the growth of the brain and to investigate the connections between brain function, development, and behavior.

The research has turned up some surprises, among them the discovery of striking changes taking place during the teen years. These findings have altered long-held assumptions about the timing of brain maturation. In key ways, the brain doesn't look like that of an adult until the early 20s.

An understanding of how the brain of an adolescent is changing may help explain a puzzling contradiction of adolescence: young people at this age are close to a lifelong peak of physical health, strength, and mental capacity, and yet, for some, this can be a hazardous age. Mortality rates jump between early and late adolescence. Rates of death by injury between ages 15 to 19 are about six times that of the rate between ages 10 and 14. Crime rates are highest among young males and rates of alcohol abuse are high relative to other ages. Even though most adolescents come through this transitional age well, it's important to understand the risk factors for behavior that can have serious consequences. Genes, childhood experience, and the environment in which a young person reaches adolescence all shape behavior. Adding to this complex picture, research is revealing how all these factors act in the context of a brain that is changing, with its own impact on behavior.

The more we learn, the better we may be able to understand the abilities and vulnerabilities of teens, and the significance of this stage for life-long mental health.

The fact that so much change is taking place beneath the surface may be something for parents to keep in mind during the ups and downs of adolescence.

The "Visible" Brain

A clue to the degree of change taking place in the teen brain came from studies in which scientists did brain scans of children as they grew from early childhood through age 20. The scans revealed unexpectedly late changes in the volume of gray matter, which forms the thin, folding outer layer or cortex of the brain. The cortex is where the processes of thought and memory are based. Over the course of childhood, the volume of gray matter in the cortex increases and then declines. A decline in volume is normal at this age and is in fact a necessary part of maturation.

The assumption for many years had been that the volume of gray matter was highest in very early childhood, and gradually fell as a child grew. The more recent scans, however, revealed that the high point of the volume of gray matter occurs during early adolescence.

17

While the details behind the changes in volume on scans are not completely clear, the results push the timeline of brain maturation into adolescence and young adulthood. In terms of the volume of gray matter seen in brain images, the brain does not begin to resemble that of an adult until the early 20s.

The scans also suggest that different parts of the cortex mature at different rates. Areas involved in more basic functions mature first: those involved, for example, in the processing of information from the senses, and in controlling movement. The parts of the brain responsible for more "top-down" control, controlling impulses, and planning ahead—the hallmarks of adult behavior—are among the last to mature.

What's Gray Matter?

The details of what is behind the increase and decline in gray matter are still not completely clear. Gray matter is made up of the cell bodies of neurons, the nerve fibers that project from them, and support cells. One of the features of the brain's growth in early life is that there is an early blooming of synapses—the connections between brain cells or neurons—followed by pruning as the brain matures. Synapses are the relays over which neurons communicate with each other and are the basis of the working circuitry of the brain. Already more numerous than an adult's at birth, synapses multiply rapidly in the first months of life. A 2-year-old has about half again as many synapses as an adult. (For an idea of the complexity of the brain: a cube of brain matter, 1 millimeter on each side, can contain between 35 and 70 million neurons and an estimated 500 billion synapses.)

Scientists believe that the loss of synapses as a child matures is part of the process by which the brain becomes more efficient. Although genes play a role in the decline in synapses, animal research has shown that experience also shapes the decline. Synapses "exercised" by experience survive and are strengthened, while others are pruned away. Scientists are working to determine to what extent the changes in gray matter on brain scans during the teen years reflect growth and pruning of synapses.

A Spectrum of Change

Research using many different approaches is showing that more than gray matter is changing:

- Connections between different parts of the brain increase throughout childhood and well into adulthood. As the brain develops, the fibers connecting nerve cells are wrapped in a

18

protein that greatly increases the speed with which they can transmit impulses from cell to cell. The resulting increase in connectivity—a little like providing a growing city with a fast, integrated communication system—shapes how well different parts of the brain work in tandem. Research is finding that the extent of connectivity is related to growth in intellectual capacities such as memory and reading ability.

- Several lines of evidence suggest that the brain circuitry involved in emotional responses is changing during the teen years. Functional brain imaging studies, for example, suggest that the responses of teens to emotionally loaded images and situations are heightened relative to younger children and adults. The brain changes underlying these patterns involve brain centers and signaling molecules that are part of the reward system with which the brain motivates behavior. These age-related changes shape how much different parts of the brain are activated in response to experience, and in terms of behavior, the urgency and intensity of emotional reactions.

- Enormous hormonal changes take place during adolescence. Reproductive hormones shape not only sex-related growth and behavior, but overall social behavior. Hormone systems involved in the brain's response to stress are also changing during the teens. As with reproductive hormones, stress hormones can have complex effects on the brain, and as a result, behavior.

- In terms of sheer intellectual power, the brain of an adolescent is a match for an adult's. The capacity of a person to learn will never be greater than during adolescence. At the same time, behavioral tests, sometimes combined with functional brain imaging, suggest differences in how adolescents and adults carry out mental tasks. Adolescents and adults seem to engage different parts of the brain to different extents during tests requiring calculation and impulse control, or in reaction to emotional content.

- Research suggests that adolescence brings with it brain-based changes in the regulation of sleep that may contribute to teens' tendency to stay up late at night. Along with the obvious effects of sleep deprivation, such as fatigue and difficulty maintaining attention, inadequate sleep is a powerful contributor to irritability and depression. Studies of children and adolescents have found that sleep deprivation can increase impulsive behavior;

some researchers report finding that it is a factor in delinquency. Adequate sleep is central to physical and emotional health.

The Changing Brain and Behavior in Teens

One interpretation of all these findings is that in teens, the parts of the brain involved in emotional responses are fully online, or even more active than in adults, while the parts of the brain involved in keeping emotional, impulsive responses in check are still reaching maturity. Such a changing balance might provide clues to a youthful appetite for novelty, and a tendency to act on impulse—without regard for risk.

While much is being learned about the teen brain, it is not yet possible to know to what extent a particular behavior or ability is the result of a feature of brain structure—or a change in brain structure. Changes in the brain take place in the context of many other factors, among them, inborn traits, personal history, family, friends, community, and culture.

Alcohol and the Teen Brain

Adults drink more frequently than teens, but when teens drink they tend to drink larger quantities than adults. There is evidence to suggest that the adolescent brain responds to alcohol differently than the adult brain, perhaps helping to explain the elevated risk of binge drinking in youth. Drinking in youth, and intense drinking are both risk factors for later alcohol dependence. Findings on the developing brain should help clarify the role of the changing brain in youthful drinking, and the relationship between youth drinking and the risk of addiction later in life.

Teens and the Brain: More Questions for Research

Scientists continue to investigate the development of the brain and the relationship between the changes taking place, behavior, and health. The following questions are among the important ones that are targets of research:

- How do experience and environment interact with genetic pre-programming to shape the maturing brain, and as a result, future abilities and behavior? In other words, to what extent does what a teen does and learns shape his or her brain over the rest of a lifetime?

- In what ways do features unique to the teen brain play a role in the high rates of illicit substance use and alcohol abuse in the late teen to young adult years? Does the adolescent capacity for learning make this a stage of particular vulnerability to addiction?

- Why is it so often the case that, for many mental disorders, symptoms first emerge during adolescence and young adulthood?

This last question has been the central reason to study brain development from infancy to adulthood. Scientists increasingly view mental illnesses as developmental disorders that have their roots in the processes involved in how the brain matures. By studying how the circuitry of the brain develops, scientists hope to identify when and for what reasons development goes off track. Brain imaging studies have revealed distinctive variations in growth patterns of brain tissue in youth who show signs of conditions affecting mental health. Ongoing research is providing information on how genetic factors increase or reduce vulnerability to mental illness; and how experiences during infancy, childhood, and adolescence can increase the risk of mental illness or protect against it.

The Adolescent and Adult Brain

It is not surprising that the behavior of adolescents would be a study in change, since the brain itself is changing in such striking ways. Scientists emphasize that the fact that the teen brain is in transition doesn't mean it is somehow not up to par. It is different from both a child's and an adult's in ways that may equip youth to make the transition from dependence to independence. The capacity for learning at this age, an expanding social life, and a taste for exploration and limit testing may all, to some extent, be reflections of age-related biology.

Understanding the changes taking place in the brain at this age presents an opportunity to intervene early in mental illnesses that have their onset at this age. Research findings on the brain may also serve to help adults understand the importance of creating an environment in which teens can explore and experiment while helping them avoid behavior that is destructive to themselves and others.

Section 2.3

The Aging Brain

Text in this section is excerpted from "Alzheimer's Disease: Unraveling
the Mystery," National Institute on Aging (NIA), January 22, 2015.

The Changing Brain in Healthy Aging

In the past several decades, investigators have learned much about
what happens in the brain when people have a neurodegenerative
disease such as Parkinson's disease, AD, or other dementias. Their
findings also have revealed much about what happens during healthy
aging. Researchers are investigating a number of changes related to
healthy aging in hopes of learning more about this process so they can
fill gaps in our knowledge about the early stages of AD.

As a person gets older, changes occur in all parts of the body, including
the brain:

- Certain parts of the brain shrink, especially the prefrontal cortex (an area at the front of the frontal lobe) and the hippocampus. Both areas are important to learning, memory, planning,
  and other complex mental activities.

- Changes in neurons and neurotransmitters affect communication between neurons. In certain brain regions, communication between neurons can be reduced because white matter
  (myelin-covered axons) is degraded or lost.

- Changes in the brain's blood vessels occur. Blood flow can be
  reduced because arteries narrow and less growth of new capillaries occurs.

- In some people, structures called plaques and tangles develop
  outside of and inside neurons, respectively, although in much
  smaller amounts than in AD.

- Damage by **free radicals** increases (free radicals are a kind of
  molecule that reacts easily with other molecules).

- Inflammation increases (inflammation is the complex process that occurs when the body responds to an injury, disease, or abnormal situation).

What effects does aging have on mental function in healthy older people? Some people may notice a modest decline in their ability to learn new things and retrieve information, such as remembering names. They may perform worse on complex tasks of attention, learning, and memory than would a younger person. However, if given enough time to perform the task, the scores of healthy people in their 70s and 80s are often similar to those of young adults. In fact, as they age, adults often improve in other cognitive areas, such as vocabulary and other forms of verbal knowledge.

It also appears that additional brain regions can be activated in older adults during cognitive tasks, such as taking a memory test. Researchers do not fully understand why this happens, but one idea is that the brain engages mechanisms to compensate for difficulties that certain regions may be having. For example, the brain may recruit alternate brain networks in order to perform a task. These findings have led many scientists to believe that major declines in mental abilities are not inevitable as people age. Growing evidence of the adaptive (what scientists call "plastic") capabilities of the older brain provide hope that people may be able to do things to sustain good brain function as they age. A variety of interacting factors, such as lifestyle, overall health, environment, and genetics also may play a role.

Another question that scientists are asking is why some people remain cognitively healthy as they get older while others develop cognitive impairment or dementia. The concept of "cognitive reserve" may provide some insights. Cognitive reserve refers to the brain's ability to operate effectively even when some function is disrupted. It also refers to the amount of damage that the brain can sustain before changes in cognition are evident. People vary in the cognitive reserve they have, and this variability may be because of differences in genetics, education, occupation, lifestyle, leisure activities, or other life experiences. These factors could provide a certain amount of tolerance and ability to adapt to change and damage that occurs during aging. At some point, depending on a person's cognitive reserve and unique mix of genetics, environment, and life experiences, the balance may tip in favor of a disease process that will ultimately lead to dementia. For another person, with a different reserve and a different mix of genetics, environment, and life experiences, the balance may result in no apparent decline in cognitive function with age.

Scientists are increasingly interested in the influence of all these factors on brain health, and studies are revealing some clues about actions people can take that may help preserve healthy brain aging. Fortunately, these actions also benefit a person's overall health. They include:

- Controlling risk factors for chronic disease, such as heart disease and diabetes (for example, keeping blood cholesterol and blood pressure at healthy levels and maintaining a healthy weight)

- Enjoying regular exercise and physical activity

- Eating a healthy diet that includes plenty of vegetables and fruits

- Engaging in intellectually stimulating activities and maintaining close social ties with family, friends, and community

Chapter 3

How Toxins Affect the Brain

Chapter Contents

Section 3.1

Impact of Drug Abuse and Addiction on the Brain

Text in this section is excerpted from "Drug Facts: Understanding Drug Abuse and Addiction," National Institute on Drug Abuse (NIDA), November 2012.

Many people do not understand why or how other people become addicted to drugs. It is often mistakenly assumed that drug abusers lack moral principles or willpower and that they could stop using drugs simply by choosing to change their behavior. In reality, drug addiction is a complex disease, and quitting takes more than good intentions or a strong will. In fact, because drugs change the brain in ways that foster compulsive drug abuse, quitting is difficult, even for those who are ready to do so. Through scientific advances, we know more about how drugs work in the brain than ever, and we also know that drug addiction can be successfully treated to help people stop abusing drugs and lead productive lives.

Drug abuse and addiction have negative consequences for individuals and for society. Estimates of the total overall costs of substance abuse in the United States, including productivity and health- and crime-related costs, exceed $600 billion annually. This includes approximately $193 billion for illicit drugs,[1] $193 billion for tobacco,[2] and $235 billion for alcohol.[3] As staggering as these numbers are, they do not fully describe the breadth of destructive public health and safety implications of drug abuse and addiction, such as family disintegration, loss of employment, failure in school, domestic violence, and child abuse.

What Is Drug Addiction?

Addiction is a chronic, often relapsing brain disease that causes compulsive drug seeking and use, despite harmful consequences to the addicted individual and to those around him or her. Although the initial decision to take drugs is voluntary for most people, the brain changes that occur over time challenge an addicted person's self-control and hamper his or her ability to resist intense impulses to take drugs.

Fortunately, treatments are available to help people counter addiction's powerful disruptive effects. Research shows that combining addiction treatment medications with behavioral therapy is the best way to ensure success for most patients. Treatment approaches that are tailored to each patient's drug abuse patterns and any co-occurring medical, psychiatric, and social problems can lead to sustained recovery and a life without drug abuse.

Similar to other chronic, relapsing diseases, such as diabetes, asthma, or heart disease, drug addiction can be managed successfully. And as with other chronic diseases, it is not uncommon for a person to relapse and begin abusing drugs again. Relapse, however, does not signal treatment failure—rather, it indicates that treatment should be reinstated or adjusted or that an alternative treatment is needed to help the individual regain control and recover.

What Happens to Your Brain When You Take Drugs?

Drugs contain chemicals that tap into the brain's communication system and disrupt the way nerve cells normally send, receive, and process information. There are at least two ways that drugs cause this disruption: (1) by imitating the brain's natural chemical messengers and (2) by overstimulating the "reward circuit" of the brain.

Some drugs (e.g., marijuana and heroin) have a similar structure to chemical messengers called neurotransmitters, which are naturally produced by the brain. This similarity allows the drugs to "fool" the brain's receptors and activate nerve cells to send abnormal messages.

Other drugs, such as cocaine or methamphetamine, can cause the nerve cells to release abnormally large amounts of natural neurotransmitters (mainly dopamine) or to prevent the normal recycling of these brain chemicals, which is needed to shut off the signaling between neurons. The result is a brain awash in dopamine, a neurotransmitter present in brain regions that control movement, emotion, motivation, and feelings of pleasure. The overstimulation of this reward system, which normally responds to natural behaviors linked to survival (eating, spending time with loved ones, etc.), produces euphoric effects in response to psychoactive drugs. This reaction sets in motion a reinforcing pattern that "teaches" people to repeat the rewarding behavior of abusing drugs.

As a person continues to abuse drugs, the brain adapts to the overwhelming surges in dopamine by producing less dopamine or by reducing the number of dopamine receptors in the reward circuit. The result is a lessening of dopamine's impact on the reward circuit, which reduces the abuser's ability to enjoy not only the drugs but also other events in life that previously brought pleasure. This decrease compels the addicted person to keep abusing drugs in an attempt to bring the dopamine function back to normal, but now larger amounts of the drug are required to achieve the same dopamine high—an effect known as tolerance.

Long-term abuse causes changes in other brain chemical systems and circuits as well. Glutamate is a neurotransmitter that influences the reward circuit and the ability to learn. When the optimal concentration of glutamate is altered by drug abuse, the brain attempts to compensate, which can impair cognitive function. Brain imaging studies of drug-addicted individuals show changes in areas of the brain that are critical to judgment, decision making, learning and memory, and behavior control. Together, these changes can drive an abuser to seek out and take drugs compulsively despite adverse, even devastating consequences—that is the nature of addiction.

Why Do Some People Become Addicted While Others Do Not?

No single factor can predict whether a person will become addicted to drugs. Risk for addiction is influenced by a combination of factors that include individual biology, social environment, and age or stage of development. The more risk factors an individual has, the greater the chance that taking drugs can lead to addiction. For example:

- **Biology**. The genes that people are born with—in combination with environmental influences—account for about half of their addiction vulnerability. Additionally, gender, ethnicity, and the presence of other mental disorders may influence risk for drug abuse and addiction.

- **Environment**. A person's environment includes many different influences, from family and friends to socioeconomic status and quality of life in general. Factors such as peer pressure, physical and sexual abuse, stress, and quality of parenting can greatly influence the occurrence of drug abuse and the escalation to addiction in a person's life.

- **Development**. Genetic and environmental factors interact with critical developmental stages in a person's life to affect addiction vulnerability. Although taking drugs at any age can lead to addiction, the earlier that drug use begins, the more likely it will progress to more serious abuse, which poses a special challenge to adolescents. Because areas in their brains that govern decision making, judgment, and self-control are still developing, adolescents may be especially prone to risk-taking behaviors, including trying drugs of abuse.

Prevention Is the Key

Drug addiction is a preventable disease. Results from NIDA-funded research have shown that prevention programs involving families, schools, communities, and the media are effective in reducing drug abuse. Although many events and cultural factors affect drug abuse trends, when youths perceive drug abuse as harmful, they reduce their drug taking. Thus, education and outreach are key in helping youth and the general public understand the risks of drug abuse. Teachers, parents, and medical and public health professionals must keep sending the message that drug addiction can be prevented if one never abuses drugs.

References

1. National Drug Intelligence Center (2011). The Economic Impact of Illicit Drug Use on American Society. Washington D.C.: United States Department of Justice. Available at: http://www.justice.gov/archive/ndic/pubs44/44731/44731p.pdf (PDF, 2.4MB).

2. Centers for Disease Control and Prevention. Smoking-Attributable Mortality, Years of Potential Life Lost, and Productivity Losses—United States, 2000–2004. Morbidity and Mortality Weekly Report. Available at: http://www.cdc.gov/mmwr/preview/mmwrhtml/mm5745a3.htm (PDF 1.4MB).

3. Rehm, J., Mathers, C., Popova, S., Thavorncharoensap, M., Teerawattananon Y., Patra, J. Global burden of disease and injury and economic cost attributable to alcohol use and alcohol-use disorders. Lancet, 373(9682):2223–2233, 2009.

Section 3.2

Dangers of Mercury Exposure

Text in this section is excerpted from "ToxFAQs™ for Mercury,"
Agency for Toxic Substances and Disease Registry, August 29, 2014.

Highlights

Exposure to mercury occurs from breathing contaminated air, ingesting contaminated water and food, and having dental and medical treatments. Mercury, at high levels, may damage the brain, kidneys, and developing fetus. This chemical has been found in at least 714 of 1,467 National Priorities List sites identified by the Environmental Protection Agency.

What is mercury?

Mercury is a naturally occurring metal which has several forms. The metallic mercury is a shiny, silver-white, odorless liquid. If heated, it is a colorless, odorless gas.

Mercury combines with other elements, such as chlorine, sulfur, or oxygen, to form inorganic mercury compounds or "salts," which are usually white powders or crystals. Mercury also combines with carbon to make organic mercury compounds. The most common one, methylmercury, is produced mainly by microscopic organisms in water and soil. More mercury in the environment can increase the amounts of methylmercury that these small organisms make.

Metallic mercury is used to produce chlorine gas and caustic soda, and is also used in thermometers, dental fillings, and batteries. Mercury salts are sometimes used in skin lightening creams and as antiseptic creams and ointments.

What happens to mercury when it enters the environment?

- Inorganic mercury (metallic mercury and inorganic mercury compounds) enters the air from mining ore deposits, burning coal and waste, and from manufacturing plants.

- It enters water or soil from natural deposits, disposal of wastes, and volcanic activity.

- Methylmercury may be formed in water and soil by small organisms called bacteria.

- Methylmercury builds up in the tissues of fish. Larger and older fish tend to have the highest levels of mercury.

How might I be exposed to mercury?

- Eating fish or shellfish contaminated with methylmercury.

- Breathing vapors in air from spills, incinerators, and industries that burn mercury-containing fuels.

- Release of mercury from dental work and medical treatments.

- Breathing contaminated workplace air or skin contact during use in the workplace.

- Practicing rituals that include mercury.

How can mercury affect my health?

The nervous system is very sensitive to all forms of mercury. Methylmercury and metallic mercury vapors are more harmful than other forms, because more mercury in these forms reaches the brain. Exposure to high levels of metallic, inorganic, or organic mercury can permanently damage the brain, kidneys, and developing fetus. Effects on brain functioning may result in irritability, shyness, tremors, changes in vision or hearing, and memory problems.

Short-term exposure to high levels of metallic mercury vapors may cause effects including lung damage, nausea, vomiting, diarrhea, increases in blood pressure or heart rate, skin rashes, and eye irritation.

How likely is mercury to cause cancer?

There are inadequate human cancer data available for all forms of mercury. Mercuric chloride has caused increases in several types of tumors in rats and mice, and methylmercury has caused kidney tumors in male mice. The EPA has determined that mercuric chloride and methylmercury are possible human carcinogens.

How does mercury affect children?

Very young children are more sensitive to mercury than adults. Mercury in the mother's body passes to the fetus and may accumulate there. It also can pass to a nursing infant through breast milk. However, the benefits of breast feeding may be greater than the possible adverse effects of mercury in breast milk.

Mercury's harmful effects that may be passed from the mother to the fetus include brain damage, mental retardation, incoordination, blindness, seizures, and inability to speak. Children poisoned by mercury may develop problems of their nervous and digestive systems, and kidney damage.

How can families reduce the risk of exposure to mercury?

- Carefully handle and dispose of products that contain mercury, such as thermometers or fluorescent light bulbs.

- Do not vacuum up spilled mercury, because it will vaporize and increase exposure. If a large amount of mercury has been spilled, contact your health department. Teach children not to play with shiny, silver liquids.

- Properly dispose of older medicines that contain mercury. Keep all mercury-containing medicines away from children.

- Pregnant women and children should keep away from rooms where liquid mercury has been used.

- Learn about wildlife and fish advisories in your area from your public health or natural resources department.

Is there a medical test to show whether I've been exposed to mercury?

Tests are available to measure mercury levels in the body. Blood or urine samples are used to test for exposure to metallic mercury and to inorganic forms of mercury. Mercury in whole blood or in scalp hair is measured to determine exposure to methylmercury. Your doctor can take samples and send them to a testing laboratory.

Has the federal government made recommendations to protect human health?

The EPA has set a limit of 2 parts of mercury per billion parts of drinking water (2 ppb).

The Food and Drug Administration (FDA) has set a maximum permissible level of 1 part of methylmercury in a million parts of seafood (1 ppm).

The Occupational Safety and Health Administration (OSHA) has set limits of 0.1 milligram of organic mercury per cubic meter of workplace air and 0.05 milligrams of metallic mercury vapor per cubic meter for 8-hour shifts and 40-hour work weeks.

Section 3.3

Dangers of Lead Exposure

Text in this section is excerpted from "ToxFAQs™ for Lead," Agency for Toxic Substances and Disease Registry, August 27, 2014.

Highlights

Exposure to lead can happen from breathing workplace air or dust, eating contaminated foods, or drinking contaminated water. Children can be exposed from eating lead-based paint chips or playing in contaminated soil. Lead can damage the nervous system, kidneys, and reproductive system. Lead has been found in at least 1,272 of the 1,684 National Priority List sites identified by the Environmental Protection Agency (EPA).

What is lead?

Lead is a naturally occurring bluish-gray metal found in small amounts in the earth's crust. Lead can be found in all parts of our environment. Much of it comes from human activities including burning fossil fuels, mining, and manufacturing.

33

Lead has many different uses. It is used in the production of batteries, ammunition, metal products (solder and pipes), and devices to shield X-rays. Because of health concerns, lead from paints and ceramic products, caulking, and pipe solder has been dramatically reduced in recent years. The use of lead as an additive to gasoline was banned in 1996 in the United States.

What happens to lead when it enters the environment?

- Lead itself does not break down, but lead compounds are changed by sunlight, air, and water.

- When lead is released to the air, it may travel long distances before settling to the ground.

- Once lead falls onto soil, it usually sticks to soil particles.

- Movement of lead from soil into groundwater will depend on the type of lead compound and the characteristics of the soil.

How might I be exposed to lead?

- Eating food or drinking water that contains lead. Water pipes in some older homes may contain lead solder. Lead can leach out into the water.

- Spending time in areas where lead-based paints have been used and are deteriorating. Deteriorating lead paint can contribute to lead dust.

- Working in a job where lead is used or engaging in certain hobbies in which lead is used, such as making stained glass.

- Using health-care products or folk remedies that contain lead.

How can lead affect my health?

The effects of lead are the same whether it enters the body through breathing or swallowing. Lead can affect almost every organ and system in your body. The main target for lead toxicity is the nervous system, both in adults and children. Long-term exposure of adults can result in decreased performance in some tests that measure functions of the nervous system. It may also cause weakness in fingers, wrists, or ankles. Lead exposure also causes small increases in blood pressure, particularly in middle-aged and older people and can cause anemia. Exposure to high lead levels can severely damage the brain and kidneys in adults or children and ultimately cause death. In pregnant women, high levels of exposure to lead may cause miscarriage. High-level exposure in men can damage the organs responsible for sperm production.

How likely is lead to cause cancer?

We have no conclusive proof that lead causes cancer in humans. Kidney tumors have developed in rats and mice that had been given large doses of some kind of lead compounds. The Department of Health and Human Services (DHHS) has determined that lead and lead compounds are reasonably anticipated to be human carcinogens and the EPA has determined that lead is a probable human carcinogen. The International Agency for Research on Cancer (IARC) has determined that inorganic lead is probably carcinogenic to humans and that there is insufficient information to determine whether organic lead compounds will cause cancer in humans.

How does lead affect children?

Small children can be exposed by eating lead-based paint chips, chewing on objects painted with lead-based paint, or swallowing house dust or soil that contains lead.

Children are more vulnerable to lead poisoning than adults. A child who swallows large amounts of lead may develop blood anemia, severe stomach ache, muscle weakness, and brain damage. If a child swallows smaller amounts of lead, much less severe effects on blood and brain function may occur. Even at much lower levels of exposure, lead can affect a child's mental and physical growth.

Exposure to lead is more dangerous for young and unborn children. Unborn children can be exposed to lead through their mothers. Harmful effects include premature births, smaller babies, decreased mental ability in the infant, learning difficulties, and reduced growth in young children. These effects are more common if the mother or baby was exposed to high levels of lead. Some of these effects may persist beyond childhood.

How can families reduce the risk of exposure to lead?

- Avoid exposure to sources of lead.

- Do not allow children to chew or mouth surfaces that may have been painted with lead-based paint.

- If you have a water lead problem, run or flush water that has been standing overnight before drinking or cooking with it.

- Some types of paints and pigments that are used as make-up or hair coloring contain lead. Keep these kinds of products away from children.

- If your home contains lead-based paint or you live in an area contaminated with lead, wash children's hands and faces often to remove lead dusts and soil, and regularly clean the house of dust and tracked in soil.

Is there a medical test to show whether I've been exposed to lead?

A blood test is available to measure the amount of lead in your blood and to estimate the amount of your recent exposure to lead. Blood tests are commonly used to screen children for lead poisoning. Lead in teeth or bones can be measured by X-ray techniques, but these methods are not widely available. Exposure to lead also can be evaluated by measuring erythrocyte protoporphyrin (EP) in blood samples. EP is a part of red blood cells known to increase when the amount of lead in the blood is high. However, the EP level is not sensitive enough to identify children with elevated blood lead levels below about 25 micrograms per deciliter. These tests usually require special analytical equipment that is not available in a doctor's office. However, your doctor can draw blood samples and send them to appropriate laboratories for analysis.

Has the federal government made recommendations to protect human health?

The Centers for Disease Control and Prevention (CDC) recommends that states test children at ages 1 and 2 years. Children should be tested at ages 3–6 years if they have never been tested for lead, if they receive services from public assistance programs for the poor such as Medicaid or the Supplemental Food Program for Women, Infants, and Children, if they live in a building or frequently visit a house built before 1950; if they visit a home (house or apartment) built before 1978 that has been recently remodeled; and/or if they have a brother, sister, or playmate who has had lead poisoning. CDC considers a blood lead level of 10 micrograms per deciliter to be a level of concern for children.

EPA limits lead in drinking water to 15 micrograms per deciliter.

Section 3.4

Dangers of Manganese Exposure

Text in this section is excerpted from "ToxFAQs™ for Manganese,"
Agency for Toxic Substances and Disease Registry, March 20, 2014.

Highlights

Manganese is a trace element and eating a small amount from food
or water is needed to stay healthy. Exposure to excess levels of manganese may occur from breathing air, particularly where manganese
is used in manufacturing, and from drinking water and eating food.
At high levels, it can cause damage to the brain. Manganese has been
found in at least 869 of the 1,669 National Priorities List sites identified by the Environmental Protection Agency (EPA).

What is manganese?

Manganese is a naturally occurring metal that is found in many
types of rocks. Pure manganese is silver-colored, but does not occur
naturally. It combines with other substances such as oxygen, sulfur,
or chlorine. Manganese occurs naturally in most foods and may be
added to some foods.

Manganese is used principally in steel production to improve hard-
ness, stiffness, and strength. It may also be used as an additive in
gasoline to improve the octane rating of the gas.

What happens to manganese when it enters the environment?

- Manganese can be released to the air, soil, and water from the
  manufacture, use, and disposal of manganese-based products.

- Manganese cannot break down in the environment. It can only
  change its form or become attached to or separated from particles.

- In water, manganese tends to attach to particles in the water or
  settle into the sediment.

- The chemical state of manganese and the type of soil determine how fast it moves through the soil and how much is retained in the soil.

- The manganese-containing gasoline additive may degrade in the environment quickly when exposed to sunlight, releasing manganese.

How might I be exposed to manganese?

- The primary way you can be exposed to manganese is by eating food or manganese-containing nutritional supplements. Vegetarians, who consume foods rich in manganese such as grains, beans and nuts, as well as heavy tea drinkers, may have a higher intake of manganese than the average person.

- Certain occupations like welding or working in a factory where steel is made may increase your chances of being exposed to high levels of manganese.

- Manganese is routinely contained in groundwater, drinking water, and soil at low levels. Drinking water containing manganese or swimming or bathing in water containing manganese may expose you to low levels of this chemical.

How can manganese affect my health?

Manganese is an essential nutrient, and eating a small amount of it each day is important to stay healthy.

The most common health problems in workers exposed to high levels of manganese involve the nervous system. These health effects include behavioral changes and other nervous system effects, which include movements that may become slow and clumsy. This combination of symptoms when sufficiently severe is referred to as "manganism". Other less severe nervous system effects such as slowed hand movements have been observed in some workers exposed to lower concentrations in the work place.

Exposure to high levels of manganese in air can cause lung irritation and reproductive effects.

Nervous system and reproductive effects have been observed in animals after high oral doses of manganese.

How likely is manganese to cause cancer?

The EPA concluded that existing scientific information cannot determine whether or not excess manganese can cause cancer.

How can manganese affect children?

Studies in children have suggested that extremely high levels of manganese exposure may produce undesirable effects on brain development, including changes in behavior and decreases in the ability to learn and remember. We do not know for certain that these changes were caused by manganese alone. We do not know if these changes are temporary or permanent. We do not know whether children are more sensitive than adults to the effects of manganese, but there is some indication from experiments in laboratory animals that they may be.

Studies of manganese workers have not found increases in birth defects or low birth weight in their offspring. No birth defects were observed in animals exposed to manganese.

How can families reduce the risk of exposure to manganese?

- Children are not likely to be exposed to harmful amounts of manganese in the diet. However, higher-than-usual amounts of manganese may be absorbed if their diet is low in iron. It is important to provide your child with a well-balanced diet.

- Workers exposed to high levels of airborne manganese in certain occupational settings may accumulate manganese dust on their work clothes. Manganese-contaminated work clothing should be removed before getting into your car or entering your home to help reduce the exposure hazard for yourself and your family.

Is there a medical test to determine whether I've been exposed to manganese?

Several tests are available to measure manganese in blood, urine, hair, or feces. Because manganese is normally present in our body, some is always found in tissues or fluids.

Because excess manganese is usually removed from the body within a few days, past exposures are difficult to measure with common laboratory tests.

Has the federal government made recommendations to protect human health?

The EPA has determined that exposure to manganese in drinking water at concentrations of 1 milligram per liter for up to 10 days is not expected to cause any adverse effects in a child.

The EPA has established that lifetime exposure to 0.3 milligrams per liter manganese is not expected to cause any adverse effects.

The FDA has determined that the manganese concentration in bottled drinking water should not exceed 0.05 milligrams per liter.

The Occupational Health and Safety Administration (OSHA) has established a ceiling limit (concentration that should not be exceeded at any time during exposure) of 5 milligrams per cubic meter for manganese in workplace air.

Chapter 4

Neurological Diagnostic Tests and Procedures

Diagnostic tests and procedures are vital tools that help physicians confirm or rule out the presence of a neurological disorder or other medical condition. A century ago, the only way to make a positive diagnosis for many neurological disorders was by performing an autopsy after a patient had died. But decades of basic research into the characteristics of disease, and the development of techniques that allow scientists to see inside the living brain and monitor nervous system activity as it occurs, have given doctors powerful and accurate tools to diagnose disease and to test how well a particular therapy may be working.

Perhaps the most significant changes in diagnostic imaging over the past 20 years are improvements in spatial resolution (size, intensity, and clarity) of anatomical images and reductions in the time needed to send signals to and receive data from the area being imaged. These advances allow physicians to simultaneously see the structure of the brain and the changes in brain activity as they occur. Scientists continue to improve methods that will provide sharper anatomical images and more detailed functional information.

Text in this chapter is excerpted from "Neurological Diagnostic Tests and Procedures," National Institute of Neurological Disorders and Stroke (NINDS), April 28, 2014.

Researchers and physicians use a variety of diagnostic imaging techniques and chemical and metabolic analyses to detect, manage, and treat neurological disease. Some procedures are performed in specialized settings, conducted to determine the presence of a particular disorder or abnormality. Many tests that were previously conducted in a hospital are now performed in a physician's office or at an outpatient testing facility, with little if any risk to the patient. Depending on the type of procedure, results are either immediate or may take several hours to process.

What are some of the more common screening tests?

Laboratory screening tests of blood, urine, or other substances are used to help diagnose disease, better understand the disease process, and monitor levels of therapeutic drugs. Certain tests, ordered by the physician as part of a regular check-up, provide general information, while others are used to identify specific health concerns. For example, blood and blood product tests can detect brain and/or spinal cord infection, bone marrow disease, hemorrhage, blood vessel damage, toxins that affect the nervous system, and the presence of antibodies that signal the presence of an autoimmune disease. Blood tests are also used to monitor levels of therapeutic drugs used to treat epilepsy and other neurological disorders. Genetic testing of DNA extracted from white cells in the blood can help diagnose Huntington's disease and other congenital diseases. Analysis of the fluid that surrounds the brain and spinal cord can detect meningitis, acute and chronic inflammation, rare infections, and some cases of multiple sclerosis. Chemical and metabolic testing of the blood can indicate protein disorders, some forms of muscular dystrophy and other muscle disorders, and diabetes. Urinalysis can reveal abnormal substances in the urine or the presence or absence of certain proteins that cause diseases including the mucopolysaccharidoses.

Genetic testing or counseling can help parents who have a family history of a neurological disease determine if they are carrying one of the known genes that cause the disorder or find out if their child is affected. Genetic testing can identify many neurological disorders, including spina bifida, in utero (while the child is inside the mother's womb). Genetic tests include the following:

- *Amniocentesis*, usually done at 14-16 weeks of pregnancy, tests a sample of the amniotic fluid in the womb for genetic defects (the fluid and the fetus have the same DNA). Under local anesthesia, a thin needle is inserted through the woman's abdomen and into the womb. About 20 milliliters of fluid (roughly 4 teaspoons) is withdrawn and sent to a lab for evaluation. Test results often take 1–2 weeks.

- *Chorionic villus sampling,* or CVS, is performed by removing and testing a very small sample of the placenta during early pregnancy. The sample, which contains the same DNA as the fetus, is removed by catheter or fine needle inserted through the cervix or by a fine needle inserted through the abdomen. It is tested for genetic abnormalities and results are usually available within 2 weeks. CVS should not be performed after the tenth week of pregnancy.

- *Uterine ultrasound* is performed using a surface probe with gel. This noninvasive test can suggest the diagnosis of conditions such as chromosomal disorders. (See ultrasound imaging, below.)

What is a neurological examination?

A *neurological examination* assesses motor and sensory skills, the functioning of one or more cranial nerves, hearing and speech, vision, coordination and balance, mental status, and changes in mood or behavior, among other abilities. Items including a tuning fork, flashlight, reflex hammer, ophthalmoscope, and needles are used to help diagnose brain tumors, infections such as encephalitis and meningitis, and diseases such as Parkinson's disease, Huntington's disease, amyotrophic lateral sclerosis (ALS), and epilepsy. Some tests require the services of a specialist to perform and analyze results.

X-rays of the patient's chest and skull are often taken as part of a neurological work-up. X-rays can be used to view any part of the body, such as a joint or major organ system. In a conventional x-ray, also called a radiograph, a technician passes a concentrated burst of low-dose ionized radiation through the body and onto a photographic plate. Since calcium in bones absorbs x-rays more easily than soft tissue or muscle, the bony structure appears white on the film. Any vertebral misalignment or fractures can be seen within minutes. Tissue masses such as injured ligaments or a bulging disc are not visible on conventional x-rays. This fast, noninvasive, painless procedure is usually performed in a doctor's office or at a clinic.

Fluoroscopy is a type of x-ray that uses a continuous or pulsed beam of low-dose radiation to produce continuous images of a body part in motion. The fluoroscope (x-ray tube) is focused on the area of interest and pictures are either videotaped or sent to a monitor for viewing. A contrast medium may be used to highlight the images. Fluoroscopy can be used to evaluate the flow of blood through arteries.

What are some diagnostic tests used to diagnose neurological disorders?

Based on the result of a neurological exam, physical exam, patient history, x-rays of the patient's chest and skull, and any previous screening or testing, physicians may order one or more of the following diagnostic tests to determine the specific nature of a suspected neurological disorder or injury. These diagnostics generally involve either *nuclear medicine imaging*, in which very small amounts of radioactive materials are used to study organ function and structure, or *diagnostic imaging*, which uses magnets and electrical charges to study human anatomy.

The following list of available procedures—in alphabetical rather than sequential order—includes some of the more common tests used to help diagnose a neurological condition.

Angiography is a test used to detect blockages of the arteries or veins. A *cerebral angiogram* can detect the degree of narrowing or obstruction of an artery or blood vessel in the brain, head, or neck. It is used to diagnose stroke and to determine the location and size of a brain tumor, aneurysm, or vascular malformation. This test is usually performed in a hospital outpatient setting and takes up to 3 hours, followed by a 6- to 8-hour resting period. The patient, wearing a hospital or imaging gown, lies on a table that is wheeled into the imaging area. While the patient is awake, a physician anesthetizes a small area of the leg near the groin and then inserts a catheter into a major artery located there. The catheter is threaded through the body and into an artery in the neck. Once the catheter is in place, the needle is removed and a guide wire is inserted. A small capsule containing a radiopaque dye (one that is highlighted on x-rays) is passed over the guide wire to the site of release. The dye is released and travels through the bloodstream into the head and neck. A series of x-rays is taken and any obstruction is noted. Patients may feel a warm to hot sensation or slight discomfort as the dye is released.

Biopsy involves the removal and examination of a small piece of tissue from the body. *Muscle* or *nerve biopsies* are used to diagnose neuromuscular disorders and may also reveal if a person is a carrier of a defective gene that could be passed on to children. A small sample of muscle or nerve is removed under local anesthetic and studied under a microscope. The sample may be removed either surgically, through a slit made in the skin, or by needle biopsy, in which a thin hollow needle is inserted through the skin and into the muscle. A small piece of muscle or nerve remains in the hollow needle when it is removed from the body. The biopsy is usually performed at an outpatient testing facility. A brain biopsy, used to determine tumor type, requires surgery to remove a small piece of the brain or tumor. Performed in a hospital, this operation is riskier than a muscle biopsy and involves a longer recovery period.

Brain scans are imaging techniques used to diagnose tumors, blood vessel malformations, or hemorrhage in the brain. These scans are used to study organ function or injury or disease to tissue or muscle. Types of brain scans include computed tomography, magnetic resonance imaging, and positron emission tomography (see descriptions, below).

Cerebrospinal fluid analysis involves the removal of a small amount of the fluid that protects the brain and spinal cord. The fluid is tested to detect any bleeding or brain hemorrhage, diagnose infection to the brain and/or spinal cord, identify some cases of multiple sclerosis and other neurological conditions, and measure intracranial pressure.

The procedure is usually done in a hospital. The sample of fluid is commonly removed by a procedure known as a *lumbar puncture*, or *spinal tap*. The patient is asked to either lie on one side, in a ball position with knees close to the chest, or lean forward while sitting on a table or bed. The doctor will locate a puncture site in the lower back, between two vertebrate, then clean the area and inject a local anesthetic. The patient may feel a slight stinging sensation from this injection. Once the anesthetic has taken effect, the doctor will insert a special needle into the spinal sac and remove a small amount of fluid (usually about three teaspoons) for testing. Most patients will feel a sensation of pressure only as the needle is inserted.

A common after-effect of a lumbar puncture is headache, which can be lessened by having the patient lie flat. Risk of nerve root injury or infection from the puncture can occur but it is rare. The entire procedure takes about 45 minutes.

Computed tomography, also known as a CT scan, is a non-invasive, painless process used to produce rapid, clear two-dimensional images of organs, bones, and tissues. Neurological CT scans are used to view the brain and spine. They can detect bone and vascular irregularities, certain brain tumors and cysts, herniated discs, epilepsy, encephalitis, spinal stenosis (narrowing of the spinal canal), a blood clot or intracranial bleeding in patients with stroke, brain damage from head injury, and other disorders. Many neurological disorders share certain characteristics and a CT scan can aid in proper diagnosis by differentiating the area of the brain affected by the disorder.

Scanning takes about 20 minutes (a CT of the brain or head may take slightly longer) and is usually done at an imaging center or hospital on an outpatient basis. The patient lies on a special table that slides into a narrow chamber. A sound system built into the chamber allows the patient to communicate with the physician or technician. As the patient lies still, x-rays are passed through the body at various angles and are detected by a computerized scanner. The data is processed and displayed as cross-sectional images, or "slices," of the internal structure of the body or organ. A light sedative may be given to patients who are unable to lie still and pillows may be used to support and stabilize the head and body. Persons who are claustrophobic may have difficulty taking this imaging test.

Occasionally a contrast dye is injected into the bloodstream to highlight the different tissues in the brain. Patients may feel a warm or cool sensation as the dye circulates through the bloodstream or they may experience a slight metallic taste.

Although very little radiation is used in CT, pregnant women should avoid the test because of potential harm to the fetus from ionizing radiation.

Discography is often suggested for patients who are considering lumbar surgery or whose lower back pain has not responded to conventional treatments. This outpatient procedure is usually performed at a testing facility or a hospital. The patient is asked to put on a metal-free hospital gown and lie on an imaging table. The physician numbs the skin with anesthetic and inserts a thin needle, using x-ray guidance, into the spinal disc. Once the needle is in place, a small amount of contrast dye is injected and CT scans are taken. The contrast dye outlines any damaged areas. More than one disc may be imaged at the same time. Patient recovery usually takes about an hour. Pain medicine may be prescribed for any resulting discomfort.

An *intrathecal contrast-enhanced CT scan* (also called cisternography) is used to detect problems with the spine and spinal nerve roots. This test is most often performed at an imaging center. The patient is asked to put on a hospital or imaging gown. Following application of a topical anesthetic, the physician removes a small sample of the spinal fluid via lumbar puncture. The sample is mixed with a contrast dye and injected into the spinal sac located at the base of the lower back. The patient is then asked to move to a position that will allow the contrast fluid to travel to the area to be studied. The dye allows the spinal canal and nerve roots to be seen more clearly on a CT scan. The scan may take up to an hour to complete. Following the test, patients may experience some discomfort and/or headache that may be caused by the removal of spinal fluid.

Electroencephalography, or EEG, monitors brain activity through the skull. EEG is used to help diagnose certain seizure disorders, brain tumors, brain damage from head injuries, inflammation of the brain and/or spinal cord, alcoholism, certain psychiatric disorders, and metabolic and degenerative disorders that affect the brain. EEGs are also used to evaluate sleep disorders, monitor brain activity when a patient has been fully anesthetized or loses consciousness, and confirm brain death.

This painless, risk-free test can be performed in a doctor's office or at a hospital or testing facility. Prior to taking an EEG, the person must avoid caffeine intake and prescription drugs that affect the nervous system. A series of cup-like electrodes are attached to the patient's scalp, either with a special conducting paste or with extremely fine needles. The electrodes (also called leads) are small devices that are attached to wires and carry the electrical energy of the brain to a machine for reading. A very low electrical current is sent through the electrodes and the baseline brain energy is recorded. Patients are then exposed to a variety of external stimuli—including bright or flashing light, noise or certain drugs—or are asked to open and close the eyes, or to change breathing patterns. The electrodes transmit the resulting changes in brain wave patterns. Since movement and nervousness can change brain wave patterns, patients usually recline in a chair or on a bed during the test, which takes up to an hour. Testing for certain disorders requires performing an EEG during sleep, which takes at least 3 hours.

In order to learn more about brain wave activity, electrodes may be inserted through a surgical opening in the skull and into the brain to reduce signal interference from the skull.

Electromyography, or EMG, is used to diagnose nerve and muscle dysfunction and spinal cord disease. It records the electrical activity from the brain and/or spinal cord to a peripheral nerve root (found in the arms and legs) that controls muscles during contraction and at rest.

During an EMG, very fine wire electrodes are inserted into a muscle to assess changes in electrical voltage that occur during movement and when the muscle is at rest. The electrodes are attached through a series of wires to a recording instrument. Testing usually takes place at a testing facility and lasts about an hour but may take longer, depending on the number of muscles and nerves to be tested. Most patients find this test to be somewhat uncomfortable.

An EMG is usually done in conjunction with a *nerve conduction velocity* (NCV) test, which measures electrical energy by assessing the nerve's ability to send a signal. This two-part test is conducted most often in a hospital. A technician tapes two sets of flat electrodes on the skin over the muscles. The first set of electrodes is used to send small pulses of electricity (similar to the sensation of static electricity) to stimulate the nerve that directs a particular muscle. The second set of electrodes transmits the responding electrical signal to a recording machine. The physician then reviews the response to verify any nerve damage or muscle disease. Patients who are preparing to take an EMG or NCV test may be asked to avoid caffeine and not smoke for 2 to 3 hours prior to the test, as well as to avoid aspirin and non-steroidal anti-inflammatory drugs for 24 hours before the EMG. There is no discomfort or risk associated with this test.

Electronystagmography (ENG) describes a group of tests used to diagnose involuntary eye movement, dizziness, and balance disorders, and to evaluate some brain functions. The test is performed at an imaging center. Small electrodes are taped around the eyes to record eye movements. If infrared photography is used in place of electrodes, the patient wears special goggles that help record the information. Both versions of the test are painless and risk-free.

Evoked potentials (also called evoked response) measure the electrical signals to the brain generated by hearing, touch, or sight. These tests are used to assess sensory nerve problems and confirm neurological conditions including multiple sclerosis, brain tumor, acoustic neuroma (small tumors of the inner ear), and spinal cord injury. Evoked potentials are also used to test sight and hearing (especially in infants and young children), monitor brain activity among coma patients, and confirm brain death.

Testing may take place in a doctor's office or hospital setting. It is painless and risk-free. Two sets of needle electrodes are used to test for nerve damage. One set of electrodes, which will be used to measure the electrophysiological response to stimuli, is attached to the patient's scalp using conducting paste. The second set of electrodes is attached to the part of the body to be tested. The physician then records the amount of time it takes for the impulse generated by stimuli to reach the brain. Under normal circumstances, the process of signal transmission is instantaneous.

Auditory evoked potentials (also called brain stem auditory evoked response) are used to assess high-frequency hearing loss, diagnose any damage to the acoustic nerve and auditory pathways in the brainstem, and detect acoustic neuromas. The patient sits in a soundproof room and wears headphones. Clicking sounds are delivered one at a time to one ear while a masking sound is sent to the other ear. Each ear is usually tested twice, and the entire procedure takes about 45 minutes.

Visual evoked potentials detect loss of vision from optic nerve damage (in particular, damage caused by multiple sclerosis). The patient sits close to a screen and is asked to focus on the center of a shifting checkerboard pattern. Only one eye is tested at a time; the other eye is either kept closed or covered with a patch. Each eye is usually tested twice. Testing takes 30–45 minutes.

Somatosensory evoked potentials measure response from stimuli to the peripheral nerves and can detect nerve or spinal cord damage or nerve degeneration from multiple sclerosis and other degenerating diseases. Tiny electrical shocks are delivered by electrode to a nerve in an arm or leg. Responses to the shocks, which may be delivered for more than a minute at a time, are recorded. This test usually lasts less than an hour.

Magnetic resonance imaging (MRI) uses computer-generated radio waves and a powerful magnetic field to produce detailed images of body structures including tissues, organs, bones, and nerves. Neurological uses include the diagnosis of brain and spinal cord tumors, eye disease, inflammation, infection, and vascular irregularities that may lead to stroke. MRI can also detect and monitor degenerative disorders such as multiple sclerosis and can document brain injury from trauma.

The equipment houses a hollow tube that is surrounded by a very large cylindrical magnet. The patient, who must remain still during the test, lies on a special table that is slid into the tube. The patient will be asked to remove jewelry, eyeglasses, removable dental work, or other items that might interfere with the magnetic imaging. The patient should wear a sweat shirt and sweat pants or other clothing free of metal eyelets or buckles. MRI scanning equipment creates a magnetic field around the body strong enough to temporarily realign water molecules in the tissues. Radio waves are then passed through the body to detect the "relaxation" of the molecules back to a random alignment and trigger a resonance signal at different angles within the body. A computer processes this resonance into either a three-dimensional picture or a two-dimensional "slice" of the tissue being scanned, and differentiates between bone, soft tissues and fluid-filled spaces by their water content and structural properties. A contrast dye may be used to enhance visibility of certain areas or tissues. The patient may hear grating or knocking noises when the magnetic field is turned on and off. (Patients may wear special earphones to block out the sounds.) Unlike CT scanning, MRI does not use ionizing radiation to produce images. Depending on the part(s) of the body to be scanned, MRI can take up to an hour to complete. The test is painless and risk-free, although persons who are obese or claustrophobic may find it somewhat uncomfortable. (Some centers also use open MRI machines that do not completely surround the person being tested and are less confining. However, open MRI does not currently provide the same picture quality as standard MRI and some tests may not be available using this equipment). Due to the incredibly strong magnetic field generated by an MRI, patients with implanted medical devices such as a pacemaker should avoid the test.

Functional MRI (fMRI) uses the blood's magnetic properties to produce real-time images of blood flow to particular areas of the brain. An fMRI can pinpoint areas of the brain that become active and note how long they stay active. It can also tell if brain activity within a region occurs simultaneously or sequentially. This imaging process is used to assess brain damage from head injury or degenerative disorders such as Alzheimer's disease and to identify and monitor other neurological disorders, including multiple sclerosis, stroke, and brain tumors.

Myelography involves the injection of a water- or oil-based contrast dye into the spinal canal to enhance x-ray imaging of the spine. *Myelograms* are used to diagnose spinal nerve injury, herniated discs, fractures, back or leg pain, and spinal tumors.

The procedure takes about 30 minutes and is usually performed in a hospital. Following an injection of anesthesia to a site between two vertebrae in the lower back, a small amount of the cerebrospinal fluid is removed by spinal tap (see *cerebrospinal fluid analysis*, above) and the contrast dye is injected into the spinal canal. After a series of x-rays is taken, most or all of the contrast dye is removed by aspiration. Patients may experience some pain during the spinal tap and when the dye is injected and removed. Patients may also experience headache following the spinal tap. The risk of fluid leakage or allergic reaction to the dye is slight.

Positron emission tomography (PET) scans provide two- and three-dimensional pictures of brain activity by measuring radioactive isotopes that are injected into the bloodstream. PET scans of the brain are used to detect or highlight tumors and diseased tissue, measure cellular and/or tissue metabolism, show blood flow, evaluate patients who have seizure disorders that do not respond to medical therapy and patients with certain memory disorders, and determine brain changes following injury or drug abuse, among other uses. PET may be ordered as a follow-up to a CT or MRI scan to give the physician a greater understanding of specific areas of the brain that may be involved with certain problems. Scans are conducted in a hospital or at a testing facility, on an outpatient basis. A low-level radioactive isotope, which binds to chemicals that flow to the brain, is injected into the bloodstream and can be traced as the brain performs different functions. The patient lies still while overhead sensors detect gamma rays in the body's tissues. A computer processes the information and displays it on a video monitor or on film. Using different compounds, more than one brain function can be traced simultaneously. PET is painless and relatively risk-free. Length of test time depends on the part of the body to be scanned. PET scans are performed by skilled technicians at highly sophisticated medical facilities.

A *polysomnogram* measures brain and body activity during sleep. It is performed over one or more nights at a sleep center. Electrodes are pasted or taped to the patient's scalp, eyelids, and/or chin. Throughout the night and during the various wake/sleep cycles, the electrodes record brain waves, eye movement, breathing, leg and skeletal muscle activity, blood pressure, and heart rate. The patient may be videotaped to note any movement during sleep. Results are then used to identify any characteristic patterns of sleep disorders, including restless legs syndrome, periodic limb movement disorder, insomnia, and breathing disorders such as obstructive sleep apnea. Polysomnograms are non-invasive, painless, and risk-free.

Single photon emission computed tomography (SPECT), a nuclear imaging test involving blood flow to tissue, is used to evaluate certain brain functions. The test may be ordered as a follow-up to an MRI to diagnose tumors, infections, degenerative spinal disease, and stress fractures. As with a PET scan, a radioactive isotope, which binds to chemicals that flow to the brain, is injected intravenously into the body. Areas of increased blood flow will collect more of the isotope. As the patient lies on a table, a gamma camera rotates around the head and records where the radioisotope has traveled. That information is converted by computer into cross-sectional slices that are stacked to produce a detailed three-dimensional image of blood flow and activity within the brain. The test is performed at either an imaging center or a hospital.

Thermography uses infrared sensing devices to measure small temperature changes between the two sides of the body or within a specific organ. Also known as digital infrared thermal imaging, ther-mography may be used to detect vascular disease of the head and neck, soft tissue injury, various neuromusculoskeletal disorders, and the presence or absence of nerve root compression. It is performed at an imaging center, using infrared light recorders to take thousands of pictures of the body from a distance of 5 to 8 feet. The information is converted into electrical signals which results in a computer-generated two-dimensional picture of abnormally cold or hot areas indicated by color or shades of black and white. Thermography does not use radi-ation and is safe, risk-free, and noninvasive.

Ultrasound imaging, also called ultrasound scanning or sonog-raphy, uses high-frequency sound waves to obtain images inside the body. *Neurosonography* (ultrasound of the brain and spinal column) analyzes blood flow in the brain and can diagnose stroke, brain tumors, hydrocephalus (build-up of cerebrospinal fluid in the brain), and vas-cular problems. It can also identify or rule out inflammatory processes causing pain. It is more effective than an x-ray in displaying soft tissue masses and can show tears in ligaments, muscles, tendons, and other soft tissue masses in the back. *Transcranial Doppler ultrasound* is used to view arteries and blood vessels in the neck and determine blood flow and risk of stroke.

During ultrasound, the patient lies on an imaging table and removes clothing around the area of the body to be scanned. A jelly-like lubricant is applied and a transducer, which both sends and receives high-frequency sound waves, is passed over the body. The sound wave echoes are recorded and displayed as a computer-generated real-time visual image of the structure or tissue being examined. Ultrasound is painless, noninvasive, and risk-free. The test is performed on an outpatient basis and takes between 15 and 30 minutes to complete.

Part Two

Degenerative Brain Disorders

Chapter 5

Dementias

Chapter Contents

Section 5.1

Dementias

Text in this section is excerpted from "Dementia: Hope through
Research," National Institute of Neurological Disorders and Stroke
(NINDS), February 23, 2015.

Introduction

A diagnosis of dementia can be frightening for those affected by
the syndrome, their family members, and caretakers. Learning more
about dementia can help. This section provides a general overview of
various types of dementia, and describes how the disorders are diagnosed and treated.

Alzheimer's disease (AD) is the most common form of dementia
in those over the age of 65. As many as 5 million Americans age 65
and older may have AD, and that number is expected to double for
every 5-year interval beyond age 65. But Alzheimer's is only one of
many dementia disorders; an estimated 20 to 40 percent of people with
dementia have some other form of the disorder. Among all people with
dementia, many are believed to have a mixed type of dementia that
can involve more than one of the disorders.

Age is the primary risk factor for developing dementia. For that
reason, the number of people living with dementia could double in
the next 40 years with an increase in the number of Americans who
are age 65 or older—from 40 million today to more than 88 million in
2050. Regardless of the form of dementia, the personal, economic, and
societal demands can be devastating.

Research over the past 30 years has helped us learn more about
dementia—possible causes, who is at risk, and how it develops and
affects the brain. This work offers the hope of better drugs and treatments for these disorders.

The Basics of Dementia

Dementia is the loss of cognitive functioning, which means the
loss of the ability to think, remember, or reason, as well as behavioral

abilities, to such an extent that it interferes with a person's daily life and activities. Signs and symptoms of dementia result when once-healthy neurons (nerve cells) in the brain stop working, lose connections with other brain cells, and die. While everyone loses some neurons as they age, people with dementia experience far greater loss.

Researchers are still trying to understand the underlying disease processes involved in the disorders. Scientists have some theories about mechanisms that may lead to different forms of dementias, but more research is needed to better understand if and how these mechanisms contribute to the development of dementia.

While dementia is more common with advanced age (as many as half of all people age 85 or older may have some form of dementia), it is not a normal part of aging. Many people live into their 90s and beyond without any signs of dementia.

Memory loss, though common, is not the only sign of dementia. For a person to be considered to have dementia, he or she must meet the following criteria:

- Two or more core mental functions must be impaired. These functions include memory, language skills, visual perception, and the ability to focus and pay attention. These also include cognitive skills such as the ability to reason and solve problems.

- The loss of brain function is severe enough that a person cannot do normal, everyday tasks.

- In addition, some people with dementia cannot control their emotions. Their personalities may change. They can have delusions, which are strong beliefs without proof, such as the idea that someone is stealing from them. They also may hallucinate, seeing or otherwise experiencing things that are not real.

Types of Dementia

Various disorders and factors contribute to the development of dementia. Neurodegenerative disorders such as AD, frontotemporal disorders, and Lewy body dementia result in a progressive and irreversible loss of neurons and brain functions. Currently, there are no cures for these progressive neurodegenerative disorders.

However, other types of dementia can be halted or even reversed with treatment. Normal pressure hydrocephalus, for example, often resolves when excess cerebrospinal fluid in the brain is drained via a shunt and rerouted elsewhere in the body. Cerebral vasculitis responds to aggressive treatment with immunosuppressive drugs. In rare cases, treatable infectious disorders can cause dementia. Some drugs, vitamin deficiencies, alcohol abuse, depression, and brain tumors can cause neurological deficits that resemble dementia. Most of these causes respond to treatment.

Some types of dementia disorders are described below.

> **Editor's Note:** For more detailed information on specific dementias and degenerative disorders, see sections 5.2 through 5.8.

Tauopathies

In some dementias, a protein called tau clumps together inside nerve cells in the brain, causing the cells to stop functioning properly and die. Disorders that are associated with an accumulation of tau are called tauopathies.

In AD, the tau protein becomes twisted and aggregates to form bundles, called neurofibrillary tangles, inside the neurons. Abnormal clumps (plaques) of another protein, called amyloid, are prominent in spaces between brain cells and are a hallmark of the disease. Both plaques and tangles are thought to contribute to reduced function and nerve-cell death in AD, but scientists do not fully understand this relationship. It is not clear, for example, if the plaques and tangles cause the disorder, or if their presence flags some other process that leads to neuronal death in AD.

Other types of tauopathies include the following disorders:

Corticobasal degeneration (CBD) is a progressive neurological disorder characterized by nerve-cell loss and atrophy (shrinkage) of specific areas of the brain, including the cerebral cortex and the basal ganglia. The disorder tends to progress gradually, with the onset of early symptoms around age 60. At first, one side of the body is affected more than the other side, but as the disease progresses both sides become impaired. An individual may have difficulty using one hand, or one's hand may develop an abnormal position.

Other signs and symptoms may include memory loss; trouble making familiar, focused movements (apraxia) such as brushing one's teeth; involuntary muscular jerks (myoclonus) and involuntary muscle contractions (dystonia); alien limb, in which the person feels as though

60

a limb is being controlled by a force other than oneself; muscle rigidity (resistance to imposed movement); postural instability; and difficulty swallowing (dysphagia). People with CBD also may have visual-spatial problems that make it difficult to interpret visual information, such as the distance between objects.

There is no cure for CBD. Supportive therapies are available to reduce the burden of certain symptoms. For example, botulinum toxin can help control muscle contractions. Speech therapy and physical therapy may help one learn how to cope with daily activities.

Frontotemporal disorders (FTD) are caused by a family of brain diseases that primarily affect the frontal and temporal lobes of the brain; they account for up to 10 percent of all dementia cases. Some, but not all, forms of FTD are considered tauopathies. In some cases, FTD is associated with mutations in the gene for tau (MAPT), and tau aggregates are present. However, other forms of FTD are associated with aggregates of the protein TDP-43, a mutated protein found among people with a type of ALS that is inherited. Mutations in a protein called progranulin may also play a role in some TDP43-opathies.

In FTD, changes to nerve cells in the brain's frontal lobes affect the ability to reason and make decisions, prioritize and multitask, act appropriately, and control movement. Some people decline rapidly over 2 to 3 years, while others show only minimal changes for many years. People can live with frontotemporal disorders for 2 to 10 years, sometimes longer, but it is difficult to predict the time course for an affected individual. In some cases, FTD is associated with progressive neuromuscular weakness otherwise known as amyotrophic lateral sclerosis (ALS, or Lou Gehrig's disease). The signs and symptoms may vary greatly among individuals as different parts of the brain are affected. No treatment that can cure or reverse FTD is currently available.

Clinically, FTD is classified into two main types of syndromes:

- *Behavioral variant frontotemporal dementia* causes a person to undergo behavior and personality changes. People with this disorder may do impulsive things that are out of character, such as steal or be rude to others. They may engage in repetitive behavior (such as singing, clapping, or echoing another person's speech). They may overeat compulsively; lose inhibitions, causing them to say or do inappropriate things (sometimes sexual in nature); or become apathetic and experience excessive sleepiness. While they may be cognitively impaired, their memory may stay relatively intact.

61

- *Primary progressive aphasia (PPA)* causes a person to have
  trouble with expressive and receptive speaking—finding and/
  or expressing thoughts and/or words. Sometimes a person with
  PPA cannot name common objects. Problems with memory, reasoning, and judgment are not apparent at first but can develop
  and progress over time. PPA is a language disorder not to be
  confused with the aphasia that can result from a stroke. Many
  people with PPA, though not all, develop symptoms of dementia.
  In one form of PPA, called semantic PPA or semantic dementia,
  a person slowly loses the ability to understand single words and
  sometimes to recognize the faces of familiar people and common
  objects.

Other types of FTDs include:

- *Frontotemporal dementia with parkinsonism linked to chromosome 17 (FTDP-17),* a rare form of dementia that is believed to
  be inherited from one parent and is linked to a defect in the gene
  that makes the tau protein. The three core features are behavioral and personality changes, cognitive impairment, and motor
  symptoms. People with this type of FTD often have delusions,
  hallucinations, and slowness of movement and tremor as seen in
  Parkinson's disease. Typical behavioral/personality characteristics include apathy, defective judgment, and compulsive and
  abusive behavior. Diagnosis of the disorder requires the confirmed presence of clinical features and genetic analysis. Palliative and symptomatic treatments such as physical therapy are
  the mainstays of management.

- *Pick's disease,* a tauopathy subtype of FTD characterized by
  hallmark Pick bodies—masses comprised of tau protein that
  accumulate inside nerve cells, causing them to appear enlarged
  or balloon-like. Some of the symptoms of this rare neurodegenerative disorder are similar to those of AD, including loss
  of speech, inappropriate behavior, and trouble with thinking.
  However, while inappropriate behavior characterizes the early
  stages of Pick's disease, memory loss is often the first symptom
  of AD. Antidepressants and antipsychotics can control some of
  the behavioral symptoms of Pick's disease, but no treatment is
  available to stop the disease from progressing.

Progressive supranuclear palsy (PSP) is a rare brain disorder
that damages the upper brain stem, including the substantia nigra

(a movement control center in the midbrain). This region also is affected in Parkinson's disease, which may explain an overlap in motor symptoms shared by these disorders. Eye movements are especially affected, causing slow and then limited mobility of the eye. The most common early signs and symptoms include loss of balance, unexplained falls, general body stiffness, apathy, and depression. A person with this type of dementia may suddenly laugh or cry very easily (known as pseudobulbar affect). As the disorder progresses, people develop blurred vision and a characteristic vacant stare that involves loss of facial expression. Speech usually becomes slurred, and swallowing solid foods or liquids becomes difficult. PSP gets progressively worse, but people can live a decade or more after the onset of symptoms. Dextromethorphan, a common ingredient in cough medicine, has been approved for the treatment of pseudobulbar affect.

Argyrophilic grain disease is a common, late-onset degenerative disease characterized by tau deposits called argyrophilic grains in brain regions involved in memory and emotion. The disease's signs and symptoms are indistinguishable from late-onset AD. Confirmation of the diagnosis can be made only at autopsy.

Synucleinopathies

In these brain disorders, a protein called alpha-synuclein accumulates inside neurons. Although it is not fully understood what role this protein plays, changes in the protein and/or its function have been linked to Parkinson's disease and other disorders.

One type of synucleinopathy, **Lewy body dementia,** involves protein aggregates called Lewy bodies, balloon-like structures that form inside of nerve cells. The initial symptoms may vary, but over time, people with these disorders develop very similar cognitive, behavioral, physical, and sleep-related symptoms. Lewy body dementia is one of the most common causes of dementia, after Alzheimer's disease and vascular disease.

Types of Lewy body dementia include:

- *Dementia with Lewy bodies (DLB),* one of the more common forms of progressive dementia. Symptoms such as difficulty sleeping, loss of smell, and visual hallucinations often precede movement and other problems by as long as 10 years, which consequently results in DLB going unrecognized or misdiagnosed as a psychiatric disorder until its later stages. Neurons in the substantia nigra that produce dopamine die or become impaired, and the brain's outer layer (cortex) degenerates. Many neurons that remain contain Lewy bodies.

- Later in the course of DLB, some signs and symptoms are similar to AD and may include memory loss, poor judgment, and confusion. Other signs and symptoms of DLB are similar to those of Parkinson's disease, including difficulty with movement and posture, a shuffling walk, and changes in alertness and attention. Given these similarities, DLB can be very difficult to diagnose. There is no cure for DLB, but there are drugs that control some symptoms. The medications used to control DLB symptoms can make motor function worse or exacerbate hallucinations.

- *Parkinson's disease dementia (PDD)*, a clinical diagnosis related to DLB that can occur in people with Parkinson's disease. PDD may affect memory, social judgment, language, or reasoning. Autopsy studies show that people with PDD often have amyloid plaques and tau tangles similar to those found in people with AD, though it is not understood what these similarities mean. A majority of people with Parkinson's disease develop dementia, but the time from the onset of movement symptoms to the onset of dementia symptoms varies greatly from person to person. Risk factors for developing PDD include the onset of Parkison's-related movement symptoms followed by mild cognitive impairment and REM sleep behavior disorder, which involves having frequent nightmares and visual hallucinations.

Vascular Dementia and Vascular Cognitive Impairment

Vascular dementia and vascular cognitive impairment (VCI) are caused by injuries to the vessels supplying blood to the brain. These disorders can be caused by brain damage from multiple strokes or any injury to the small vessels carrying blood to the brain. Dementia risk can be significant even when individuals have suffered only small strokes. Vascular dementia and VCI arise as a result of risk factors that similarly increase the risk for cerebrovascular disease (stroke), including atrial fibrillation, hypertension, diabetes, and high cholesterol. Vascular dementia also has been associated with a condition called amyloid angiopathy, in which amyloid plaques accumulate in the blood-vessel walls, causing them to break down and rupture. Symptoms of vascular dementia and VCI can begin suddenly and progress or subside during one's lifetime.

Some types of vascular dementia include:

Cerebral autosomal dominant arteriopathy with subcortical infarcts and leukoencephalopathy (CADASIL). This inherited form of cardiovascular disease results in a thickening of the walls of small- and medium-sized blood vessels, eventually stemming the flow of blood to the brain. It is associated with mutations of a specific gene called Notch3, which gives instructions to a protein on the surface of the smooth muscle cells that surround blood vessels. CADASIL is associated with multi-infarct dementia, stroke, migraine with aura (migraine preceded by visual symptoms), and mood disorders. The first symptoms can appear in people between ages 20 and 40. Many people with CADASIL are undiagnosed. People with first-degree relatives who have CADASIL can be tested for genetic mutations to the Notch3 gene to determine their own risk of developing CADASIL.

Multi-infarct dementia. This type of dementia occurs when a person has had many small strokes that damage brain cells. One side of the body may be disproportionally affected, and multi-infarct dementia may impair language or other functions, depending on the region of the brain that is affected. Doctors call these "local" or "focal" symptoms, as opposed to the "global" symptoms seen in AD that tend to affect several functions and both sides of the body. When the strokes occur on both sides of the brain, however, dementia is more likely than when stroke occurs on one side of the brain. In some cases, a single stroke can damage the brain enough to cause dementia. This so-called single-infarct dementia is more common when stroke affects the left side of the brain—where speech centers are located—and/or when it involves the hippocampus, the part of the brain that is vital for memory.

Subcortical vascular dementia, also called Binswanger's disease. This is a rare form of dementia that involves extensive microscopic damage to the small blood vessels and nerve fibers that make up white matter, the "network" part of the brain believed to be critical for relaying messages between regions. The symptoms of Binswanger's are related to the disruption of subcortical neural circuits involving short-term memory, organization, mood, attention, decision making, and appropriate behavior. A characteristic feature of this disease is psychomotor slowness, such as an increase in the time it takes for a person to think of a letter and then write it on a piece of paper.

Other symptoms include urinary incontinence that is unrelated to a urinary tract condition, trouble walking, clumsiness, slowness, lack of facial expression, and speech difficulties. Symptoms tend to begin after age 60, and they progress in a stepwise manner. People with subcortical vascular disease often have high blood pressure, a history of stroke, or evidence of disease of the large blood vessels in the neck or heart valves. Treatment is aimed at preventing additional strokes and may include drugs to control blood pressure.

Mixed Dementia

Autopsy studies looking at the brains of people who had dementia suggest that a majority of those age 80 and older probably had "mixed dementia," caused by both AD-related neurodegenerative processes and vascular disease-related processes. In fact, some studies indicate that mixed vascular-degenerative dementia is the most common cause of dementia in the elderly. In a person with mixed dementia, it may not be clear exactly how many of a person's symptoms are due to AD or another type of dementia. In one study, approximately 40 percent of people who were thought to have AD were found after autopsy to also have some form of cerebrovascular disease. Several studies have found that many of the major risk factors for vascular disease also may be risk factors for AD.

Researchers are still working to understand how underlying disease processes in mixed dementia influence each other. It is not clear, for example, if symptoms are likely to be worse when a person has brain changes reflecting multiple types of dementia. Nor do we know if a person with multiple dementias can benefit from treating one type, for example, when a person with AD controls high blood pressure and other vascular disease risk factors.

Other Conditions That Cause Dementia

Doctors have identified many other conditions that can cause dementia or dementia-like symptoms.

Other Brain Diseases

Creutzfeldt-Jakob disease (CJD). A rare brain disorder that affects about one in every million people worldwide each year, CJD belongs to a family of diseases known as the transmissible spongiform encephalopathies, or TSEs. Spongiform refers to the fact that the brain becomes filled with microscopic swellings that give the appearance of holes, like a sponge. CJD and other TSEs are believed to be caused by infectious proteins called prions that become misfolded. Scientists believe that the presence of misfolded prions can trigger normal proteins to misfold as well, causing a chain reaction. These abnormal prion proteins tend to clump together, which is believed to be related to the brain damage.

Symptoms usually begin after age 60, and most people die within a year of onset. In most cases, CJD occurs in people who have no known risk factors for the disease; however, an estimated 5 to 10 percent of cases in the U.S. are associated with genetic mutations. In addition, a type of CJD, called variant CJD (vCJD), has been found in Great Britain and several other European countries. vCJD has been observed to affect people who are younger than those with other forms of CJD and is believed to be caused by eating beef from cattle infected with a TSE called bovine spongiform encephalopathy, more commonly known as "mad cow disease." Inherited forms of CJD include:

- *Fatal familial insomnia.* This prion disease causes a part of the brain involved in sleep to slowly degenerate. People with the disease have trouble sleeping and may show signs of poor reflexes and hallucinations.

- *Gerstmann-Straussler-Scheinker disease.* Symptoms include a loss of coordination (ataxia) and dementia that begin when people are 50 to 60 years old.

Huntington's disease. This hereditary disorder is caused by a faulty gene for a protein called huntingtin. Symptoms begin around age 30 or 40 years and include abnormal and uncontrollable movements called chorea, as well as gait changes and lack of coordination. Huntington's disease may affect a person's judgment, memory, and other cognitive functions. As the disease progresses, these cognitive problems worsen, and motor difficulties lead to complete loss of ability for self-care. Children of people with Huntington's have a 50 percent chance of having the disorder.

Secondary dementias. These dementias occur in people with disorders that damage brain tissue. Such disorders may include multiple sclerosis; meningitis; encephalitis; and Wilson's disease, in which excessive amounts of copper build up to cause brain damage. In rare cases, people with brain tumors may develop dementia because of damage to their brain circuits or a buildup of pressure inside the skull. Symptoms may include changes in personality, psychotic episodes, or problems with speech, language, thinking, and memory.

Head Injury

Chronic traumatic encephalopathy, initially known as dementia pugilistica, is caused by repeated traumatic brain injury (TBI), such as in boxers or in people who suffered multiple concussions while playing a contact sport. People with this condition often develop poor coordination, slurred speech, and other symptoms similar to those seen in Parkinson's disease, along with dementia, 20 years or more after the TBI events. This form of dementia also is characterized by brain atrophy and widespread deposits of tau aggregates. In some individuals, even just 5 to 10 years beyond the TBI events, behavioral and mood changes may occur. Dementia may not yet be present and the brain may not have atrophied, but small focal deposits of tau are seen in the brain at autopsy.

Subdural hematoma, or bleeding between the brain's surface and its outer covering (the dura), is common in the elderly after a fall. Subdural hematomas can cause dementia-like symptoms and changes in mental function. With treatment, some symptoms can be reversed.

Reversible Dementias

Many conditions that cause dementia can be reversed with the appropriate treatment.

- Cerebral vasculitis, an inflammation and necrosis (tissue death) of blood vessel walls, can cause a form of dementia that may resolve when the person is treated with immune suppressants.

- Some studies have shown that people with depression are at increased risk of developing dementia. Severe depression can cause dementia and can be treated.

- Infections can cause confusion or delirium due to related fever or other side effects associated with the body's response to a foreign entity.

- Metabolic disorders of the nervous system, such as mitochondrial disorders, leukodystrophies, and lysosomal storage diseases, can lead to dementia.

- Metabolic problems and endocrine abnormalities such as thyroid problems, low blood sugar levels (called hypoglycemia), and low or high levels of sodium or calcium also may also cause dementia.

- Normal pressure hydrocephalus is an abnormal buildup of cerebro-spinal fluid in the brain. Elderly individuals with the condition usually have trouble with walking and bladder control before onset of dementia. Normal pressure hydrocephalus can be treated or even reversed by implanting a shunt system to divert fluid from the brain.

• Nutritional deficiencies of vitamin B1 (thiamine), caused by chronic alcoholism, and vitamin B12 deficiencies can be reversed with treatment.

• Paraneoplastic syndromes (a group of symptoms that may develop when substances released by some cancer cells disrupt the normal function of surrounding cells and tissue) can cause symptoms that resemble dementia. Such symptoms generally occur in people with cancer when the body's immune response to the cancer also ends up targeting proteins in the central nervous system. In many cases, the neurologic condition occurs before the cancer is detected. Circulating antibodies against brain proteins are common in both neurologic and cancer conditions.

• Side effects of medications or drug combinations may cause dementias that arise quickly or develop slowly over time.

Environmental Factors

Environmental factors may play a role in the development of certain types of dementia. This relationship is complex, however, since a person may carry genetic mutations that influence his or her response to environmental factors. Examples of environmental factors include:

Anoxia. Anoxia and a related condition, hypoxia, are terms often used to describe a state in which there is a curtailed supply of oxygen to an organ's tissues. Anoxia and hypoxia can lead to the loss of neurons and diffuse brain injury. Characteristics of the resulting dementia include confusion, personality changes, hallucinations, or memory loss. This type of dementia commonly occurs in people who survive cardiac arrest.

Poisoning. Exposure to lead, mercury, other heavy metals, or poisonous substances can lead to symptoms of dementia. These symptoms may or may not resolve after treatment, depending on how severely the brain is damaged.

Editor's Note: For further information on exposure to toxins, see Chapter 3: How Toxins Affect the Brain.

Substance abuse. People who have abused substances such as alcohol and recreational drugs sometimes display signs of dementia even after the substance abuse has stopped. This condition is known as substance- induced persisting dementia.

Infectious Disease

HIV-associated dementia (HAD) can occur in people who are positive for the human immunodeficiency virus, the virus that causes AIDS. HAD damages the brain's white matter and leads to a type of dementia associated with memory problems, social withdrawal, and trouble concentrating. People with HAD may develop movement problems as well. The incidence of HAD has dropped dramatically with the availability of effective antiviral therapies for managing the underlying HIV infection.

Risk Factors for Dementia

The following risk factors can increase a person's chance of developing one or more kinds of dementia. Some of these factors can be modified, while others cannot.

- **Age.** The risk goes up with advanced age.

- **Alcohol use.** Most studies suggest that drinking large amounts of alcohol increases the risk of dementia, while drinking a moderate amount may be protective.

- **Atherosclerosis.** The accumulation of fats and cholesterol in the lining of arteries, coupled with an inflammatory process that leads to a thickening of the vessel walls (known as atherosclerosis), can hinder blood from getting to the brain, which can lead to stroke or another brain injury. For example, high levels of low-density lipoprotein (LDL, or "bad" cholesterol) can raise the risk for vascular dementia. High LDL levels also have been linked to AD.

- **Diabetes.** People with diabetes appear to have a higher risk for dementia, although the evidence for this association is modest. Poorly controlled diabetes, however, is a well-proven risk factor for stroke and cardiovascular disease-related events, which in turn increase the risk for vascular dementia.

- **Down syndrome.** Many people with Down syndrome develop early-onset AD, with signs of dementia by the time they reach middle age.

- **Genetics.** One's likelihood of developing a genetically linked form of dementia increases when more than one family member has the disorder. But in some cases, such as with CADASIL, having just one parent who carries a mutation increases the risk of inheriting the condition. In other instances, genetic mutations may underlie dementias in specific populations. For example, a mutation of the gene TREM2 has been found to be common among people with a form of very early onset frontotemporal dementia that runs in Turkish families.

- **Hypertension.** High blood pressure has been linked to cognitive decline, stroke, and types of dementia that affect the white matter regions of the brain.

- **Mental illness.** Depression has been associated with mild mental impairment and cognitive function decline.

- **Smoking.** Smokers are prone to diseases that slow or stop blood from getting to the brain.

Diagnosis

Doctors first assess whether the individual has an underlying treatable condition such as depression, abnormal thyroid function, drug-induced encephalopathy, normal pressure hydrocephalus, or vitamin B12 deficiency. Early diagnosis is important, as some causes for symptoms can be treated. In many cases, the specific type of dementia that a person has may not be confirmed until after the person has died and the brain is examined.

An assessment generally includes:

- **Patient history.** Typical questions about a person's medical and family history might include asking about whether dementia runs in the family, how and when symptoms began, and if the person is taking certain medications that might cause or exacerbate symptoms.

- **Physical exam.** Measuring blood pressure and other vital signs may help physicians detect conditions that might cause or occur with dementia. Such conditions may be treatable.

- **Neurological evaluations.** Assessing balance, sensory function, reflexes, vision, eye movements, and other functions helps identify signs of conditions that may affect the diagnosis or are treatable with drugs. Doctors also might use an electroencephalogram, a test that records patterns of electrical activity in the brain, to check for abnormal electrical brain activity.

The following procedures also may be used when diagnosing dementia:

- **Brain scans.** These tests can identify strokes, tumors, and other problems that can cause dementia. Scans also identify changes in the brain's structure and function. The most common scans are computed tomographic (CT) scans and Magnetic Resonance Imaging (MRI). CT scans use X-rays to produce images of the brain and other organs. MRI scans use a computer, magnetic fields, and radio waves to produce detailed images of body structures, including tissues, organs, bones, and nerves.

- Other types of scans let doctors watch the brain as it functions. Two of these tests are single photon-emission computed tomography, which can be used to measure blood flow to the brain, and positron emission tomography (PET), which uses radioactive isotopes to provide pictures of brain activity. These scans are used to look for patterns of altered brain activity that are common in dementia. Researchers also use PET imaging with compounds that bind to beta-amyloid to detect levels of the protein, a hallmark of AD, in the living brain.

- **Cognitive and neuropsychological tests.** These tests measure memory, language skills, math skills, and other abilities related to mental functioning. For example, people with AD often show impairment in problem-solving, memory, and the ability to perform once-automatic tasks.

- **Laboratory tests.** Many tests help rule out other conditions. They include measuring levels of sodium and other electrolytes in the blood, a complete blood count, a blood sugar test, urine analysis, a check of vitamin B12 levels, cerebrospinal fluid analysis, drug and alcohol tests, and an analysis of thyroid function.

- **Presymptomatic tests.** Some dementias are associated with a known gene defect. In these cases, a genetic test could help people know if they are at risk for dementia. People should talk with family members, their primary health care professional, and a genetic counselor before getting tested.

- **Psychiatric evaluation.** This will help determine if depression or another mental health condition is causing or contributing to a person's symptoms.

Treatment

Some dementias are treatable. However, therapies to stop or slow common neurodegenerative diseases such as AD have largely been unsuccessful, though some drugs are available to manage certain symptoms.

Most drugs for dementia are used to treat symptoms in AD. One class of drugs, called cholinesterase inhibitors, includes donepezil, rivastigmine, and galantamine. These drugs can temporarily improve or stabilize memory and thinking skills in some people by increasing the activity of the cholinergic brain network. The drug memantine is in another class of medications called NMDA receptor agonists, which prevents declines in learning and memory. NMDA receptor agonists work by regulating the activity of the neurotransmitter gluta-mate. When glutamate activity levels are excessive, neurons may die. Memantine may be combined with a cholinesterase inhibitor for added benefits. These drugs are sometimes used to treat other dementias as well. None of these drugs can stop or reverse the course of the disease.

- **Creutzfeldt-Jakob disease.** There are no treatments to cure or control CJD. Management focuses on reducing symptoms and making people comfortable.

- **Dementia with Lewy bodies.** Drugs available for managing DLB are aimed at relieving symptoms such as stiffness, halluci-nations, and delusions. However, many of the agents for treating the physical symptoms, particularly antipsychotics, can make the mental health symptoms worse. Conversely, drugs used to treat mental health symptoms can exacerbate physical symptoms. Studies suggest that AD drugs may benefit people with DLB.

- **Frontotemporal disorders.** There are no medications approved to treat or prevent FTD and most other types of pro-gressive dementia. Sedatives, antidepressants, and other drugs used to treat Parkinson's and Alzheimer's symptoms may help manage certain symptoms and behavioral problems associated with the disorders.

- **Parkinson's disease dementia.** Some studies suggest that the cholin-esterase inhibitors used in people with AD might improve cognitive, behavioral, and psychotic symptoms in people with Parkinson's disease dementia. The U.S. Food and Drug Administration has approved one Alzheimer's drug, rivastigmine, to treat cognitive symptoms in PDD.

- **Vascular dementia.** This type of dementia is often managed with drugs to prevent strokes. The aim is to reduce the risk of additional brain damage. Some studies suggest that drugs that improve memory in AD might benefit people with early vascular dementia. Most of the modifiable risk factors that influence development of vascular dementia and VCI are the same risk factors for cerebrovascular disease, such as hypertension, atrial fibrillation, diabetes, and high cholesterol. Interventions that address these risk factors may be incorporated into the management of vascular dementia.

Conclusion

Currently, there are no cures for the common dementias caused by progressive neurodegeneration, including AD, frontotemporal disorders, and Lewy body dementia. However, some forms of dementia are treatable. A better understanding of dementia disorders, as well as their diagnosis and treatment, will make it possible for affected individuals and their caretakers to live their lives more fully and meet daily challenges. NIH, primarily through research activities funded by NINDS and NIA, continues to make discoveries in the lab, design therapeutic approaches to dementias, and create tools and resources to help speed the development of treatments that can be used in practice. These discoveries may eventually lead to ways to slow disease progression or even cure and prevent the dementias.

Section 5.2

Frontotemporal Dementia

Text in this section is excerpted from "Frontotemporal Disorders:
Information for Patients, Families, and Caregivers," National
Institute on Aging (NIA), January 22, 2015.

Introduction

Few people have heard of frontotemporal disorders, which lead to
dementias that affect personality, behavior, language, and movement.
These disorders are little known outside the circles of researchers,
clinicians, patients, and caregivers who study and live with them.
Although frontotemporal disorders remain puzzling in many ways,
researchers are finding new clues that will help them solve this medical
mystery and better understand other common dementias.

The symptoms of frontotemporal disorders gradually rob people of
basic abilities—thinking, talking, walking, and socializing—that most
of us take for granted. They often strike people in the prime of life,
when they are working and raising families. Families suffer, too, as
they struggle to cope with the person's daily needs as well as changes
in relationships and responsibilities.

This section is meant to help people with frontotemporal disorders,
their families, and caregivers learn more about these conditions and
resources for coping. It explains what is known about the different
types of disorders and how they are diagnosed. Most importantly, it
describes how to treat and manage these difficult conditions, with
practical advice for caregivers.

The Basics of Frontotemporal Disorders

Frontotemporal disorders are the result of damage to neurons
(nerve cells) in parts of the brain called the frontal and temporal lobes.
As neurons die in the frontal and temporal regions, these lobes atrophy, or shrink. Gradually, this damage causes difficulties in thinking
and behaviors normally controlled by these parts of the brain. Many
possible symptoms can result, including unusual behaviors, emotional

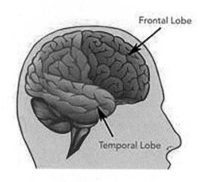

Figure 5.1. *The Frontal and Temporal Lobes*

Damage to the brain's frontal and temporal lobes causes forms of dementia called frontotemporal disorders.

problems, trouble communicating, difficulty with work, or difficulty with walking.

A Form of Dementia

Frontotemporal disorders are forms of dementia caused by a family of brain diseases known as frontotemporal lobar degeneration (FTLD). Dementia is a severe loss of thinking abilities that interferes with a person's ability to perform daily activities such as working, driving, and preparing meals. Other brain diseases that can cause dementia include Alzheimer's disease and multiple strokes. Scientists estimate that FTLD may cause up to 10 percent of all cases of dementia and may be about as common as Alzheimer's among people younger than age 65. Roughly 60 percent of people with FTLD are 45 to 64 years old.

People can live with frontotemporal disorders for up to 10 years, sometimes longer, but it is difficult to predict the time course for an individual patient. The disorders are progressive, meaning symptoms get worse over time. In the early stages, people may have just one type of symptom. As the disease progresses, other types of symptoms appear as more parts of the brain are affected.

No cure or treatments that slow or stop the progression of frontotemporal disorders are available today. However, research is improving awareness and understanding of these challenging conditions. This progress is opening doors to better diagnosis, improved care, and, eventually, new treatments.

Changes in the Brain

Frontotemporal disorders affect the frontal and temporal lobes of the brain. They can begin in the frontal lobe, the temporal lobe, or

FTD? FTLD? Understanding Terms

One of the challenges shared by patients, families, clinicians, and researchers is confusion about how to classify and label frontotemporal disorders. A diagnosis by one doctor may be called something else by a second, and the same condition or syndrome referred to by another name by a pathologist who examines the brain after death.

For many years, scientists and physicians used the term *frontotemporal dementia* (FTD) to describe this group of illnesses. After further research, FTD is now understood to be just one of several possible variations and is more precisely called behavioral variant frontotemporal dementia, or bvFTD.

This section uses the term *frontotemporal* disorders to refer to changes in behavior and thinking that are caused by underlying brain diseases collectively called *frontotemporal lobar degeneration* (FTLD). FTLD is not a single brain disease but rather a family of neurodegenerative diseases, any one of which can cause a frontotemporal disorder. Frontotemporal disorders are diagnosed by physicians and psychologists based on a person's symptoms and results of brain scans and genetic tests. With the exception of known genetic causes, FTLD can be identified definitively only by brain autopsy after death.

both. Initially, frontotemporal disorders leave other brain regions untouched, including those that control short-term memory.

The frontal lobes, situated above the eyes and behind the forehead both on the right and left sides of the brain, direct executive functioning. This includes planning and sequencing (thinking through which steps come first, second, third, and so on), prioritizing (doing more important activities first and less important activities last), multitasking (shifting from one activity to another as needed), and monitoring and correcting errors.

When functioning well, the frontal lobes also help manage emotional responses. They enable people to avoid inappropriate social behaviors, such as shouting loudly in a library or at a funeral. They help people make decisions that make sense for a given situation. When the frontal lobes are damaged, people may focus on insignificant details and ignore important aspects of a situation or engage in purposeless activities. The frontal lobes are also involved in language, particularly linking words to form sentences, and in motor functions, such as moving the arms, legs, and mouth.

The temporal lobes, located below and to the side of each frontal lobe on the right and left sides of the brain, contain essential areas for memory but also play a major role in language and emotions. They help people understand words, speak, read, write, and connect words with their meanings. They allow people to recognize objects and to relate appropriate emotions to objects and events. When the temporal lobes are dysfunctional, people may have difficulty recognizing emotions and responding appropriately to them.

Which lobe—and part of the lobe—is affected first determines which symptoms appear first. For example, if the disease starts in the part of the frontal lobe responsible for decision-making, then the first symptom might be trouble managing finances. If it begins in the part of the temporal lobe that connects emotions to objects, then the first symptom might be an inability to recognize potentially dangerous objects—a person might reach for a snake or plunge a hand into boiling water, for example.

Types of Frontotemporal Disorders

Frontotemporal disorders can be grouped into three types, defined by the earliest symptoms physicians identify when they examine patients.

- **Progressive behavior/personality decline**—characterized by changes in personality, behavior, emotions, and judgment (called behavioral variant frontotemporal dementia).

- **Progressive language decline**—marked by early changes in language ability, including speaking, understanding, reading, and writing (called primary progressive aphasia).

- **Progressive motor decline**—characterized by various difficulties with physical movement, including the use of one or more limbs, shaking, difficulty walking, frequent falls, and poor coordination (called corticobasal syndrome, supranuclear palsy, or amyotrophic lateral sclerosis).

In the early stages it can be hard to know which of these disorders a person has because symptoms and the order in which they appear can vary widely from one person to the next. Also, the same symptoms can appear in different disorders. For example, language problems are

Table 5.1. Types of Frontotemporal Disorders

Diagnostic Terms	Main Early Symptoms
Progressive Behavior/Personality Decline	
• **Behavioral variant frontotemporal dementia (bvFTD)** • **Temporal/frontal variant FTD (tvFTD, fvFTD)** • **Pick's disease**	• Apathy, reduced initiative • Inappropriate and impulsive behaviors • Emotional flatness or excessive emotions • Memory generally intact
Progressive Language Decline	
• **Primary progressive aphasia (PPA)** • **Progressive nonfluent aphasia** • **Semantic dementia**	• Semantic PPA (also called semantic dementia): can't understand words or recognize familiar people and objects • Agrammatic PPA (also called progressive nonfluent aphasia): omits words that link nouns and verbs (such as to, from, the) • Logopenic PPA: trouble finding the right words while speaking, hesitation, and/or pauses in speech
Progressive Motor Decline	
• **Corticobasal syndrome (CBS)**	• Muscle rigidity • Difficulty closing buttons, operating simple appliances; difficulty swallowing • Language or spatial orientation problems
• **Progressive supranuclear palsy (PSP)**	• Progressive problems with balance and walking • Slow movement, falling, body stiffness • Restricted eye movements
• **FTD with parkinsonism**	• Movement problems similar to Parkinson's disease, such as slowed movement and stiffness • Changes in behavior or language
• **FTD with amyotrophic lateral sclerosis (FTD-ALS)**	• Combination of FTD and ALS (Lou Gehrig's disease) • Changes in behavior and/or language • Muscle weakness and loss, fine jerks, wiggling in muscles

most typical of primary progressive aphasia but can also appear later in the course of behavioral variant frontotemporal dementia. The table below summarizes the three types of frontotemporal disorders and lists the various terms that could be used when clinicians diagnose these disorders.

Behavioral Variant Frontotemporal Dementia

The most common frontotemporal disorder, behavioral variant fronto-temporal dementia (bvFTD), involves changes in personality, behavior, and judgment. People with this dementia can act strangely around other people, resulting in embarrassing social situations. Often, they don't know or care that their behavior is unusual and don't show any consideration for the feelings of others. Over time, language and/or movement problems may occur, and the person needs more care and supervision.

What's going on?

Brian, an attorney, began having trouble organizing his cases. In time, his law firm assigned him to do paperwork only. Brian's wife thought he was depressed because his father had died 2 years earlier. Brian, 56, was treated for depression, but his symptoms got worse. He became more disorganized and began making sexual comments to his wife's female friends. Even more unsettling, he neither understood nor cared that his behavior disturbed his family and friends. As time went on, Brian had trouble paying bills and was less affectionate toward his wife and young son. Three years after Brian's symptoms began, his counselor recommended a neurological evaluation. Brian was diagnosed with bvFTD.

In the past, bvFTD was called Pick's disease, named after Arnold Pick, the German scientist who first described it in 1892. The term Pick's disease is now used to describe abnormal collections in the brain of the protein tau, called "Pick bodies." Some patients with bvFTD have Pick bodies in the brain, and some do not.

Primary Progressive Aphasia

Primary progressive aphasia (PPA) involves changes in the ability to communicate—to use language to speak, read, write, and understand what others are saying. Problems with memory, reasoning, and judgment are not apparent at first but can develop over time. In addition, some people with PPA may experience significant behavioral changes, similar to those seen in bvFTD, as the disease progresses.

There are three types of PPA, categorized by the kind of language problems seen at first. Researchers do not fully understand the biological basis of the different types of PPA. But they hope one day to link specific language problems with the abnormalities in the brain that cause them.

> **"What do you mean by salt?"**
>
> Jane, 62, a university professor, began having trouble remembering the names of common objects while she lectured. She also had a hard time following conversations, especially when more than one person was involved. Her family and co-workers were unaware of Jane's difficulties—until she had a hard time recognizing longtime colleagues. One night at the dinner table, when Jane's husband asked her to pass the salt, she said, "Salt? What do you mean by salt?" He took her to a neurologist, who diagnosed semantic PPA. As her illness progressed, Jane developed behavioral symptoms and had to retire early.

In *semantic PPA*, also called semantic dementia, a person slowly loses the ability to understand single words and sometimes to recognize the faces of familiar people and common objects.

In *agrammatic PPA*, also called progressive nonfluent aphasia, a person has more and more trouble producing speech. Eventually, the person may no longer be able to speak at all. He or she may eventually develop movement symptoms similar to those seen in corticobasal syndrome.

In *logopenic PPA*, a person has trouble finding the right words during conversation but can understand words and sentences. The person does not have problems with grammar.

Movement Disorders

Two rare neurological disorders associated with FTLD, corticobasal syndrome (CBS) and progressive supranuclear palsy (PSP), occur when the parts of the brain that control movement are affected. The disorders may affect thinking and language abilities, too.

CBS can be caused by corticobasal degeneration—gradual atrophy and loss of nerve cells in specific parts of the brain. This degeneration causes progressive loss of the ability to control movement, typically beginning around age 60. The most prominent symptom may be the inability to use the hands or arms to perform a movement despite normal strength (called apraxia). Symptoms may appear first on one side of the body, but eventually both sides are affected. Occasionally, a person with CBS first has language problems or trouble orienting objects in space and later develops movement symptoms.

Confusing symptoms

Carol had a tingling sensation and numbness in her upper right arm. Then her arm became stiff. She had to change from cursive handwriting to printing. Carol, 61, told her doctor that she had trouble getting her thoughts out and described her speech as "stumbling." She had increasing trouble talking but could still understand others. Eventually, she was diagnosed with CBS.

PSP causes problems with balance and walking. People with the disorder typically move slowly, experience unexplained falls, lose facial expression, and have body stiffness, especially in the neck and upper body—symptoms similar to those of Parkinson's disease. A hallmark sign of PSP is trouble with eye movements, particularly looking down. These symptoms may give the face a fixed stare. Behavior problems can also develop.

Other movement-related frontotemporal disorders include *frontotemporal dementia with parkinsonism* and *frontotemporal dementia with amyotrophic lateral sclerosis (FTD-ALS)*.

Frontotemporal dementia with parkinsonism can be an inherited disease caused by a genetic tau mutation. Symptoms include movement problems similar to those of Parkinson's disease, such as slowed movement, stiffness, and balance problems, and changes in behavior or language.

FTD-ALS is a combination of bvFTD and ALS, commonly called Lou Gehrig's disease. Symptoms include the behavioral and/or language changes seen in bvFTD as well as the progressive muscle weakness seen in ALS. Symptoms of either disease may appear first, with other symptoms developing over time. Mutations in certain genes have been found in some patients with FTD-ALS.

> **Trouble with walking**
>
> For a year and a half, John had trouble walking and fell several times. He also had trouble concentrating. He couldn't read because the words merged together on the page. John, 73, also seemed less interested in social activities and projects around the house. His wife noticed that he was more irritable than usual and sometimes said uncharacteristically inappropriate things. John's primary care doctor did several tests, then referred him to a neurologist, who noted abnormalities in his eye movements and diagnosed PSP.

Causes

Frontotemporal lobar degeneration (FTLD) is not a single brain disease but rather a family of brain diseases that share some common molecular features. Scientists are beginning to understand the biological and genetic basis for the changes observed in brain cells that lead to FTLD.

Scientists describe FTLD in terms of patterns of change in the brain seen in an autopsy after death. These changes include loss of neurons and abnormal amounts or forms of proteins called tau and TDP-43. These proteins occur naturally in the body and help cells function properly. When the proteins don't work properly, for reasons not yet fully understood, neurons in specific brain regions are damaged.

In most cases, the cause of a frontotemporal disorder is unknown. In about 15 to 40 percent of people, a genetic (hereditary) cause can be identified. Individuals with a family history of frontotemporal disorders are more likely to have a genetic form of the disease than those without such a history.

Familial and inherited forms of frontotemporal disorders are often related to mutations (permanent changes) in certain genes. Genes are basic units of heredity that tell cells how to make the proteins the body needs to function. Even small changes in a gene may produce an abnormal protein, which can lead to changes in the brain and, eventually, disease.

Scientists have discovered several different genes that, when mutated, can lead to frontotemporal disorders:

- **Tau gene (also called the MAPT gene)**—A mutation in this gene causes abnormalities in a protein called tau, which forms tangles inside neurons and ultimately leads to the destruction of brain cells. Inheriting a mutation in this gene means a person will almost surely develop a frontotemporal disorder, usually bvFTD, but the exact age of onset and symptoms cannot be predicted.

- **PGRN gene**—A mutation in this gene can lead to lower production of the protein progranulin, which in turn causes TDP-43, a cellular protein, to go awry in brain cells. Many frontotemporal disorders can result, though bvFTD is the most common. The PGRN gene can cause different symptoms in different family members and cause the disease to begin at different ages.

- **VCP, CHMP2B, TARDBP, and FUS genes**—Mutations in these genes lead to very rare familial types of frontotemporal disorders.

- **C9ORF72 gene**—An unusual mutation in this gene appears to be the most common genetic abnormality in familial frontotemporal disorders and familial ALS. This mutation can cause a frontotemporal disorder, ALS, or both conditions in a person.

Diagnosis

No single test, such as a blood test, can be used to diagnose a frontotemporal disorder. A definitive diagnosis can be confirmed only by a genetic test in familial cases or a brain autopsy after a person dies. To diagnose a probable frontotemporal disorder in a living person, a doctor—usually a neurologist, psychiatrist, or psychologist—will:

- record a person's symptoms, often with the help of family members or friends

- compile a personal and family medical history

- perform a physical exam and order blood tests to help rule out other similar conditions

- if appropriate, order testing to uncover genetic mutations

- conduct a neuropsychological evaluation to assess behavior, language, memory, and other cognitive functions

- use brain imaging to look for changes in the frontal and temporal lobes.

Different types of brain imaging may be used. A magnetic resonance imaging (MRI) scan shows changes in the size and shape of the brain, including the frontal and temporal lobes. It may reveal other potentially treatable causes of the person's symptoms, such as a stroke or tumor. In the early stage of disease, the MRI may appear normal. In this case, other types of imaging, such as positron emission tomography (PET) or single photon emission computed tomography (SPECT), may be useful. PET and SPECT scans measure activity in the brain by monitoring blood flow, glucose usage, and oxygen usage. Other PET scans can help rule out a diagnosis of Alzheimer's.

> **Is it depression?**
>
> Ana's husband was the first to notice a change in his 55-year-old wife's personality. Normally active in her community, she became less interested in her volunteer activities. She wanted to stay home, did not initiate conversations, and went on her daily walks only if her husband suggested it. Ana's family thought she might be depressed. A psychologist recognized that her cognition was impaired and referred her to a neurologist, who diagnosed bvFTD.

Frontotemporal disorders can be hard to diagnose because their symptoms—changes in personality and behavior and difficulties with speech and movement—are similar to those of other conditions. For example, bvFTD is sometimes misdiagnosed as a mood disorder, such as depression, or as a stroke, especially when there are speech or movement problems. To make matters more confusing, a person can have both a frontotemporal disorder and another type of dementia such as Alzheimer's disease. Also, since these disorders are rare, physicians may be unfamiliar with the relevant symptoms and signs.

Getting the wrong diagnosis can be frustrating. Without knowing their true condition, people with frontotemporal disorders may not get appropriate treatment to manage their symptoms. Families may not get the help they need. People lose valuable time needed to plan treatment and future care. The medical centers listed in Resources are places where people with frontotemporal disorders can be diagnosed and treated.

Researchers are studying ways to diagnose frontotemporal disorders earlier and more accurately. One area of research involves biomarkers, such as proteins or other substances in the blood or cerebrospinal fluid, which can be used to measure the progress of disease or the effects of treatment. Also being studied are ways to improve brain imaging, including seeing the tau protein, and neuropsychological testing, which assesses learning, language, problem solving, memory, and other thinking skills.

Common Symptoms

Symptoms of frontotemporal disorders vary from person to person and from one stage of the disease to the next as different parts of the frontal and temporal lobes are affected. In general, changes in the frontal lobe are associated with behavioral symptoms, while changes in the temporal lobe lead to language and emotional disorders.

Symptoms are often misunderstood. Family members and friends may think that a person is misbehaving, leading to anger and conflict. For example, a person with bvFTD may neglect personal hygiene or start shoplifting. It is important to understand that people with these disorders cannot control their behaviors and other symptoms. Moreover, they lack any awareness of their illness, making it difficult to get help.

Behavioral Symptoms

- **Problems with executive functioning**—Problems with planning and sequencing (thinking through which steps come first, second, third, and so on), prioritizing (doing more important activities first and less important activities last), multitasking (shifting from one activity to another as needed), and self-monitoring and correcting behavior.

- **Perseveration**—A tendency to repeat the same activity or to say the same word over and over, even when it no longer makes sense.

- **Social disinhibition**—Acting impulsively without considering how others perceive the behavior. For example, a person might hum at a business meeting or laugh at a funeral.

- **Compulsive eating**—Gorging on food, especially starchy foods like bread and cookies, or taking food from other people's plates.

- **Utilization behavior**—Difficulty resisting impulses to use or touch objects that one can see and reach. For example, a person picks up the telephone receiver while walking past it when the phone is not ringing and the person does not intend to place a call.

Language Symptoms

- **Aphasia**—A language disorder in which the ability to use or understand words is impaired but the physical ability to speak properly is normal.

- **Dysarthria**—A language disorder in which the physical ability to speak properly is impaired (e.g., slurring) but the message is normal.

People with PPA may have only problems using and understanding words or also problems with the physical ability to speak. People with both kinds of problems have trouble speaking and writing. They may become mute, or unable to speak. Language problems usually get worse, while other thinking and social skills may remain normal for longer before deteriorating.

> **Embarrassing behavior**
>
> David and his wife ran a successful store until he began to act strangely. He intruded on his teenaged daughters' gatherings with friends, standing and staring at them but not realizing how embarrassed they were. He took food from other people's plates. A year later, David, 47, and his wife lost their business. After a misdiagnosis of depression and no improvement, David's wife took him to a neurologist, who diagnosed bvFTD.

Emotional Symptoms

- **Apathy**—A lack of interest, drive, or initiative. Apathy is often confused with depression, but people with apathy may not be sad. They often have trouble starting activities but can participate if others do the planning.

- **Emotional changes**—Emotions are flat, exaggerated, or improper. Emotions may seem completely disconnected from a situation or are expressed at the wrong times or in the wrong circumstances. For example, a person may laugh at sad news.

- **Social-interpersonal changes**—Difficulty "reading" social signals, such as facial expressions, and understanding personal

relationships. People may lack empathy—the ability to understand how others are feeling—making them seem indifferent,
uncaring, or selfish. For example, the person may show no
emotional reaction to illnesses or accidents that occur to family
members.

Movement Symptoms

- **Dystonia**—Abnormal postures of body parts such as the hands
  or feet. A limb may be bent stiffly or not used when performing
  activities that are normally done with two hands.

- **Gait disorder**—Abnormalities in walking, such as walking
  with a shuffle, sometimes with frequent falls.

- **Tremor**—Shakiness, usually of the hands.

- **Clumsiness**—Dropping of small objects or difficulty manipulat-
  ing small items like buttons or screws.

- **Apraxia**—Loss of ability to make common motions, such as
  combing one's hair or using a knife and fork, despite normal
  strength.

- **Neuromuscular weakness**—Severe weakness, cramps, and
  rippling movements in the muscles.

Treatment and Management

So far, there is no cure for frontotemporal disorders and no way
to slow down or prevent them. However, there are ways to manage
symptoms. A team of specialists—doctors, nurses, and speech, physical, and occupational therapists—familiar with these disorders can
help guide treatment.

Managing Behavior

The behaviors of a person with bvFTD can upset and frustrate
family members and other caregivers. It is natural to grieve for the
"lost person," but it is also important to learn how to best live with the
person he or she has become. Understanding changes in personality
and behavior and knowing how to respond can reduce caregivers' frustration and help them cope with the challenges of caring for a person
with a frontotemporal disorder.

Changing the schedule

Matthew, 53, diagnosed with bvFTD, insisted on playing the card game solitaire on the computer for hours every morning. He did not care that this activity interfered with his wife's schedule. His wife figured out how to rearrange her day to stay home in the morning and take Matthew on errands and appointments in the afternoon. A portable device for solitaire in the car helped distract him.

Managing behavioral symptoms can involve several approaches. To ensure the safety of a person and his or her family, caregivers may have to take on new responsibilities or arrange care that was not needed before. For example, they may have to drive the person to appointments and errands, care for young children, or arrange for help at home.

It is helpful, though often difficult, to accept rather than challenge people with behavioral symptoms. Arguing or reasoning with them will not help because they cannot control their behaviors or even see that they are unusual or upsetting to others. Instead, be as sensitive as possible and understand that it's the illness "talking." Frustrated caregivers can take a "timeout"—take deep breaths, count to 10, or leave the room for a few minutes.

To deal with apathy, limit choices and offer specific choices. Open-ended questions ("What would you like to do today?") are more difficult to answer than specific ones ("Do you want to go to the movies or the shopping center today?").

Maintaining the person's schedule and modifying the environment can also help. A regular schedule is less confusing and can help people sleep better. If compulsive eating is an issue, caregivers may have to supervise eating, limit food choices, lock food cabinets and the refrigerator, and distract the person with other activities. To deal with other compulsive behaviors, caregivers may have to change schedules or offer new activities.

Medications are available to treat certain behavioral symptoms. Antidepressants called selective serotonin reuptake inhibitors are commonly prescribed to treat social disinhibition and impulsive behavior. Patients with aggression or delusions sometimes take low doses of antipsychotic medications. The use of Alzheimer's disease medications to improve behavioral and cognitive symptoms in people with bvFTD and related disorders is being studied, though results so far have been mixed, with some medications making symptoms worse. If a particular medication is not working, a doctor may try another. Always consult a doctor before changing, adding, or stopping a drug.

Treating Language Problems

Treatment of primary progressive aphasia (PPA) has two goals— maintaining language skills and using new tools and other ways to communicate. Treatment tailored to a person's specific language problem and stage of PPA generally works best. Since language ability declines over time, different strategies may be needed as the illness progresses.

To communicate without talking, a person with PPA may use a communication notebook (an album of photos labeled with names of people and objects), gestures, and drawings. Some people find it helpful to use or point to lists of words or phrases stored in a computer or personal digital assistant.

Finding a new way to communicate

Mary Ann, a television news anchor for 20 years, began having trouble reading the nightly news. At first, her doctor thought she had a vision problem, but tests showed that her eyesight was normal. Although normally creative and energetic, Mary Ann, 52, had trouble finishing assignments and voicing her ideas at staff meetings. In time, she was let go from her job. Mary Ann applied for Social Security disability benefits, which required a medical exam. Her symptoms puzzled several doctors until a neurologist diagnosed logopenic PPA. A speech therapist taught Mary Ann to use a personal digital assistant to express words and phrases. For emergencies, Mary Ann carries a card in her wallet that explains her condition.

Caregivers can also learn new ways of talking to someone with PPA. For example, they can speak slowly and clearly, use simple sentences, wait for responses, and ask for clarification if they don't understand something.

A speech-language pathologist who knows about PPA can test a person's language skills and determine the best tools and strategies to use. Note that many speech-language pathologists are trained to treat aphasia caused by stroke, which requires different strategies from those used with PPA.

Managing Movement Problems

No treatment can slow down or stop frontotemporal-related movement disorders, though medications and physical and occupational therapy may provide modest relief.

For people with corticobasal syndrome (CBS), movement difficulties are sometimes treated with medications for Parkinson's disease. But these medicines offer only minimal or temporary improvement. Physical and occupational therapy may help people with CBS move more easily. Speech therapy may help them manage language symptoms.

For people with progressive supranuclear palsy (PSP), sometimes Parkinson's disease drugs provide temporary relief for slowness, stiffness, and balance problems. Exercises can keep the joints limber, and weighted walking aids—such as a walker with sandbags over the lower front rung—can help maintain balance. Speech, vision, and swallowing difficulties usually do not respond to any drug treatment. Antidepressants have shown modest success. For people with abnormal eye movements, bifocals or special glasses called prisms are sometimes prescribed.

People with FTD-ALS typically decline quickly over the course of 2 to 3 years. During this time, physical therapy can help treat muscle symptoms, and a walker or wheelchair may be useful. Speech therapy may help a person speak more clearly at first. Later on, other ways of communicating, such as a speech synthesizer, can be used. The ALS symptoms of the disorder ultimately make it impossible to stand, walk, eat, and breathe on one's own.

For any movement disorder caused by FTLD, a team of experts can help patients and their families address difficult medical and caregiving issues. Physicians, nurses, social workers, and physical, occupational, and speech therapists who are familiar with frontotemporal disorders can ensure that people with movement disorders get appropriate medical treatment and that their caregivers can help them live as well as possible.

The Future of Treatment

Researchers are continuing to explore the genetic and biological actions in the body that lead to frontotemporal disorders. In particular, they seek more information about genetic mutations that cause FTLD, as well as the disorders' natural history and disease pathways. They also want to develop better ways, such as specialized brain imaging, to track its progression, so that treatments, when they become available, can be directed to the right people. The ultimate goal is to identify possible new drugs and other treatments to test.

Researchers are also looking for better treatments for frontotemporal disorders. Possible therapies that target the abnormal proteins found in the brain are being tested in the laboratory and in animals. Clinical trials and studies are testing a number of possible treatments in humans.

Caring for a Person with a Frontotemporal Disorder

In addition to managing the medical and day-to-day care of people with frontotemporal disorders, caregivers can face a host of other challenges. These challenges may include changing family relationships, loss of work, poor health, decisions about long-term care, and end-of-life concerns.

Family Issues

People with frontotemporal disorders and their families often must cope with changing relationships, especially as symptoms get worse. For example, the wife of a man with bvFTD not only becomes her husband's caregiver, but takes on household responsibilities he can no longer perform. Children may suffer the gradual "loss" of a parent at a critical time in their lives. The symptoms of bvFTD often embarrass family members and alienate friends. Life at home can become very stressful.

Work Issues

Frontotemporal disorders disrupt basic work skills, such as organizing, planning, and following through on tasks. Activities that were easy before the illness began might take much longer or become impossible. People lose their jobs because they can no longer perform them. As a result, the caregiver might need to take a second job to make ends meet—or reduce hours or even quit work to provide care and run the household. An employment attorney can offer information and advice about employee benefits, family leave, and disability if needed.

Workers diagnosed with any frontotemporal disorder can qualify quickly for Social Security disability benefits through the "compassionate allowances" program. For more information, see www.socialsecurity .gov/compassionateallowances or call 1-800-772-1213.

Caregiver Health and Support

Caring for someone with a frontotemporal disorder can be very hard, both physically and emotionally. To stay healthy, caregivers can do the following:

- Get regular health care.

- Ask family and friends for help with child care, errands, and other tasks.

- Spend time doing enjoyable activities, away from the demands of caregiving. Arrange for respite care—short-term caregiving services that give the regular caregiver a break—or take the person to an adult day care center, a safe, supervised environment for adults with dementia or other disabilities.

- Join a support group for caregivers of people with frontotemporal disorders. Such groups allow caregivers to learn coping strategies and share feelings with others in the same position.

Long-Term Care

For many caregivers, there comes a point when they can no longer take care of the person with a frontotemporal disorder without help. The caregiving demands are simply too great, perhaps requiring around-the-clock care. As the disease progresses, caregivers may want to get home healthcare services or look for a residential care facility, such as a group home, assisted living facility, or nursing home. The decision to move the person with a frontotemporal disorder to a care facility can be difficult, but it can also give caregivers peace of mind to know that the person is safe and getting good care. The decreased level of stress may also improve the caregivers' relationship with his or her loved one.

End-of-Life Concerns

People with frontotemporal disorders typically live 6 to 8 years with their conditions, sometimes longer, sometimes less. Most people die of problems related to advanced disease. For example, as movement skills decline, a person can have trouble swallowing, leading to aspiration pneumonia, in which food or fluid gets into the lungs and causes infection. People with balance problems may fall and seriously injure themselves.

It is difficult, but important, to plan for the end of life. Legal documents, such as a will, living will, and durable powers of attorney for health care and finances, should be created or updated as soon as possible after a diagnosis of bvFTD, PPA, or a related disorder. Early on, many people can understand and participate in legal decisions. But as their illness progresses, it becomes harder to make such decisions.

A physician who knows about frontotemporal disorders can help determine the person's mental capacity. An attorney who specializes in elder law, disabilities, or estate planning can provide legal advice, prepare documents, and make financial arrangements for the caregiving spouse or partner and dependent children. If necessary, the person's access to finances can be reduced or eliminated.

Conclusion

It is impossible to predict the exact course of frontotemporal disorders. These disorders are not easy to live with, but with help, people can meet the challenges and prepare for the future. Getting an early, accurate diagnosis and the right medical team are crucial first steps. Researchers and clinicians are working toward a deeper understanding of frontotemporal disorders and better diagnosis and treatment to help people manage these difficult conditions.

Section 5.3

Progressive Supranuclear Palsy (PSP)

Text in this section is excerpted from "Progressive Supranuclear
Palsy Fact Sheet," National Institute of Neurological Disorders and
Stroke (NINDS), February 6, 2015.

What is progressive supranuclear palsy?

Progressive supranuclear palsy (PSP) is a rare brain disorder that
causes serious and progressive problems with control of gait and balance, along with complex eye movement and thinking problems. One of
the classic signs of the disease is an inability to aim the eyes properly,
which occurs because of lesions in the area of the brain that coordinates
eye movements. Some individuals describe this effect as a blurring.
Affected individuals often show alterations of mood and behavior,
including depression and apathy as well as progressive mild dementia.

The disorder's long name indicates that the disease begins slowly
and continues to get worse (*progressive*), and causes weakness (*palsy*)
by damaging certain parts of the brain above pea-sized structures
called nuclei that control eye movements (*supranuclear*).

PSP was first described as a distinct disorder in 1964, when three
scientists published a paper that distinguished the condition from
Parkinson's disease. It is sometimes referred to as Steele-Richard-
son-Olszewski syndrome, reflecting the combined names of the scientists who defined the disorder. Although PSP gets progressively worse,
no one dies from PSP itself.

Who gets PSP?

Approximately 20,000 Americans—or one in every 100,000 people
over the age of 60—have PSP, making it much less common than Parkinson's disease, which affects more than 500,000 Americans. Affected
individuals are usually middle-aged or elderly, and men are affected
more often than women. PSP is often difficult to diagnose because its
symptoms can be very much like those of other, more common movement disorders, and because some of the most characteristic symptoms
may develop late or not at all.

What are the symptoms?

The most frequent first symptom of PSP is a loss of balance while walking. Individuals may have unexplained falls or a stiffness and awkwardness in gait. Sometimes the falls are described by the person experiencing them as attacks of dizziness.

Other common early symptoms are changes in personality such as a loss of interest in ordinary pleasurable activities or increased irritability, cantankerousness, and forgetfulness. Individuals may suddenly laugh or cry for no apparent reason, they may be apathetic, or they may have occasional angry outbursts, also for no apparent reason. It must be emphasized that the pattern of signs and symptoms can be quite different from person to person.

As the disease progresses, most people will begin to develop a blurring of vision and problems controlling eye movement. In fact, eye problems usually offer the first definitive clue that PSP is the proper diagnosis. Individuals affected by PSP have trouble voluntarily shifting their gaze downward, and also can have trouble controlling their eyelids. This can lead to involuntary closing of the eyes, prolonged or infrequent blinking, or difficulty in opening the eyes.

Another common visual problem is an inability to maintain eye contact during a conversation. This can give the mistaken impression that the person is hostile or uninterested.

Speech usually becomes slurred and swallowing solid foods or liquids can be difficult.

In rare cases, the symptoms will be more similar to those of Parkinson disease, and some individuals may even have tremors. This version is often referred to as "Parkinsonian PSP" or PSP-P.

What causes PSP?

We know that the symptoms of PSP are caused by a gradual deterioration of brain cells in a few specific areas in the brain, mainly in the region called the brainstem. One of these areas, the substantia nigra, is also affected in Parkinson's disease, and damage to this region of the brain accounts in part for the motor symptoms that PSP and Parkinson's have in common.

Scientists do not fully know what causes these brain cells to degenerate, but it is known that a hallmark of the disease is the accumulation of an abnormal protein called tau. There is no evidence that PSP is contagious, and genetic factors have not been implicated in most individuals. No ethnic or racial groups have been affected more often than any others, and PSP is no more likely to occur in some geographic areas than in others.

There are, however, several theories about PSP's cause. One possibility is that an unconventional virus-like agent infects the body and takes years or decades to start producing visible effects. Another possibility is that random genetic mutations, of the kind that occur in all of us all the time, happen to occur in particular cells or certain genes, in just the right combination to injure these cells. A third possibility is that there is exposure to some unknown chemical in the food, air, or water which slowly damages certain vulnerable areas of the brain. This theory stems from a clue found on the Pacific island of Guam, where a common neurological disease occurring only there and on a few neighboring islands shares some of the characteristics of PSP, Alzheimer's disease, Parkinson's disease, and amyotrophic lateral sclerosis (Lou Gehrig's disease). Its cause is thought to be a dietary factor or toxic substance found only in that area.

Another possible cause of PSP is cellular damage caused by free radicals, reactive molecules produced continuously by all cells during normal metabolism. Although the body has built-in mechanisms for clearing free radicals from the system, scientists suspect that, under certain circumstances, free radicals can react with and damage other molecules. A great deal of research is directed at understanding the role of free radical damage in human diseases.

How is PSP diagnosed?

Initial complaints in PSP are typically vague and an early diagnosis is always difficult. The primary complaints fall into these categories: 1) symptoms of disequilibrium, such as unsteady walking or abrupt and unexplained falls without loss of consciousness; 2) visual complaints, including blurred vision, difficulties in looking up or down, double vision, light sensitivity, burning eyes, or other eye trouble; 3) slurred speech; and 4) various mental complaints such as slowness of thought, impaired memory, personality changes, and changes in mood.

PSP is often misdiagnosed because some of its symptoms are very much like those of Parkinson's disease, Alzheimer's disease, and more rare neurodegenerative disorders, such as Creutzfeldt-Jakob disease. In fact, PSP is most often misdiagnosed as Parkinson's disease early in the course of the illness. Memory problems and personality changes may also lead a physician to mistake PSP for depression, or even attribute symptoms to some form of dementia. The key to diagnosing PSP is identifying early gait instability and difficulty moving the eyes, the hallmark of the disease, as well as ruling out other similar disorders, some of which are treatable.

How is PSP different from Parkinson's disease?

Both PSP and Parkinson's disease cause stiffness, movement difficulties, and clumsiness. However, people with PSP usually stand straight or occasionally even tilt their heads backward (and tend to fall backward), while those with Parkinson's disease usually bend forward. Problems with speech and swallowing are much more common and severe in PSP than in Parkinson's disease, and tend to show up earlier in the course of the disease. Eye movements are abnormal in PSP but close to normal in Parkinson's disease. Both diseases share other features: onset in late middle age, bradykinesia (slow movement), and rigidity of muscles. Tremor, very common in individuals with Parkinson's disease, is rare in PSP. Although individuals with Parkinson's disease markedly benefit from the drug levodopa, people with PSP respond poorly and only transiently to this drug.

What is the prognosis?

PSP gets progressively worse but is not itself directly life-threatening. It does, however, predispose individuals to serious complications such as pneumonia secondary to difficulty in swallowing (dysphagia). The most common complications are choking and pneumonia, head injury, and fractures caused by falls. The most common cause of death is pneumonia. With good attention to medical and nutritional needs, it is possible for most individuals with PSP to live a decade or more after the first symptoms of the disease.

Is there any treatment?

There is currently no effective treatment for PSP, although scientists are searching for better ways to manage the disease. In some individuals the slowness, stiffness, and balance problems of PSP may respond to antiparkinsonian agents such as levodopa, but the effect is usually temporary.

Excessive eye closing can respond to botulinum injections.

Non-drug treatment for PSP can take many forms. Individuals frequently use weighted walking aids because of their tendency to fall backward. Bifocals or special glasses called prisms are sometimes prescribed for people with PSP to remedy the difficulty of looking down.

Formal physical therapy is of no proven benefit in PSP, but certain exercises can be done to keep the joints limber.

A gastrostomy (or a jejunostomy) may be necessary when there are swallowing disturbances or the definite risk of severe choking. This minimally invasive surgical procedure involves the placement of a tube through the skin of the abdomen into the stomach (intestine) for feeding purposes. Deep brain stimulation and other surgical procedures used in individuals with Parkinson's disease have not been proven effective in PSP.

What research is being done?

Studies to improve the diagnosis of PSP have recently been conducted at the National Institute of Neurological Disorders and Stroke (NINDS). Experiments to find the cause or causes of PSP are currently under way. Clinical trials are testing medications used for other conditions in PSP, but the results so far have not been very encouraging.

In addition, there is a great deal of ongoing research on Parkinson's and Alzheimer's diseases at the National Institutes of Health and at university medical centers throughout the country. Better understanding of those common related disorders will go a long way toward solving the problem of PSP, just as studying PSP may help shed light on Parkinson's and Alzheimer's diseases.

Section 5.4

Lewy Body Dementia (LBD)

Text in this section is excerpted from "Lewy Body Dementia: Information for Patients, Families, and Professionals," National Institute of Aging (NIA), January 22, 2015.

Introduction

Lewy body dementia (LBD) is a complex, challenging, and surprisingly common type of brain disorder. It is complex because it affects many parts of the brain in ways that scientists are trying to understand more fully. It is challenging because its many possible symptoms make it hard to do everyday tasks that once came easily.

Although less known than its "cousins" Alzheimer's disease and Parkinson's disease, LBD is not a rare disorder. More than 1 million Americans, most of them older adults, are affected by its disabling changes in the ability to think and move.

As researchers seek better ways to treat LBD—and ultimately to find a cure—people with LBD and their families struggle day to day to get an accurate diagnosis, find the best treatment, and manage at home.

The Basics of Lewy Body Dementia

LBD is a disease associated with abnormal deposits of a protein called alpha-synuclein in the brain. These deposits, called Lewy bodies, affect chemicals in the brain whose changes, in turn, can lead to problems with thinking, movement, behavior, and mood. LBD is one of the most common causes of dementia, after Alzheimer's disease and vascular disease.

Dementia is a severe loss of thinking abilities that interferes with a person's capacity to perform daily activities such as household tasks, personal care, and handling finances. Dementia has many possible causes, including stroke, tumor, depression, and vitamin deficiency, as well as disorders such as LBD, Parkinson's, and Alzheimer's.

Diagnosing LBD can be challenging for a number of reasons. Early LBD symptoms are often confused with similar symptoms found in brain diseases like Alzheimer's. Also, LBD can occur alone or along with Alzheimer's or Parkinson's disease.

There are two types of LBD—dementia with Lewy bodies and Parkinson's disease dementia. The earliest signs of these two diseases differ but reflect the same biological changes in the brain. Over time, people with dementia with Lewy bodies or Parkinson's disease dementia may develop similar symptoms.

Who Is Affected by LBD?

LBD affects an estimated 1.3 million individuals in the United States and accounts for up to 20 percent of people with dementia worldwide. LBD typically begins at age 50 or older, although sometimes younger people have it. LBD appears to affect slightly more men than women.

LBD is a progressive disease, meaning symptoms start slowly and worsen over time. The disease lasts an average of 5 to 7 years from the time of diagnosis to death, but the time span can range from 2 to 20 years. How quickly symptoms develop and change varies greatly from person to person, depending on overall health, age, and severity of symptoms.

In the early stage of LBD, usually before a diagnosis is made, symptoms can be mild, and people can function fairly normally. As the disease advances, people with LBD require more and more help due to a decline in thinking and movement abilities. In the late stage of the disease, they may depend entirely on others for assistance and care.

Some LBD symptoms may respond to treatment for a period of time. Currently, there is no cure for the disease. Research is improving our understanding of this challenging condition, and advances in science may one day lead to better diagnosis, improved care, and new treatments.

Understanding Terms

The terms used to describe Lewy body dementia (LBD) can be confusing. Doctors and researchers may use different terms to describe the same condition. In this booklet, the term Lewy body dementia is used to describe all dementias whose primary cause is abnormal deposits of Lewy bodies in the brain.

The two types of LBD are:

- dementia with Lewy bodies, in which cognitive (thinking) symptoms appear within a year of movement problems
- Parkinson's disease dementia, in which cognitive symptoms develop more than a year after the onset of movement problems

As LBD progresses, symptoms of both types of LBD are very similar.

What Are Lewy Bodies?

Lewy bodies are named for Dr. Friederich Lewy, a German neurologist. In 1912, he discovered abnormal protein deposits that disrupt the brain's normal functioning in people with Parkinson's disease. These abnormal deposits are now called "Lewy bodies."

Lewy bodies are made of a protein called alpha-synuclein. In the healthy brain, a protein associated with alpha-synuclein plays a number of important roles in neurons (nerve cells) in the brain, especially at synapses, where brain cells communicate with each other. In LBD, alpha-synuclein forms into clumps inside neurons throughout the brain. This process may cause neurons to work less effectively and, eventually, to die. The activities of brain chemicals important to brain function are also affected. The result is widespread damage to certain parts of the brain and a decline in abilities affected by those brain regions.

Lewy bodies affect a few different brain regions in LBD:

- the cerebral cortex, which controls many functions, including information processing, perception, thought, and language

- the limbic cortex, which plays a major role in emotions and behavior

- the hippocampus, which is essential to forming new memories

- the midbrain, including the substantia nigra, which is involved in movement

- areas of the brain stem important in regulating sleep and maintaining alertness

- brain regions important in recognizing smells (olfactory pathways)

Types of Lewy Body Dementia

Lewy body dementia includes two related conditions—dementia with Lewy bodies and Parkinson's disease dementia. The difference between them lies largely in the timing of cognitive (thinking) and movement symptoms. In dementia with Lewy bodies, cognitive symptoms are noted within a year of parkinsonism, any condition that involves the types of movement changes seen in Parkinson's disease. In Parkinson's disease dementia, movement symptoms are most pronounced, with cognitive symptoms developing years later.

Dementia with Lewy Bodies

People with dementia with Lewy bodies first have a decline in cognitive skills that may look somewhat like Alzheimer's disease. But over time they also develop movement and other distinctive symptoms that suggest dementia with Lewy bodies.

Symptoms that distinguish this form of dementia from others may include:

- visual hallucinations early in the course of dementia
- fluctuations in cognitive ability, attention, and alertness
- slowness of movement, difficulty walking, or rigidity (parkinsonism)
- sensitivity to medications used to treat hallucinations
- REM sleep behavior disorder, in which people physically act out their dreams
- more trouble with complex mental activities, such as multitasking, problem solving, and analytical thinking, than with memory

Parkinson's Disease Dementia

This type of LBD starts as a movement disorder, with symptoms such as slowed movement, muscle stiffness, tremor, or a shuffling walk. These symptoms lead to a diagnosis of Parkinson's disease. Later on, cognitive symptoms of dementia and changes in mood and behavior may arise.

Not all people with Parkinson's develop dementia, and it is difficult to predict who will. Being diagnosed with Parkinson's late in life is a risk factor for Parkinson's disease dementia.

Causes and Risk Factors

The precise cause of LBD is unknown, but scientists are learning more about its biology and genetics. For example, they know that an accumulation of Lewy bodies is associated with a loss of certain neurons in the brain that produce two important neurotransmitters, chemicals that act as messengers between brain cells. One of these messengers, acetylcholine, is important for memory and learning. The other, dopamine, plays an important role in behavior, cognition, movement, motivation, sleep, and mood.

Scientists are also learning about risk factors for LBD. Age is considered the greatest risk factor. Most people who develop the disorder are over age 50.

Other known risk factors for LBD include the following:

- **Diseases and health conditions**—Certain diseases and health conditions, particularly Parkinson's disease and REM sleep behavior disorder, are linked to a higher risk of LBD.

- **Genetics**—While having a family member with LBD may increase a person's risk, LBD is not normally considered a genetic disease. A small percentage of families with dementia with Lewy bodies has a genetic association, but in most cases, the cause is unknown. At this time, no genetic test can accurately predict whether someone will develop LBD. Future genetic research may reveal more information about causes and risk.

- **Lifestyle**—No specific lifestyle factor has been proven to increase one's risk for LBD. However, some studies suggest that a healthy lifestyle—including regular exercise, mental stimulation, and a healthy diet—might reduce the chance of developing age-associated dementias.

Common Symptoms

People with LBD may not have every LBD symptom, and the severity of symptoms can vary greatly from person to person. Throughout the course of the disease, any sudden, major change in functional ability or behavior should be reported to a doctor.

The most common symptoms include changes in cognition, movement, sleep, and behavior.

Cognitive Symptoms

LBD causes changes in thinking abilities. These changes may include:

- **Dementia**—Severe loss of thinking abilities that interferes with a person's capacity to perform daily activities. Dementia is a primary symptom in LBD and usually includes trouble with visual and spatial abilities (judging distance and depth or misidentifying objects), multitasking, problem solving, and reasoning. Memory problems may not be evident at first but often arise as LBD progresses. Dementia can also include changes in mood and behavior, poor judgment, loss of initiative, confusion about time and place, and difficulty with language and numbers.

- **Cognitive fluctuations**—Unpredictable changes in concentration, attention, alertness, and wakefulness from day to day and sometimes throughout the day. A person with LBD may stare into space for periods of time, seem drowsy and lethargic, and sleep for several hours during the day despite getting enough sleep the night before. His or her flow of ideas may be disorganized, unclear, or illogical at times. The person may seem better one day, then worse the next day. These cognitive fluctuations are common in LBD but are not always easy for a doctor to identify.

- **Hallucinations**—Seeing or hearing things that are not present. Visual hallucinations occur in up to 80 percent of people with LBD, often early on. They are typically realistic and detailed, such as images of children or animals. Auditory hallucinations are less common than visual ones but may also occur. Hallucinations that are not disruptive may not require treatment. However, if they are frightening or dangerous (for example, if the person attempts to fight a perceived intruder), then a doctor may prescribe medication.

Table 5.2. Main Symptoms of Lewy Body Dementia

Symptom	Dementia with Lewy Bodies	Parkinson's Disease Dementia
Dementia	Appears within a year of movement problems (primary symptom)	Appears later in the disease, after movement problems (primary symptom)
Movement problems (parkinsonism)	Appear at the same time as or after dementia (primary symptom)	Appear before dementia (primary symptom)
Fluctuating cognition, attention, alertness	Primary symptom	Common symptom
Visual hallucinations	Primary symptom	Primary symptom
REM sleep behavior disorder	May develop years before other symptoms (common symptom)	May develop years before other symptoms (common symptom)
Extreme sensitivity to antipsychotic medications	Common symptom	Common symptom
Changes in personality and mood (depression, delusions, apathy)	Common symptom	Common symptom
Changes in autonomic (involuntary) nervous system (blood pressure, bladder and bowel control)	Common symptom	Common symptom

Source: Adapted from the Lewy Body Dementia Association, DLB and PDD Diagnostic Criteria, www.lbda.org/node/470.

Movement Symptoms

Some people with LBD may not experience significant movement problems for several years. Others may have them early on. At first, signs of movement problems, such as a change in handwriting, may be very mild and thus overlooked. Parkinsonism is seen early on in Parkinson's disease dementia but can also develop later on in dementia with Lewy bodies. Specific symptoms of parkinsonism may include:

- muscle rigidity or stiffness
- shuffling gait, slow movement, or frozen stance
- tremor or shaking, most commonly in the hands and usually at rest
- balance problems and falls
- stooped posture
- loss of coordination
- smaller handwriting than was usual for the person
- reduced facial expression
- difficulty swallowing or a weak voice

Sleep Disorders

Sleep disorders are common in people with LBD but are often undiagnosed. A sleep specialist can play an important role on a treatment team, helping to diagnose and treat sleep disorders.

Sleep-related disorders seen in people with LBD may include:

- **REM sleep behavior disorder**—A condition in which a person seems to act out dreams. It may include vivid dreaming, talking in one's sleep, violent movements, or falling out of bed. Sometimes only the bed partner of the person with LBD is aware of these symptoms. REM sleep behavior disorder appears in some people years before other LBD symptoms.

- **Excessive daytime sleepiness**—Sleeping 2 or more hours a day.

- **Insomnia**—Difficulty falling or staying asleep, or waking up too early.

- **Restless leg syndrome**—A condition in which a person, while resting, feels the urge to move his or her legs to stop unpleasant or unusual sensations. Walking or moving usually relieves the discomfort.

Behavioral and Mood Symptoms

Changes in behavior and mood are possible in LBD. These changes may include:

- **Depression**—A persistent feeling of sadness, inability to enjoy activities, and trouble with sleeping, eating, and other normal activities.

- **Apathy**—A lack of interest in normal daily activities or events, and less social interaction.

- **Anxiety**—Intense apprehension, uncertainty, or fear about a future event or situation. A person may ask the same questions over and over or be angry or fearful when a loved one is not present.

- **Agitation**—Restlessness, as seen by pacing, hand wringing, an inability to get settled, constant repeating of words or phrases, or irritability.

- **Delusions**—Strongly held false beliefs or opinions not based on evidence. For example, a person may think his or her spouse is having an affair or that relatives long dead are still living. A delusion that may be seen in LBD is Capgras syndrome, in which the person believes a relative or friend has been replaced by an imposter.

- **Paranoia**—An extreme, irrational distrust of others, such as suspicion that people are taking or hiding things.

Other LBD Symptoms

People with LBD can also experience significant changes in the part of the nervous system that regulates automatic actions such as those of the heart, glands, and muscles. The person may have:

- frequent changes in body temperature
- problems with blood pressure
- dizziness
- fainting
- frequent falls
- sensitivity to heat and cold
- sexual dysfunction

- urinary incontinence

- constipation

- a poor sense of smell

Diagnosis

It's important to know which type of LBD a person has, both to tailor treatment to particular symptoms and to understand how the disease will likely progress. Clinicians and researchers use the "1-year rule" to diagnose which form of LBD a person has. If cognitive symptoms appear within a year of movement problems, the diagnosis is dementia with Lewy bodies. If cognitive problems develop more than a year after the onset of movement problems, the diagnosis is Parkinson's disease dementia.

Regardless of the initial symptoms, over time all people with LBD will develop similar symptoms due to the presence of Lewy bodies in the brain. But there are some differences. For example, dementia with Lewy bodies may progress more quickly than Parkinson's disease dementia.

Dementia with Lewy bodies is often hard to diagnose because its early symptoms may resemble those of Alzheimer's or Parkinson's disease. As a result, it is often misdiagnosed or missed altogether. As additional symptoms appear, it is often easier to make an accurate diagnosis.

The good news is that doctors are increasingly able to diagnose LBD earlier and more accurately as researchers identify which symptoms help distinguish it from similar disorders.

Difficult as it is, getting an accurate diagnosis of LBD early on is important so that a person:

- gets the right medical treatment and avoids potentially harmful treatment

- has time to plan medical care and arrange legal and financial affairs

- can build a support team to stay independent and maximize quality of life

While a diagnosis of LBD can be distressing, some people are relieved to know the reason for their troubling symptoms. It is important to allow time to adjust to the news. Talking about a diagnosis can help shift the focus toward developing a treatment plan.

Who Can Diagnose LBD?

Many physicians and other medical professionals are not familiar with LBD, so patients may consult several doctors before receiving a diagnosis. Visiting a family doctor is often the first step for people who are experiencing changes in thinking, movement, or behavior. However, neurologists—doctors who specialize in disorders of the brain and nervous system—generally have the expertise needed to diagnose LBD. Geriatric psychiatrists, neuropsychologists, and geriatricians may also be skilled in diagnosing the condition.

If a specialist cannot be found in your community, ask the neurology department of the nearest medical school for a referral. A hospital affiliated with a medical school may also have a dementia or movement disorders clinic that provides expert evaluation.

Tests Used to Diagnose LBD

Doctors perform physical and neurological examinations and various tests to distinguish LBD from other illnesses. A thorough evaluation includes:

- Medical history and examination—A review of previous and current illnesses, medications, and current symptoms and tests of movement and memory give the doctor valuable information.

- Medical tests—Laboratory studies can help rule out other diseases and hormonal or vitamin deficiencies that can cause dementia.

- Brain imaging—Computed tomography or magnetic resonance imaging can detect brain shrinkage or structural abnormalities and help rule out other possible causes of dementia or movement symptoms. A single photon emission computed tomography (SPECT) scan can help support a diagnosis of LBD.

- Neuropsychological tests—These tests are used to assess memory and other cognitive functions and can help identify affected brain regions.

There are no brain scans or medical tests that can definitively diagnose LBD. Currently, LBD can be diagnosed with certainty only by a brain autopsy after death.

However, researchers are studying ways to diagnose LBD more accurately in the living brain. Certain types of neuroimaging—positron emission tomography and SPECT—have shown promise in detecting differences between dementia with Lewy bodies and Alzheimer's disease. These methods may help diagnose certain features of the disorder, such as dopamine deficiencies. Researchers are also investigating the use of lumbar puncture (spinal tap) to measure proteins in cerebrospinal fluid that might distinguish dementia with Lewy bodies from Alzheimer's disease and other brain disorders.

Other Helpful Information

It is important for the patient and a close family member or friend to tell the doctor about any symptoms involving thinking, movement, sleep, behavior, or mood. Also, discuss other health problems and provide a list of all current medications, including prescriptions, over-the-counter drugs, vitamins, and supplements. Certain medications can worsen LBD symptoms.

Caregivers may be reluctant to talk about a person's symptoms when that person is present. Ask to speak with the doctor privately if necessary. The more information a doctor has, the more accurate a diagnosis can be.

Treatment and Management

While LBD currently cannot be prevented or cured, some symptoms may respond to treatment for a period of time. A comprehensive treatment plan may involve medications, physical and other types of therapy, and counseling. Changes to make the home safer, equipment to make everyday tasks easier, and social support are also very important.

A skilled care team often can provide suggestions to help improve quality of life for both people with LBD and their caregivers.

Building a Care Team

After receiving a diagnosis, a person with LBD will benefit from seeing a neurologist who specializes in dementia and/or movement disorders. A good place to start is an academic medical center in your community. Ask if it has a dementia or movement disorders clinic, which is where you may find LBD specialists. If such a specialist cannot be found, a general neurologist should be part of the care team. Ask a primary care physician for a referral.

A doctor can work with other types of healthcare providers. Depending on an individual's particular symptoms, other professionals may be helpful:

- **Physical therapists** can help with movement problems through cardiovascular, strengthening, and flexibility exercises, as well as gait training and general physical fitness programs.

- **Speech therapists** may help with low voice volume and voice projection, poor speaking ability, and swallowing difficulties.

- **Occupational therapists** help identify ways to more easily carry out everyday activities, such as eating and bathing, to promote independence.

- **Music or expressive arts therapists** may provide meaningful activities that can reduce anxiety and improve well-being.

- **Mental health counselors** can help people with LBD and their families learn how to manage difficult emotions and behaviors and plan for the future.

Support groups are another valuable resource for both people with LBD and caregivers. Sharing experiences and tips with others in the same situation can help people identify practical solutions to day-to-day challenges and get emotional and social support.

The Role of Palliative Care

The goal of palliative care (comfort care) is to improve a person's quality of life by relieving disease symptoms at any stage of illness. Palliative care can help manage LBD symptoms such as constipation, sleep disorders, and behavioral problems. Typically, a team of nurses, social workers, physical therapists, dieticians, and pharmacists works with doctors to:

- relieve troubling symptoms
- assist with medical decisions
- offer emotional and spiritual support
- coordinate care

To find a palliative medicine specialist, ask a physician or local hospital for a referral, or consult Caring Connections, a service of the National Hospice and Palliative Care Organization.

Medications

Several drugs and other treatments are available to treat LBD symptoms. It is important to work with a knowledgeable health professional because certain medications can make some symptoms worse. Some symptoms can improve with nondrug treatments.

Cognitive Symptoms

Some medications used to treat Alzheimer's disease are also used to treat the cognitive symptoms of LBD. These drugs, called cholinesterase inhibitors, act on a chemical in the brain that is important for memory and thinking. They may also improve behavioral symptoms.

The U.S. Food and Drug Administration (FDA) approves specific drugs for certain uses after rigorous testing and review. However, doctors can prescribe a drug for any use if they think it will help a patient. The FDA has approved one Alzheimer's drug, rivastigmine (Exelon®), to treat cognitive symptoms in Parkinson's disease dementia. This and other Alzheimer's drugs can have side effects such as nausea and diarrhea.

Movement Symptoms

LBD-related movement symptoms may be treated with a Parkinson's medication called carbidopa-levodopa (Sinemet®). This drug can help improve functioning by making it easier to walk, get out of bed, and move around. However, it cannot stop or reverse the progress of the disease.

Side effects of this medication can include hallucinations and other psychiatric or behavioral problems. Because of this risk, physicians may recommend not treating mild movement symptoms with medication. If prescribed, carbidopa-levodopa usually begins at a low dose and is increased gradually. Other Parkinson's medications are less commonly used in people with LBD due to a higher frequency of side effects.

A surgical procedure called deep brain stimulation, which can be very effective in treating the movement symptoms of Parkinson's disease, is not recommended for people with LBD because it can result in greater cognitive impairment.

People with LBD may benefit from physical therapy and exercise. Talk with your doctor about what physical activities are best.

Sleep Disorders

Sleep problems may increase confusion and behavioral problems in people with LBD and add to a caregiver's burden. To help alleviate sleeplessness in people with LBD, a physician can order a sleep study to identify any underlying sleep disorders such as sleep apnea, restless leg syndrome, and REM sleep behavior disorder.

REM sleep behavior disorder, a common LBD symptom, involves acting out one's dreams, leading to lost sleep and even injuries to sleep partners. Clonazepam (Klonopin®), a drug used to control seizures and relieve panic attacks, is often effective for the disorder at very low dosages. However, it can have side effects such as dizziness, unsteadiness, and problems with thinking. Melatonin, a naturally occurring hormone used to treat insomnia, may also offer some benefit when taken alone or with clonazepam.

Excessive daytime sleepiness is also common in LBD. If it is severe, a sleep specialist may prescribe a stimulant to help the person stay awake during the day.

Some people with LBD may have difficulty falling asleep. If trouble sleeping at night (insomnia) persists, a physician may recommend a prescription medication to promote sleep. It is important to note that treating insomnia and other sleep problems in people with LBD has not been extensively studied, and that treatments may worsen daytime sleepiness and should be used with caution.

Certain sleep problems can be addressed without medications. Increasing daytime exercise or activities and avoiding lengthy or frequent naps can promote better sleep. Avoiding alcohol, caffeine, or chocolate late in the day can help, too. Some over-the-counter medications can also affect sleep, so review all medications and supplements with a physician.

Behavioral and Mood Problems

Behavioral and mood problems in people with LBD can arise from hallucinations or delusions. They may also be a result of pain, illness, stress or anxiety, and the inability to express frustration, fear, or feeling overwhelmed. The person may resist care or lash out verbally or physically.

Caregivers must try to be patient and use a variety of strategies to handle such challenging behaviors. Some behavioral problems can be managed by making changes in the person's environment and/or treating medical conditions. Other problems may require medication.

The first step is to visit a doctor to see if a medical condition unrelated to LBD is causing the problem. Injuries, fever, urinary tract or pulmonary infections, pressure ulcers (bed sores), and constipation can cause behavioral problems to suddenly grow worse. Increased confusion can also occur.

Certain medications used to treat LBD symptoms or other diseases may also cause behavioral problems. For example, some over-the-counter sleep aids, strong pain medications, bladder control medications, and drugs used to treat LBD-related movement symptoms can cause confusion, agitation, hallucinations, and delusions. Similarly, some anti-anxiety medicines can actually increase anxiety in people with LBD. Review your medications with your doctor to determine if any changes are needed.

Not all behavior problems are caused by illness or medication. A person's surroundings—including levels of stimulation or stress, lighting, daily routines, and relationships—can lead to behavior issues. Caregivers can alter the home environment to try to minimize anxiety and stress for the person with LBD. In general, people with LBD benefit from having simple tasks, consistent schedules, regular exercise, and adequate sleep. Large crowds or overly stimulating environments can increase confusion and anxiety.

Coping with Behavior Problems

Follow these steps in consultation with a physician to address behavioral problems:

- Rule out physical causes, like infection, pain, or other medical conditions.
- Review current prescription and over-the-counter medications.
- Look for environmental or social factors that contribute to behavioral problems.
- Consider treating with medications if necessary and watch for side effects.

Hallucinations and delusions are among the biggest challenges for LBD caregivers. The person with LBD may not understand or accept that the hallucinations are not real and become agitated or anxious. Caregivers can help by responding to the fears expressed instead of arguing or responding factually to comments that may not be true. By tuning in to the person's emotions, caregivers can offer empathy and concern, maintain the person's dignity, and limit further tension.

Cholinesterase inhibitors may reduce hallucinations and other psychiatric symptoms of LBD. These medications may have side effects, such as nausea, and are not always effective. However, they can be a good first choice to treat behavioral symptoms. Cholinesterase inhibitors do not affect behavior immediately, so they should be considered part of a long-term strategy.

Antidepressants can be used to treat depression and anxiety, which are common in LBD. Two types of antidepressants, called selective serotonin reuptake inhibitors and norepinephrine reuptake inhibitors, are often well tolerated by people with LBD.

In some cases, antipsychotic medications are necessary to treat LBD-related behavioral symptoms to improve both the quality of life and safety of the person with LBD and his or her caregiver. But these types of medications must be used with caution because they can cause severe side effects and can worsen movement symptoms. Consult a doctor before using these types of medications.

If antipsychotics are prescribed, it is very important to use the newer kind, called atypical antipsychotics. These medications should

---

Warning About Antipsychotics

People with LBD may have severe reactions to or side effects from antipsychotics, medications used to treat delusions, hallucinations, or agitation. These side effects include increased confusion, worsened parkinsonism, extreme sleepiness, and low blood pressure that can result in fainting (orthostatic hypotension). Caregivers should contact the doctor if these side effects continue after a few days.

Some antipsychotics, including olanzapine (Zyprexa®) and risperidone (Risperdal®), should be avoided, if possible, because they are more likely than others to cause serious side effects.

In rare cases, a potentially deadly condition called neuroleptic malignant syndrome can occur. Symptoms of this condition include high fever, muscle rigidity, and muscle tissue breakdown that can lead to kidney failure. Report these symptoms to your doctor immediately.

Antipsychotic medications increase the risk of death in elderly people with dementia, including those with LBD. Doctors, patients, and family members must weigh the risks of antipsychotic use against the risks of physical harm and distress that may occur as a result of untreated behavioral symptoms.

be used at the lowest dose possible and for the shortest time possible to control symptoms. Many LBD experts prefer quetiapine (Seroquel®) or clozapine (Clozaril®) to control difficult behavioral symptoms.

Older drugs called typical (or traditional) antipsychotics, such as haloperidol (Haldol®), generally should not be prescribed for people with LBD. They can cause dangerous side effects.

Other Treatment Considerations

LBD affects the part of the nervous system that regulates automatic actions like blood pressure and digestion. One common symptom is orthostatic hypotension, low blood pressure that can cause dizziness and fainting. Simple measures such as leg elevation, elastic stockings, and, when recommended by a doctor, increasing salt and fluid intake can help. If these measures are not enough, a doctor may prescribe medication.

Urinary incontinence (inability to control urinary movements) should be treated cautiously because certain medications may worsen cognition. Consider seeing a urologist. Constipation can usually be treated by exercise and changes in diet, though laxatives and stool softeners may be necessary.

People with LBD are often sensitive to prescription and over-the-counter medications for other medical conditions. Talk with your doctor about any side effects seen in a person with LBD.

If surgery is planned and the person with LBD is told to stop taking all medications beforehand, ask the doctor to consult the person's neurologist in developing a plan for careful withdrawal. In addition, be sure to talk with the anesthesiologist in advance to discuss medication sensitivities and risks unique to LBD. People with LBD who receive certain anesthetics often become confused or delirious and may have a sudden, significant decline in functional abilities, which may become permanent.

Vitamins and Supplements

The use of vitamins and supplements to treat LBD symptoms has not been studied extensively and is not recommended as part of standard treatment. Vitamins and supplements can be dangerous when taken with other medicines. People with LBD should tell their doctors about every medication they take. Be sure to list prescription and over-the-counter medicines, as well as vitamins and supplements.

Depending on the procedure, possible alternatives to general anesthesia include a spinal or regional block. These methods are less likely to result in confusion after surgery.

Advice for People Living with Lewy Body Dementia

Coping with a diagnosis of LBD and all that follows can be challenging. Getting support from family, friends, and professionals is critical to ensuring the best possible quality of life. Creating a safe environment and preparing for the future are important, too. Take time to focus on your strengths, enjoy each day, and make the most of your time with family and friends. Here are some ways to live with LBD day to day.

Getting Help

Your family and close friends are likely aware of changes in your thinking, movement, or behavior. You may want to tell others about your diagnosis so they can better understand the reason for these changes and learn more about LBD. For example, you could say that you have been diagnosed with a brain disorder called Lewy body dementia, which can affect thinking, movement, and behavior. You can say that you will need more help over time. By sharing your diagnosis with those closest to you, you can build a support team to help you manage LBD.

As LBD progresses, you will likely have more trouble managing everyday tasks such as taking medication, paying bills, and driving. You will gradually need more assistance from family members, friends, and perhaps professional caregivers. Although you may be reluctant to get help, try to let others partner with you so you can manage responsibilities together. Remember, LBD affects your loved ones, too. You can help reduce their stress when you accept their assistance.

Finding someone you can talk with about your diagnosis—a trusted friend or family member, a mental health professional, or a spiritual advisor—may be helpful. See the Directory of organizations section to find supportive services in your area.

Consider Safety

The changes in thinking and movement that occur with LBD require attention to safety issues. Consider these steps:

- Fill out and carry the LBD Medical Alert Wallet Card and present it any time you are hospitalized, require emergency medical care, or meet with your doctors. It contains important information about medication sensitivities.

- Consider subscribing to a medical alert service, in which you push a button on a bracelet or necklace to access 911 if you need emergency help.

- Address safety issues in your home, including areas of fall risk, poor lighting, stairs, or cluttered walkways. Think about home modifications that may be needed, such as installing grab bars in the bathroom or modifying stairs with ramps. Ask your doctor to refer you to a home health agency for a home safety evaluation.

- Talk with your doctor about LBD and driving, and have your driving skills evaluated, if needed.

Plan for Your Future

There are many ways to plan ahead. Here are some things to consider:

- If you are working, consult with a legal and financial expert about planning for disability leave or retirement. Symptoms of LBD will interfere with work performance over time, and it is essential to plan now to obtain benefits you are entitled to.

- Consult with an attorney who specializes in elder law or estate planning to help you write or update important documents, such as a living will, healthcare power of attorney, and will.

- Identify local resources for home care, meals, and other services before you need them so you know whom to call when the time comes.

- Explore moving to a retirement or continuing care community where activities and varying levels of care can be provided over time, as needed. Ask about staff members' experience caring for people with LBD.

Find Enjoyment Every Day

It is important to focus on living with LBD. Your attitude can help you find enjoyment in daily life. Despite the many challenges and adjustments, you can have moments of humor, tenderness, and gratitude with the people closest to you.

Make a list of events and activities you can still enjoy—then find a way to do them! For example, listening to music, exercising, or going out for a meal allows you to enjoy time with family and friends. If you can't find pleasure in daily life, consult your doctor or another health-care professional to discuss effective ways to cope and move forward. Let your family know if you are struggling emotionally so they can offer support.

Caring for a Person with Lewy Body Dementia

As someone who is caring for a person with LBD, you will take on many different responsibilities over time. You do not have to face these responsibilities alone. Many sources of help are available, from adult day centers and respite care to online and in-person support groups.

Below are some important actions you can take to adjust to your new roles, be realistic about your situation, and care for yourself.

Educate Others About LBD

Most people, including many healthcare professionals, are not famil-iar with LBD. In particular, emergency room physicians and other hospital workers may not know that people with LBD are extremely sensitive to antipsychotic medications. Caregivers can educate health-care professionals and others by:

- Informing hospital staff of the LBD diagnosis and medication sensitivities, and requesting that the person's neurologist be consulted before giving any drugs to control behavior problems.

- Sharing educational pamphlets and other materials with doc-tors, nurses, and other healthcare professionals who care for the person with LBD. Materials are available from the Lewy Body Dementia Association.

- Teaching family and friends about LBD so they can better understand your situation.

Adjust Expectations

You will likely experience a wide range of emotions as you care for the person with LBD. Sometimes, caregiving will feel loving and rewarding. Other times, it will lead to anger, impatience, resentment, or fatigue. You must recognize your strengths and limitations, espe-cially in light of your past relationship with the person. Roles may change between a husband and wife or between a parent and adult children. Adjusting expectations can allow you to approach your new roles realistically and to seek help as needed.

Prepare for Emergencies

People with LBD may experience sudden declines in functioning or unpredictable behaviors that can result in visits to the emergency room. Infections, pain, or other medical conditions often cause increased confusion or behavioral problems. Caregivers can prepare for emergencies by having available:

- a list of the person's medications and dosages
- a list of the person's health conditions, including allergies to medicines or foods
- copies of health insurance card(s)
- copies of healthcare advance directives, such as a living will
- contact information for doctors, family members, and friends

---

People approach challenges at varied paces. Some people want to learn everything possible and be prepared for every scenario, while others manage best by taking one day at a time. Caring for someone with LBD requires a balance. On one hand, you should plan for the future. On the other hand, you may want to make each day count in personal ways and focus on creating enjoyable and meaningful moments.

Care for Yourself

As a caregiver, you play an essential role in the life of the person with LBD, so it is critical for you to maintain your own health and well-being. You may be at increased risk for poor sleep, depression, or illness as a result of your responsibilities. Watch for signs of physical or emotional fatigue such as irritability, withdrawal from friends and family, and changes in appetite or weight.

All caregivers need time away from caregiving responsibilities to maintain their well-being. Learn to accept help when it's offered and learn to ask family and friends for help. One option is professional respite care, which can be obtained through home care agencies and adult day programs. Similarly, friends or family can come to the home or take the person with LBD on an outing to give you a break.

Address Family Concerns

Not all family members may understand or accept LBD at the same time, and this can create conflict. Some adult children may deny that parents have a problem, while others may be supportive. It can take a while to learn new roles and responsibilities.

Family members who visit occasionally may not see the symptoms that primary caregivers see daily and may underestimate or minimize your responsibilities or stress. Professional counselors can help with family meetings or provide guidance on how families can work together to manage LBD.

Helping Children and Teens Cope with LBD

When someone has Lewy body dementia, it affects the whole family, including children and grandchildren. Children notice when something "doesn't seem right." Telling them in age-appropriate language that someone they know or love has been diagnosed with a brain disorder can help them make sense of the changes they see. Give them enough information to answer questions or provide explanations without overwhelming them.

Children and teens may feel a loss of connection with the person with LBD who has problems with attention or alertness. They may also resent the loss of a parent caregiver's attention and may need special time with him or her. Look for signs of stress in children, such as poor grades at school, withdrawal from friendships, or unhealthy behaviors at home. Parents may want to notify teachers or counselors of the LBD diagnosis in the family so they can watch for changes in the young person that warrant attention.

Here are some other ways parents can help children and teens adjust to a family member with LBD:

- Help them keep up with normal activities such as sports, clubs, and other hobbies outside the home. Suggest ways for kids to engage with the relative with LBD through structured activities or play. For example, the child or teen can make a cup of tea for the person with LBD.
- Find online resources for older children and teens so they can learn about dementia and LBD.

It is important for families to make time for fun. Many challenges can be faced when they are balanced with enjoyable times. While LBD creates significant changes in family routines, children and teens will cope more effectively if the disorder becomes part of, but not all of, their lives.

Research—The Road Ahead

LBD is of increasing interest to the Alzheimer's and Parkinson's disease research communities. It represents an important link between these other brain disorders, and research into one disease often contributes to better understanding of the others. However, there is a great deal to learn about LBD. At a basic level, why does alpha-synuclein accumulate into Lewy bodies, and how do Lewy bodies cause the symptoms of LBD?

Many avenues of research focus on improving our understanding of LBD. Some researchers are working to identify the specific differences in the brain between dementia with Lewy bodies and Parkinson's disease dementia. Others are looking at the disease's underlying biology, genetics, and environmental risk factors. Still other scientists are trying to identify biomarkers (biological indicators of disease) and improve screening tests to aid diagnosis.

Scientists hope that new knowledge about LBD will one day lead to more effective treatments and even ways to cure and prevent the disorder. Until then, researchers need volunteers with and without LBD for clinical studies. People with LBD who volunteer for these important studies may receive highly specialized care and access to medications that are not otherwise available.

Section 5.5

Multi-Infarct Dementia (MID)

Text in this section is excerpted from "Multi-Infarct Dementia
Information Page," National Institute of Neurological Disorders and
Stroke (NINDS), May 22, 2014.

What is Multi-Infarct Dementia?

Multi-infarct dementia (MID) is a common cause of memory loss in the elderly. MID is caused by multiple strokes (disruption of blood flow to the brain). Disruption of blood flow leads to damaged brain tissue. Some of these strokes may occur without noticeable clinical symptoms. Doctors refer to these as "silent strokes." An individual having a silent stroke may not even know it is happening, but over time, as more areas of the brain are damaged and more small blood vessels are blocked, the symptoms of MID begin to appear. MID can be diagnosed by an MRI or CT of the brain, along with a neurological examination. Symptoms include confusion or problems with short-term memory; wandering, or getting lost in familiar places; walking with rapid, shuffling steps; losing bladder or bowel control; laughing or crying inappropriately; having difficulty following instructions; and having problems counting money and making monetary transactions. MID, which typically begins between the ages of 60 and 75, affects men more often than women. Because the symptoms of MID are so similar to Alzheimer's disease, it can be difficult for a doctor to make a firm diagnosis. Since the diseases often occur together, making a single diagnosis of one or the other is even more problematic.

Is there any treatment?

There is no treatment available to reverse brain damage that has been caused by a stroke. Treatment focuses on preventing future strokes by controlling or avoiding the diseases and medical conditions that put people at high risk for stroke: high blood pressure, diabetes, high cholesterol, and cardiovascular disease. The best treatment for MID is prevention early in life – eating a healthy diet, exercising, not smoking, moderately using alcohol, and maintaining a healthy weight.

What is the prognosis?

The prognosis for individuals with MID is generally poor. The symptoms of the disorder may begin suddenly, often in a step-wise pattern after each small stroke. Some people with MID may even appear to improve for short periods of time, then decline after having more silent strokes. The disorder generally takes a downward course with intermittent periods of rapid deterioration. Death may occur from stroke, heart disease, pneumonia, or other infection.

Section 5.6

Subcortical Dementia—Binswanger's Disease

Text in this section is excerpted from "Binswanger's Disease
Information Page," National Institute of Neurological Disorders and
Stroke (NINDS), May 22, 2014.

What is Binswanger's Disease?

Binswanger's disease (BD), also called *subcortical vascular dementia*, is a type of dementia caused by widespread—microscopic areas of damage to the deep layers of white matter in the brain. The damage is the result of the thickening and narrowing (atherosclerosis) of arteries that feed the subcortical areas of the brain. Atherosclerosis (commonly known as "hardening of the arteries") is a systemic process that affects blood vessels throughout the body. It begins late in the fourth decade of life and increases in severity with age. As the arteries become more and more narrowed, the blood supplied by those arteries decreases and brain tissue dies. A characteristic pattern of BD-damaged brain tissue can be seen with modern brain imaging techniques such as CT scans or Magnetic Resonance Imaging (MRI). The symptoms associated with BD are related to the disruption of subcortical neural circuits that control what neuroscientists call *executive cognitive functioning*: short-term memory, organization, mood, the regulation of attention, the ability to act or make decisions, and appropriate behavior. The most characteristic feature of BD is psychomotor slowness - an increase in the length of time it takes, for example, for the fingers to turn the thought of a letter into the shape of a letter on a piece of paper. Other symptoms include forgetfulness (but not as severe as the forgetfulness of Alzheimer's disease), changes in speech, an unsteady gait, clumsiness or frequent falls, changes in personality or mood (most likely in the form of apathy, irritability, and depression), and urinary symptoms that aren't caused by urological disease. Brain imaging, which reveals the characteristic brain lesions of BD, is essential for a positive diagnosis.

Is there any treatment?

There is no specific course of treatment for BD. Treatment is symptomatic. People with depression or anxiety may require antidepressant medications such as the Serotonin-Specific Reuptake Inhibitors (SSRI) sertraline or citalopram. A typical antipsychotic drugs, such as risperidone and olanzapine, can be useful in individuals with agitation and disruptive behavior. Recent drug trials with the drug memantine have shown improved cognition and stabilization of global functioning and behavior. The successful management of hypertension and diabetes can slow the progression of atherosclerosis, and subsequently slow the progress of BD. Because there is no cure, the best treatment is preventive, early in the adult years, by controlling risk factors such as hypertension, diabetes, and smoking.

What is the prognosis?

BD is a progressive disease; there is no cure. Changes may be sudden or gradual and then progress in a stepwise manner. BD can often coexist with Alzheimer's disease. Behaviors that slow the progression of high blood pressure, diabetes, and atherosclerosis—such as eating a healthy diet and keeping healthy wake/sleep schedules, exercising, and not smoking or drinking too much alcohol—can also slow the progression of BD.

Section 5.7

Creutzfeldt-Jakob Disease (CJD)

Text in this section is excerpted from "Creutzfeldt-Jakob Disease Fact Sheet," National Institute of Neurological Disorders and Stroke (NINDS), February 2, 2015.

What is Creutzfeldt-Jakob Disease?

Creutzfeldt-Jakob Disease (CJD) is a rare, degenerative, invariably fatal brain disorder. It affects about one person in every one million people per year worldwide; in the United States there are about 300 cases per year. CJD usually appears in later life and runs a rapid course. Typically, onset of symptoms occurs about age 60, and about 90 percent of individuals die within 1 year. In the early stages of disease, people may have failing memory, behavioral changes, lack of coordination and visual disturbances. As the illness progresses, mental deterioration becomes pronounced and involuntary movements, blindness, weakness of extremities, and coma may occur.

There are three major categories of CJD:

- In sporadic CJD, the disease appears even though the person has no known risk factors for the disease. This is by far the most common type of CJD and accounts for at least 85 percent of cases.

- In hereditary CJD, the person has a family history of the disease and/or tests positive for a genetic mutation associated with CJD. About 5 to 10 percent of cases of CJD in the United States are hereditary.

- In acquired CJD, the disease is transmitted by exposure to brain or nervous system tissue, usually through certain medical procedures. There is no evidence that CJD is contagious through casual contact with a CJD patient. Since CJD was first described in 1920, fewer than 1 percent of cases have acquired CJD.

CJD belongs to a family of human and animal diseases known as the Transmissible Spongiform Encephalopathies (TSEs). Spongiform refers to the characteristic appearance of infected brains, which become filled with holes until they resemble sponges under a microscope. CJD is the most common of the known human TSEs. Other human TSEs include Kuru, Fatal Familial Insomnia (FFI), and Gerstmann-Straussler-Scheinker disease (GSS). Kuru was identified in people of an isolated tribe in Papua New Guinea and has now almost disappeared. FFI and GSS are extremely rare hereditary diseases, found in just a few families around the world. Other TSEs are found in specific kinds of animals. These include Bovine Spongiform Encephalopathy (BSE), which is found in cows and is often referred to as "mad cow" disease; scrapie, which affects sheep and goats; mink encephalopathy; and feline encephalopathy. Similar diseases have occurred in elk, deer, and exotic zoo animals.

What are the Symptoms of the Disease?

CJD is characterized by rapidly progressive dementia. Initially, individuals experience problems with muscular coordination; personality changes—including impaired memory, judgment, and thinking; and impaired vision. People with the disease also may experience insomnia, depression, or unusual sensations. CJD does not cause a fever or other flu-like symptoms. As the illness progresses, mental impairment becomes severe. Individuals often develop involuntary muscle jerks called myoclonus, and they may go blind. They eventually lose the ability to move and speak and enter a coma. Pneumonia and other infections often occur in these individuals and can lead to death.

There are several known variants of CJD. These variants differ somewhat in the symptoms and course of the disease. For example, a variant form of the disease-called new variant or variant (nv-CJD, v-CJD), described in Great Britain and France-begins primarily with psychiatric symptoms, affects younger individuals than other types of CJD, and has a longer than usual duration from onset of symptoms to death. Another variant, called the panencephalopathic form, occurs primarily in Japan and has a relatively long course, with symptoms often progressing for several years. Scientists are trying to learn what causes these variations in the symptoms and course of the disease.

Some symptoms of CJD can be similar to symptoms of other progressive neurological disorders, such as Alzheimer's or Huntington's disease. However, CJD causes unique changes in brain tissue which can be seen at autopsy. It also tends to cause more rapid deterioration of a person's abilities than Alzheimer's disease or most other types of dementia.

How is CJD Diagnosed?

There is currently no single diagnostic test for CJD. When a doctor suspects CJD, the first concern is to rule out treatable forms of dementia such as encephalitis (inflammation of the brain) or chronic meningitis. A neurological examination will be performed and the doctor may seek consultation with other physicians. Standard diagnostic tests will include a spinal tap to rule out more common causes of dementia and an electroencephalogram (EEG) to record the brain's electrical pattern, which can be particularly valuable because it shows a specific type of abnormality in CJD. Computerized tomography of the brain can help rule out the possibility that the symptoms result from other problems such as stroke or a brain tumor. Magnetic Resonance Imaging (MRI) brain scans also can reveal characteristic patterns of brain degeneration that can help diagnose CJD.

The only way to confirm a diagnosis of CJD is by brain biopsy or autopsy. In a brain biopsy, a neurosurgeon removes a small piece of tissue from the patient's brain so that it can be examined by a neuropathologist. This procedure may be dangerous for the individual, and the operation does not always obtain tissue from the affected part of the brain. Because a correct diagnosis of CJD does not help the person, a brain biopsy is discouraged unless it is needed to rule out a treatable disorder. In an autopsy, the whole brain is examined after death. Both brain biopsy and autopsy pose a small, but definite, risk that the surgeon or others who handle the brain tissue may become accidentally infected by self-inoculation. Special surgical and disinfection procedures can minimize this risk.

Scientists are working to develop laboratory tests for CJD. One such test, developed at NINDS, is performed on a person's cerebrospinal fluid and detects a protein marker that indicates neuronal degeneration. This can help diagnose CJD in people who already show the clinical symptoms of the disease. This test is much easier and safer than a brain biopsy. The false positive rate is about 5 to 10 percent. Scientists are working to develop this test for use in commercial laboratories. They are also working to develop other tests for this disorder.

How is the Disease Treated?

There is no treatment that can cure or control CJD. Researchers have tested many drugs, including amantadine, steroids, interferon, acyclovir, antiviral agents, and antibiotics. Studies of a variety of other drugs are now in progress. However, so far none of these treatments has shown any consistent benefit in humans.

Current treatment for CJD is aimed at alleviating symptoms and making the individual as comfortable as possible. Opiate drugs can help relieve pain if it occurs, and the drugs clonazepam and sodium valproate may help relieve myoclonus. During later stages of the disease, changing the person's position frequently can keep him or her comfortable and helps prevent bedsores. A catheter can be used to drain urine if the individual cannot control bladder function, and intravenous fluids and artificial feeding also may be used.

What Causes Creutzfeldt-Jakob Disease?

Some researchers believe an unusual "slow virus" or another organism causes CJD. However, they have never been able to isolate a virus or other organism in people with the disease. Furthermore, the agent that causes CJD has several characteristics that are unusual for known organisms such as viruses and bacteria. It is difficult to kill, it does not appear to contain any genetic information in the form of nucleic acids (DNA or RNA), and it usually has a long incubation period before symptoms appear. In some cases, the incubation period may be as long as 50 years. The leading scientific theory at this time maintains that CJD and the other TSEs are caused by a type of protein called prion.

Prion proteins occur in both a normal form, which is a harmless protein found in the body's cells, and in an infectious form, which causes disease. The harmless and infectious forms of the prion protein have the same sequence of amino acids (the "building blocks" of proteins) but the infectious form of the protein takes a different folded shape than the normal protein. Sporadic CJD may develop because some of a person's normal prions spontaneously change into the infectious form of the protein and then alter the prions in other cells in a chain reaction.

Once they appear, abnormal prion proteins aggregate, or clump together. Investigators think these protein aggregates may lead to the neuron loss and other brain damage seen in CJD. However, they do not know exactly how this damage occurs.

About 5 to 10 percent of all CJD cases are inherited. These cases arise from a mutation, or change, in the gene that controls formation of the normal prion protein. While prions themselves do not contain genetic information and do not require genes to reproduce themselves, infectious prions can arise if a mutation occurs in the gene for the body's normal prion protein. If the prion protein gene is altered in a person's sperm or egg cells, the mutation can be transmitted to the person's offspring. All mutations in the prion protein gene are inherited as dominant traits. Therefore, family history is helpful in considering the diagnosis. Several different mutations in the prion gene have been identified. The particular mutation found in each family affects how frequently the disease appears and what symptoms are most noticeable. However, not all people with mutations in the prion protein gene develop CJD.

How is CJD Transmitted?

CJD cannot be transmitted through the air or through touching or most other forms of casual contact. Spouses and other household members of sporadic CJD patients have no higher risk of contracting the disease than the general population. However, exposure to brain tissue and spinal cord fluid from infected individuals should be avoided to prevent transmission of the disease through these materials.

In some cases, CJD has spread to other people from grafts of dura mater (a tissue that covers the brain), transplanted corneas, implantation of inadequately sterilized electrodes in the brain, and injections of contaminated pituitary growth hormone derived from human pituitary glands taken from cadavers. Doctors call these cases that are linked to medical procedures iatrogenic cases. Since 1985, all human growth hormone used in the United States has been synthesized by recombinant DNA procedures, which eliminates the risk of transmitting CJD by this route.

The appearance of the new variant of CJD (nv-CJD or v-CJD) in several younger than average people in Great Britain and France has led to concern that BSE may be transmitted to humans through consumption of contaminated beef. Although laboratory tests have shown a strong similarity between the prions causing BSE and v-CJD, there is no direct proof to support this theory.

Many people are concerned that it may be possible to transmit CJD through blood and related blood products such as plasma. Some animal studies suggest that contaminated blood and related products may transmit the disease, although this has never been shown in humans. If there are infectious agents in these fluids, they are probably in very low concentrations. Scientists do not know how many abnormal prions a person must receive before he or she develops CJD, so they do not know whether these fluids are potentially infectious or not. They do know that, even though millions of people receive blood transfusions each year, there are no reported cases of someone contracting CJD from a transfusion. Even among people with hemophilia, who sometimes receive blood plasma concentrated from thousands of donors, there are no reported cases of CJD.

While there is no evidence that blood from people with sporadic CJD is infectious, studies have found that infectious prions from BSE and vCJD may accumulate in the lymph nodes (which produce white blood cells), the spleen, and the tonsils. These findings suggest that blood transfusions from people with vCJD might transmit the disease. The possibility that blood from people with vCJD may be infectious has led to a policy preventing people in the United States from donating blood if they have resided for more than 3 months in a country or countries where BSE is common.

How Can People Avoid Spreading the Disease?

To reduce the already very low risk of CJD transmission from one person to another, people should never donate blood, tissues, or organs if they have suspected or confirmed CJD, or if they are at increased risk because of a family history of the disease, a dura mater graft, or other factor.

Normal sterilization procedures such as cooking, washing, and boiling do not destroy prions. Caregivers, healthcare workers, and undertakers should take the following precautions when they are working with a person with CJD:

- Cover cuts and abrasions with waterproof dressings.

- Wear surgical gloves when handling a patient's tissues and fluids or dressing the patient's wounds.

- Avoid cutting or sticking themselves with instruments contaminated by the patient's blood or other tissues.

- Use disposable bedclothes and other cloth for contact with the patient. If disposable materials are not available, regular cloth should be soaked in undiluted chlorine bleach for an hour or more, and then washed in a normal fashion after each use.

- Use face protection if there is a risk of splashing contaminated material such as blood or cerebrospinal fluid.

- Soak instruments that have come in contact with the patient in undiluted chlorine bleach for an hour or more, then use an autoclave (pressure cooker) to sterilize them in distilled water for at least one hour at 132–134 degrees Centigrade.

Fact sheets listing additional precautions for healthcare workers and morticians are available from the NINDS and the World Health Organization.

What Research Is Taking Place?

Many researchers are studying CJD. They are examining whether the transmissible agent is, in fact, a prion or a product of the infection, and are trying to discover factors that influence prion infectivity and how the disorder damages the brain. Using rodent models of the disease and brain tissue from autopsies, they are also trying to identify factors that influence susceptibility to the disease and that govern when in life the disease appears. They hope to use this knowledge to develop improved tests for CJD and to learn what changes ultimately kill the neurons so that effective treatments can be developed.

Section 5.8

Variant Creutzfeldt-Jakob Disease (vCJD)

Text in this section is excerpted from "Fact Sheet: Variant
Creutzfeldt-Jakob Disease," Centers for Disease Control and
Prevention (CDC), June 3, 2014.

Background

Variant CJD (vCJD) is a rare, degenerative, fatal brain disorder
in humans. Although experience with this new disease is limited,
evidence to date indicates that there has never been a case of vCJD
transmitted through direct contact of one person with another. However, a case of probable transmission of vCJD through transfusion
of blood components from an asymptomatic donor who subsequently
developed the disease has been reported.

Since variant CJD was first reported in 1996, a total of 229 patients
with this disease from 12 countries have been identified. As of June 2,
2014, variant CJD cases have been reported from the following countries: 177 from the United Kingdom, 27 from France, 5 from Spain, 4
from Ireland, 4 from the United States, 3 in the Netherlands, 2 in Portu-
gal, 2 in Italy, 2 in Canada and one each from Japan, Saudi Arabia, and
Taiwan. Two of the four U.S. cases, two of the four cases from Ireland,
one of the two cases from Canada, and the single case from Japan were
likely exposed to the BSE agent while residing in the United Kingdom.

There has never been a case of vCJD that did not have a history of
exposure within a country where the cattle disease, BSE, was occurring.

It is believed that the persons who have developed vCJD became
infected through their consumption of cattle products contaminated
with the agent of BSE or in three cases, each reported from the United
Kingdom, through receipt of blood from an asymptomatic, infected
donor. There is no known treatment of vCJD and it is invariably fatal.

vCJD Differs from Classic CJD

This variant form of CJD should not be confused with the classic form of CJD that is endemic throughout the world, including the

United States. There are several important differences between these two forms of the disease. The median age at death of patients with classic CJD in the United States, for example, is 68 years, and very few cases occur in persons under 30 years of age. In contrast, the median age at death of patients with vCJD in the United Kingdom is 28 years.

vCJD can be confirmed only through examination of brain tissue obtained by biopsy or at autopsy, but a "probable case" of vCJD can be diagnosed on the basis of clinical criteria developed in the United Kingdom.

The incubation period for vCJD is unknown because it is a new disease. However, it is likely that ultimately this incubation period will be measured in terms of many years or decades. In other words, whenever a person develops vCJD from consuming a BSE-contaminated product, he or she likely would have consumed that product many years or a decade or more earlier.

In contrast to classic CJD, vCJD in the United Kingdom predominantly affects younger people, has atypical clinical features, with prominent psychiatric or sensory symptoms at the time of clinical presentation and delayed onset of neurologic abnormalities, including ataxia within weeks or months, dementia and myoclonus late in the illness, a duration of illness of at least 6 months, and a diffusely abnormal non-diagnostic electroencephalogram.

The BSE epidemic in the United Kingdom reached its peak incidence in January 1993 at almost 1,000 new cases per week. The outbreak may have resulted from the feeding of scrapie-containing sheep meat-and-bone meal to cattle. There is strong evidence and general agreement that the outbreak was amplified by feeding rendered bovine meat-and-bone meal to young calves.

U.S. Surveillance for variant CJD

The possibility that BSE can spread to humans has focused increased attention on the desirability of enhancing national surveillance for Creutzfeldt-Jakob Disease (CJD) in the United States in order to detect variant CJD. Improving methods to detect classic CJD, such as increasing the number of autopsies on patients with suspected prion disease, enhances the ability to identify cases of variant CJD.

The Centers for Disease Control and Prevention (CDC) monitors the trends and current incidence of classic CJD in the United States through several surveillance mechanisms. The oldest and most systematic method includes analyzing death certificate information from U.S. multiple cause-of-death data, compiled by the National Center for Health Statistics, CDC. During 1979-2003 the average annual age adjusted death rates of classic CJD have remained relatively stable. Moreover, deaths from non-iatrogenic CJD in persons aged <30 years in the United States remain extremely rare (<5 cases per 1 billion per year). In contrast, in the United Kingdom, over half of the patients who died with vCJD were in this young age group.

In addition, CDC collects, reviews and when indicated, actively investigates reports by health care personnel or institutions of possible iatrogenic CJD and variant CJD cases. Finally and very importantly, in 1996-97, CDC established, in collaboration with the American Association of Neuropathologists, the National Prion Disease Pathology Surveillance Center at Case Western Reserve University, which performs special diagnostic tests for prion diseases, including post-mortem tests that can detect vCJD.

vCJD Cases Reported in the US

Four cases of vCJD have been reported from the United States. By convention, variant CJD cases are ascribed to the country of initial symptom onset, regardless of where the exposure occurred. There is strong evidence that suggests that two of the four cases were exposed to the BSE agent in the United Kingdom and that the third was exposed while living in Saudi Arabia. The history of the fourth patient, including extensive travel to Europe and the Middle East, supports the likelihood that infection occurred outside the United States.

The first patient was born in the United Kingdom in the late 1970s and lived there until a move to Florida in 1992. The patient had onset of symptoms in November 2001 and died in June of 2004. The patient never donated or received blood, plasma, or organs, never received human growth hormone, nor did the patient ever have major surgery other than having wisdom teeth extracted in 2001. Additionally, there was no family history of CJD.

The second patient resided in Texas during 2001–2005. Symptoms began in early 2005 while the patient was in Texas. He then returned to the United Kingdom, where his illness progressed, and a diagnosis of variant CJD was made. The diagnosis was confirmed neuropathologically at the time of the patient's death. While living in the United States, the patient had no history of hospitalization, of having invasive medical procedures, or of donation or receipt of blood and blood products. The patient almost certainly acquired the disease in the United Kingdom. He was born in the United Kingdom and lived there throughout the defined period of risk (1980–1996) for human exposure to the agent of bovine spongiform encephalopathy (BSE, commonly known as "mad cow" disease). His stay in the United States was too brief relative to what is known about the incubation period for variant CJD.

The third patient was born and raised in Saudi Arabia and has lived in the United States since late 2005. The patient occasionally stayed in the United States for up to 3 months at a time since 2001 and there was a shorter visit in 1989. The patient's onset of symptoms occurred in Spring 2006. In late November 2006, the Clinical Prion Research Team at the University of California San Francisco Memory and Aging Center confirmed the vCJD clinical diagnosis by pathologic study of adenoid and brain biopsy tissues. The patient has no history of receipt of blood, a past neurosurgical procedure, or residing in or visiting countries of Europe. Based on the patient's history, the occurrence of a previously reported Saudi case of vCJD attributed to likely consumption of BSE-contaminated cattle products in Saudi Arabia, and the expected greater than 7-year incubation period for food-related vCJD, this U.S. case-patient was most likely infected from contaminated cattle products consumed as a child when living in Saudi Arabia. The patient has no history of donating blood and the public health investigation has identified no known risk of transmission to U.S. residents from this patient.

The fourth patient died in Texas in May 2014. Laboratory tests confirmed a diagnosis of variant CJD. The confirmation was made when laboratory results from an autopsy of the patient's brain tested positive for variant CJD.

Prevention Measures against BSE Spread

To prevent BSE from entering the United States, severe restrictions were placed on the importation of live ruminants, such as cattle, sheep, and goats, and certain ruminant products from countries where BSE was known to exist. These restrictions were later extended to include importation of ruminants and certain ruminant products from all European countries.

Because the use of ruminant tissue in ruminant feed was probably a necessary factor responsible for the BSE outbreak in the United Kingdom and because of the current evidence for possible transmission of BSE to humans, the U.S. Food and Drug Administration instituted a ruminant feed ban in June 1997 that became fully effective as of October 1997. As of October 26, 2009, a regulation issued by FDA in April 2009 came into effect establishing an enhanced BSE-related feed ban in the U.S. This enhanced feed ban will further harmonize BSE feed control measures in the U.S. with those in Canada (see below). In addition, FDA continues to enforce its important 1997 mammalian-to-ruminant feed ban through its BSE inspection and BSE feed testing programs.

As of July 12, 2007, an enhanced BSE-related feed ban came into effect in Canada. The Canadian Food Inspection Agency (CFIA) established this ban to more effectively prevent and quickly eliminate BSE from Canada. The enhanced ban prohibits most proteins, including potentially BSE infectious tissues known as "specified risk materials" (SRM) from all animal feeds, pet foods, and fertilizers, not just from cattle feed as required by the ban instituted in 1997. The 1997 feed ban in Canada was similar to the feed ban instituted in the United States that same year. As recently reported by CFIA, removing SRM from the entire animal feed system addresses risks associated with the potential contamination of cattle feed during production, distribution, storage, and use. Applying the same measure to pet food and fertilizer materials addresses the possible exposure of cattle and other susceptible animals to these products. With this ban in place, CFIA expects BSE should be eliminated from the Canadian cattle herd by about the year 2017.

In late 2001, the Harvard Center for Risk Assessment study of various scenarios involving BSE in the U.S. concluded that the FDA ruminant feed rule provides a major defense against this disease.

BSE/TSE Action Plan of the Department of Health and Human Services (DHHS)

On August 23, 2001, the Department of Health and Human Services (HHS) issued a department-wide action plan outlining steps to improve scientific understanding of BSE and other transmissible spongiform encephalopathies (TSEs). The action plan has four major components:

Surveillance for human disease is primarily the responsibility of CDC.

Protection is primarily the responsibility of the Food and Drug Administration (FDA).

Research is primarily the responsibility of the National Institutes of Health (NIH).

Oversight is primarily the responsibility of the Office of the Secretary of DHHS.

Section 5.9

Current Research on Dementias

Text in this section is excerpted from "Dementia: Hope Through
Research," National Institute of Neurological Disorders and Stroke
(NINDS), February 23, 2015.

In 2012, the President announced the National Plan to Address
Alzheimer's Disease, a national effort to expand research in Alzheimer's
and related dementias prevention and treatment and to move the most
promising drugs from discovery into clinical trials. The Plan aims to prevent and effectively treat Alzheimer's and related dementias by 2025. Its
foundation is the 2011 National Alzheimer's Project Act (NAPA), which
was developed to create and maintain a national strategy to overcome
the disease. The National Plan calls for increased federal funding for AD
research, support for those affected by AD and their families, increased
public awareness about AD, and improved data collection and analysis to better understand the impact of AD on people with the disease,
families, and the health and long-term care systems. These goals also
apply to AD-related dementias, including dementia with Lewy bodies
as well as frontotemporal, mixed (characteristics of more than one type
of dementia occur simultaneously), and vascular dementias. For more
information, see *http://aspe.hhs.gov/daltcp/napa/NatlPlan.pdf.*

The National Institute of Neurological Disorders and Stroke
(NINDS), a component of NIH, is the leading federal funder of research
on nervous system disorders. Another NIH Institute, the National
Institute on Aging (NIA), is the leading federal funder of research
on AD. Together, these Institutes are world leaders in supporting
research on the dementias, including Lewy body dementia, frontotemporal disorders, and vascular dementia.

Although scientists have some understanding of these dementias
and the mechanisms involved, ongoing research may lead to new ways
to diagnose, treat, or perhaps prevent or block disease development.
Current areas of research include:

Clinical studies. Clinical studies offer an opportunity to help
researchers find better ways to safely detect, treat, or prevent

dementias. Various NIH Institutes support clinical studies on AD and related dementias at the NIH research campus in Bethesda, MD, and at medical research centers throughout the U.S. For information about participating in clinical studies for AD, related dementias, and other disorders, visit "NIH Clinical Research Trials and You" at www. nih.gov/health/clinicaltrials. For a list of AD clinical trials and studies, see www.nia.nih.gov/alzheimers/clinical-trials. For a comprehensive list of all trials, go to www.clinicaltrials.gov.

Drugs. A number of agents that might slow the progression of AD and other dementias are in various stages of testing.

The NIA-supported Alzheimer's Disease Cooperative Study (ADCS) (*www.adcs.org*) is a consortium of academic medical centers and clinics set up by NIH in 1991 to collaborate on the development of promising Alzheimer's treatments and diagnostic tools. In the latest round of studies, the ADCS will test drug and exercise interventions in people in the early stages of the disease, examine a medication to reduce agitation in people with Alzheimer's dementia, and test a cutting-edge approach to speed testing of drugs in clinical trials. Because Alzheimer's-related brain changes begin years before symptoms appear, the A4 (Anti-amyloid Treatment in Asymptomatic Alzheimer's Disease) trial is testing a promising therapy in the early stages of the disorder. This secondary prevention trial will test an amyloid-clearing drug in the symptom-free stage of the disease in 1,000 cognitively healthy older volunteers whose brain scans show abnormal levels of amyloid accumulation. Another of the newly funded ADCS drug trials is the Prazosin for Treating Agitation trial, which will test the use of the generic drug prazosin as a treatment for agitation that may also be well-tolerated in frail and elderly people.

Exercise. Researchers are assessing the effectiveness of a supervised aerobic exercise program to enhance general cognition in adults with age-related cognitive decline. They predict that greater cognitive gains will be made by individuals with more fitness gains. Another study will determine if exercise prevents memory loss from getting worse, and if it improves daily functioning and attitudes of those with probable AD. Researchers also hope to gain a better understanding of the effects of exercise and cognitive training on improving brain function in healthy older adults who may be at risk for developing AD.

Genetics. Several genes—most notably ApoE and the gene for tau (MAPT)—have been implicated in AD and other forms of dementia. Many dementia- related disorders share genetic and other characteristics of AD. Some families share a particular genetic mutation that causes dementia. Researchers are using samples of a person's genetic material, or genome, to identify genes that may be responsible for the development of dementia and AD. For example, NIH-funded researchers recently examined ApoE's role in the development of late-onset AD and found that one of the three forms of the ApoE gene triggers an inflammatory reaction and damages the blood vessels that feed the brain. Other researchers have identified a gene variant of TREM2 that is involved with a form of frontotemporal dementia that runs in families. Additional research may identify novel genes involved with FTD and other neurodegenerative diseases, perhaps leading to therapeutic approaches where delivery of normal genes would improve or restore normal brain function.

Imaging. Clinical imaging may help researchers better understand changes in the brains of people with dementia, as well as help diagnose these disorders. Magnetic resonance imaging may reveal structural and functional differences in the brains of individuals with Parkinson's disease dementia and AD and identify small vessel disease. PET scanning uses ligands—radioactive molecules that bind to proteins to show chemical functions of tissues and organs in the body—to help produce images of brain activity. Scientists funded by NIA are testing new PET ligands that bind to beta-amyloid for early detection of Alzheimer's-type pathology and cognitive decline. Studies of PET ligands that bind to aggregates of tau are ongoing in people with very early-stage AD.

International efforts. The International Alzheimer's Disease Research Portfolio (IADRP) helps individuals learn about AD research at public and private organizations in the U.S. and abroad. It also helps organizations leverage resources and avoid duplication of effort. The Common Alzheimer's Disease Research Ontology—a classification system that allows organizations to integrate and compare research portfolios—was developed by NIA, NIH, and the Alzheimer's Association. For more information about IADRP, see *http://iadrp.nia.nih. gov/cadro-web/about.*

Proteins. One feature that several major dementias have in common is an excess in the brain of certain proteins or protein fragments that have taken abnormal forms thought to be toxic to brain cells. NIH-funded research projects are aimed at better understanding the toxic effects of protein buildup and how it is related to the development of AD and related dementias. Some of these protein abnormalities can be detected in cerebrospinal fluid.

For example, an abnormally high accumulation of beta-amyloid protein in the brain is a hallmark of AD. NINDS-funded researchers are determining which neural pathways are affected by beta-amyloid and contribute to the development of Alzheimer's pathology and symptoms. NINDS funding also led to a genetically engineered rat model of AD that has the full array of brain changes associated with the human disease and may be used to better define causes and effects of AD related to beta-amyloid accumulation. Funding also was provided by NIA, the National Institute of Mental Health (also part of NIH), and other organizations.

In FTD, AD, and other neurodegenerative diseases, the protein tau collects in abnormal tangled masses of filaments that disrupt nerve signaling, cause cell death, and impair cognition. NINDS-funded researchers are determining whether specific forms of tau interfere with nerve cell signaling and decrease memory function. Others are studying how tau pathology spreads from cell to cell. Tau-related investigations are aimed at identifying common mechanisms of FTD, as well as biomarkers (signs that may indicate disease risk and progression, and improve diagnosis) that will speed the development of novel therapeutics for PDD and other forms of dementia.

Similarly, the abnormal accumulation of the protein alpha-synuclein is a hallmark of Parkinson's disease and Lewy body dementia. Scientists hope to identify what causes alpha-synuclein to form abnormal aggregates and become toxic to nerve cells, and to understand why the aggregation is an age-related phenomenon in Parkinson's disease and other synuclein-related disorders.

Sleep. The sleep and wakefulness cycle plays an integral, but not well understood, role in many dementias, including dementia with Lewy bodies, AD, prion dementias, and PDD. Sleep studies in individuals during periods of excessive daytime sleepiness and nocturnal sleep can help determine if fluctuations in mental status among people with DLB are related to excessive daytime sleepiness. Sleep studies also can assess whether declining cognition is predicted by sleep-related and neurobehavioral markers in parkinsonism.

Stem cells. Scientists are exploring various types of cells, including stem cells, to discover nerve cell mechanisms that lead to the initiation and progression of AD and other forms of dementia. Significant research efforts have focused on induced pluripotent stem cells (iPSC), which can be "reprogrammed" from skin cells into any cell type in the body, including nerve cells. NINDS funds three research consortia to develop well-characterized iPSC for amyotrophic lateral sclerosis (ALS), Huntington's disease, and Parkinson's disease. These cells can then be used by the research community to study the effects of mutant genes and misfolded proteins on nerve cell function and health, as well as to test potential drugs and therapies for AD and related dementias.

Chapter 6

Huntington's Disease

Introduction

In 1872, the American physician George Huntington wrote about an illness that he called "an heirloom from generations away back in the dim past." He was not the first to describe the disorder, which has been traced back to the Middle Ages at least. One of its earliest names was *chorea*, which, as in "choreography," is the Greek word for dance. The term chorea describes how people affected with the disorder writhe, twist, and turn in a constant, uncontrollable dance-like motion. Later, other descriptive names evolved. "Hereditary chorea" emphasizes how the disease is passed from parent to child. "Chronic progressive chorea" stresses how symptoms of the disease worsen over time. Today, physicians commonly use the simple term Huntington's Disease (HD) to describe this highly complex disorder that causes untold suffering for thousands of families.

More than 15,000 Americans have HD. At least 150,000 others have a 50 percent risk of developing the disease and thousands more of their relatives live with the possibility that they, too, might develop HD.

Until recently, scientists understood very little about HD and could only watch as the disease continued to pass from generation to generation. Families saw the disease destroy their loved ones' ability to

Text in this chapter is excerpted from "Huntington's Disease: Hope Through Research," National Institute of Neurological Disorders and Stroke (NINDS), January 5, 2015.

feel, think, and move. In the last several years, scientists working with support from the National Institute of Neurological Disorders and Stroke (NINDS) have made several breakthroughs in the area of HD research. With these advances, our understanding of the disease continues to improve.

This chapter presents information about HD, and about current research progress, to health professionals, scientists, caregivers, and, most important, to those already too familiar with the disorder: the many families who are affected by HD.

What Causes Huntington's Disease?

HD results from genetically programmed degeneration of nerve cells, called neurons, in certain areas of the brain. This degeneration causes uncontrolled movements, loss of intellectual faculties, and emotional disturbance. Specifically affected are cells of the basal ganglia, structures deep within the brain that have many important functions, including coordinating movement. Within the basal ganglia, HD especially targets neurons of the striatum, particularly those in the caudate nuclei and the pallidum. Also affected is the brain's outer surface, or cortex, which controls thought, perception, and memory.

How is HD Inherited?

HD is found in every country of the world. It is a familial disease, passed from parent to child through a mutation or misspelling in the normal gene.

A single abnormal gene, the basic biological unit of heredity, produces HD. Genes are composed of deoxyribonucleic acid (DNA), a molecule shaped like a spiral ladder. Each rung of this ladder is composed of two paired chemicals called bases. There are four types of bases—adenine, thymine, cytosine, and guanine—each abbreviated by the first letter of its name: A, T, C, and G. Certain bases always "pair" together, and different combinations of base pairs join to form coded messages. A gene is a long string of this DNA in various combinations of A, T, C, and G. These unique combinations determine the gene's function, much like letters join together to form words. Each person has about 30,000 genes—a billion base pairs of DNA or bits of information repeated in the nuclei of human cells—which determine individual characteristics or traits.

Genes are arranged in precise locations along 23 rod-like pairs of chromosomes. One chromosome from each pair comes from an individual's mother, the other from the father. Each half of a chromosome pair is similar to the other, except for one pair, which determines the sex of the individual. This pair has two X chromosomes in females and one X and one Y chromosome in males. The gene that produces HD lies on chromosome 4, one of the 22 non-sex-linked, or "autosomal," pairs of chromosomes, placing men and women at equal risk of acquiring the disease.

The impact of a gene depends partly on whether it is dominant or recessive. If a gene is dominant, then only one of the paired chromosomes is required to produce its called-for effect. If the gene is recessive, both parents must provide chromosomal copies for the trait to be present. HD is called an autosomal dominant disorder because only one copy of the defective gene, inherited from one parent, is necessary to produce the disease.

The genetic defect responsible for HD is a small sequence of DNA on chromosome 4 in which several base pairs are repeated many, many times. The normal gene has three DNA bases, composed of the sequence CAG. In people with HD, the sequence abnormally repeats itself dozens of times. Over time—and with each successive generation—the number of CAG repeats may expand further.

Each parent has two copies of every chromosome but gives only one copy to each child. Each child of an HD parent has a 50-50 chance of inheriting the HD gene. If a child does not inherit the HD gene, he or she will not develop the disease and cannot pass it to subsequent generations. A person who inherits the HD gene, and survives long enough, will sooner or later develop the disease. In some families, all the children may inherit the HD gene; in others, none do. Whether one child inherits the gene has no bearing on whether others will or will not share the same fate.

A small number of cases of HD are sporadic, that is, they occur even though there is no family history of the disorder. These cases are thought to be caused by a new genetic mutation-an alteration in the gene that occurs during sperm development and that brings the number of CAG repeats into the range that causes disease.

What are the Major Effects of the Disease?

Early signs of the disease vary greatly from person to person. A common observation is that the earlier the symptoms appear, the faster the disease progresses.

Family members may first notice that the individual experiences mood swings or becomes uncharacteristically irritable, apathetic, passive, depressed, or angry. These symptoms may lessen as the disease progresses or, in some individuals, may continue and include hostile outbursts or deep bouts of depression.

HD may affect the individual's judgment, memory, and other cognitive functions. Early signs might include having trouble driving, learning new things, remembering a fact, answering a question, or making a decision. Some may even display changes in handwriting. As the disease progresses, concentration on intellectual tasks becomes increasingly difficult.

In some individuals, the disease may begin with uncontrolled movements in the fingers, feet, face, or trunk. These movements—which are signs of chorea—often intensify when the person is anxious. HD can also begin with mild clumsiness or problems with balance. Some people develop choreic movements later, after the disease has progressed. They may stumble or appear uncoordinated. Chorea often creates serious problems with walking, increasing the likelihood of falls.

The disease can reach the point where speech is slurred and vital functions, such as swallowing, eating, speaking, and especially walking, continue to decline. Some individuals cannot recognize other family members. Many, however, remain aware of their environment and are able to express emotions.

Some physicians have employed a recently developed Unified HD Rating Scale, or UHDRS, to assess the clinical features, stages, and course of HD. In general, the duration of the illness ranges from 10 to 30 years. The most common causes of death are infection (most often pneumonia), injuries related to a fall, or other complications.

At What Age Does HD Appear?

The rate of disease progression and the age at onset vary from person to person. Adult-onset HD, with its disabling, uncontrolled movements, most often begins in middle age. There are, however, other variations of HD distinguished not just by age at onset but by a distinct array of symptoms. For example, some persons develop the disease as adults, but without chorea. They may appear rigid and move very little, or not at all, a condition called akinesia.

Some individuals develop symptoms of HD when they are very young—before age 20. The terms "early-onset" or "juvenile" HD are often used to describe HD that appears in a young person. A common sign of HD in a younger individual is a rapid decline in school performance. Symptoms can also include subtle changes in handwriting and slight problems with movement, such as slowness, rigidity, tremor, and rapid muscular twitching, called myoclonus. Several of these symptoms are similar to those seen in Parkinson's disease, and they differ from the chorea seen in individuals who develop the disease as adults. These young individuals are said to have "akinetic-rigid" HD or the Westphal variant of HD. People with juvenile HD may also have seizures and mental disabilities. The earlier the onset, the faster the disease seems to progress. The disease progresses most rapidly in individuals with juvenile or early-onset HD, and death often follows within 10 years.

Individuals with juvenile HD usually inherit the disease from their fathers. These individuals also tend to have the largest number of CAG repeats. The reason for this may be found in the process of sperm production. Unlike eggs, sperm are produced in the millions. Because DNA is copied millions of times during this process, there is an increased possibility for genetic mistakes to occur. To verify the link between the number of CAG repeats in the HD gene and the age at onset of symptoms, scientists studied a boy who developed HD symptoms at the age of two, one of the youngest and most severe cases ever recorded. They found that he had the largest number of CAG repeats of anyone studied so far—nearly 100. The boy's case was central to the identification of the HD gene and at the same time helped confirm that juveniles with HD have the longest segments of CAG repeats, the only proven correlation between repeat length and age at onset.

A few individuals develop HD after age 55. Diagnosis in these people can be very difficult. The symptoms of HD may be masked by other health problems, or the person may not display the severity of symptoms seen in individuals with HD of earlier onset. These individuals may also show symptoms of depression rather than anger or irritability, or they may retain sharp control over their intellectual functions, such as memory, reasoning, and problem-solving.

There is also a related disorder called senile chorea. Some elderly individuals display the symptoms of HD, especially choreic movements, but do not become demented, have a normal gene, and lack a family history of the disorder. Some scientists believe that a different gene mutation may account for this small number of cases, but this has not been proven.

How is HD Diagnosed?

The great American folk singer and composer Woody Guthrie died on October 3, 1967, after suffering from HD for 13 years. He had been misdiagnosed, considered an alcoholic, and shuttled in and out of mental institutions and hospitals for years before being properly diagnosed. His case, sadly, is not extraordinary, although the diagnosis can be made easily by experienced neurologists.

A neurologist will interview the individual intensively to obtain the medical history and rule out other conditions. A tool used by physicians to diagnose HD is to take the family history, sometimes called a pedigree or genealogy. It is extremely important for family members to be candid and truthful with a doctor who is taking a family history.

The doctor will also ask about recent intellectual or emotional problems, which may be indications of HD, and will test the person's hearing, eye movements, strength, coordination, involuntary movements (chorea), sensation, reflexes, balance, movement, and mental status, and will probably order a number of laboratory tests as well.

People with HD commonly have impairments in the way the eye follows or fixes on a moving target. Abnormalities of eye movements vary from person to person and differ, depending on the stage and duration of the illness.

The discovery of the HD gene in 1993 resulted in a direct genetic test to make or confirm a diagnosis of HD in an individual who is exhibiting HD-like symptoms. Using a blood sample, the genetic test analyzes DNA for the HD mutation by counting the number of repeats in the HD gene region. Individuals who do not have HD usually have 28 or fewer CAG repeats. Individuals with HD usually have 40 or more repeats. A small percentage of individuals, however, have a number of repeats that fall within a borderline region (see table 6.1.).

The physician may ask the individual to undergo a brain imaging test. Computed tomography (CT) and magnetic resonance imaging (MRI) provide excellent images of brain structures with little if any discomfort. Those with HD may show shrinkage of some parts of the brain—particularly two areas known as the caudate nuclei and putamen—and enlargement of fluid-filled cavities within the brain

Table 6.1. Number of CAG Repeats and Outcome

No. of CAG repeats	Outcome
≤ 28	Normal range; individual will not develop HD
29–34	Individual will not develop HD but the next generation is at risk
35–39	Some, but not all, individuals in this range will develop HD; next generation is also at risk
≥ 40	Individual will develop HD

called ventricles. These changes do not definitely indicate HD, however, because they can also occur in other disorders. In addition, a person can have early symptoms of HD and still have a normal CT scan. When used in conjunction with a family history and record of clinical symptoms, however, CT can be an important diagnostic tool.

Another technology for brain imaging includes positron emission tomography (PET,) which is important in HD research efforts but is not often needed for diagnosis.

What is Presymptomatic Testing?

Presymptomatic testing is used for people who have a family history of HD but have no symptoms themselves. If either parent had HD, the person's chance would be 50-50. In the past, no laboratory test could positively identify people carrying the HD gene—or those fated to develop HD—before the onset of symptoms. That situation changed in 1983, when a team of scientists supported by the NINDS located the first genetic marker for HD—the initial step in developing a laboratory test for the disease.

A marker is a piece of DNA that lies near a gene and is usually inherited with it. Discovery of the first HD marker allowed scientists to locate the HD gene on chromosome 4. The marker discovery quickly led to the development of a presymptomatic test for some individuals, but this test required blood or tissue samples from both affected and unaffected family members in order to identify markers unique to that particular family. For this reason, adopted individuals, orphans, and people who had few living family members were unable to use the test.

Discovery of the HD gene has led to a less expensive, scientifically simpler, and far more accurate presymptomatic test that is applicable to the majority of at-risk people. The new test uses CAG repeat length to detect the presence of the HD mutation in blood. This is discussed further in the next section.

There are many complicating factors that reflect the complexity of diagnosing HD. In a small number of individuals with HD—1 to 3 percent—no family history of HD can be found. Some individuals may not be aware of their genetic legacy, or a family member may conceal a genetic disorder from fear of social stigma. A parent may not want to worry children, scare them, or deter them from marrying. In other cases, a family member may die of another cause before he or she begins to show signs of HD. Sometimes, the cause of death for a relative may not be known, or the family is not aware of a relative's death. Adopted children may not know their genetic heritage, or early symptoms in an individual may be too slight to attract attention.

How is the Presymptomatic Test Conducted?

An individual who wishes to be tested should contact the nearest testing center. (A list of such centers can be obtained from the Huntington Disease Society of America at 1-800-345-HDSA.) The testing process should include several components. Most testing programs include a neurological examination, pretest counseling, and follow-up. The purpose of the neurological examination is to determine whether or not the person requesting testing is showing any clinical symptoms of HD. It is important to remember that if an individual is showing even slight symptoms of HD, he or she risks being diagnosed with the disease during the neurological examination, even before the genetic test. During pretest counseling, the individual will learn about HD, and about his or her own level of risk, about the testing procedure. The person will be told about the test's limitations, the accuracy of the test, and possible outcomes. He or she can then weigh the risks and benefits of testing and may even decide at that time against pursuing further testing.

If a person decides to be tested, a team of highly trained specialists will be involved, which may include neurologists, genetic counselors, social workers, psychiatrists, and psychologists. This team of professionals helps the at-risk person decide if testing is the right thing to do and carefully prepares the person for a negative, positive, or inconclusive test result.

Individuals who decide to continue the testing process should be accompanied to counseling sessions by a spouse, a friend, or a relative who is not at risk. Other interested family members may participate in the counseling sessions if the individual being tested so desires.

The genetic testing itself involves donating a small sample of blood that is screened in the laboratory for the presence or absence of the HD mutation. Testing may require a sample of DNA from a closely related affected relative, preferably a parent, for the purpose of confirming the diagnosis of HD in the family. This is especially important if the family history for HD is unclear or unusual in some way.

Results of the test should be given only in person and only to the individual being tested. Test results are confidential. Regardless of test results, follow-up is recommended.

In order to protect the interests of minors, including confidentiality, testing is not recommended for those under the age of 18 unless there is a compelling medical reason (for example, the child is exhibiting symptoms).

Testing of a fetus (prenatal testing) presents special challenges and risks; in fact some centers do not perform genetic testing on fetuses. Because a positive test result using direct genetic testing means the at-risk parent is also a gene carrier, at-risk individuals who are considering a pregnancy are advised to seek genetic counseling prior to conception.

Some at-risk parents may wish to know the risk to their fetus but not their own. In this situation, parents may opt for prenatal testing using linked DNA markers rather than direct gene testing. In this case, testing does not look for the HD gene itself but instead indicates whether or not the fetus has inherited a chromosome 4 from the affected grandparent or from the unaffected grandparent on the side of the family with HD. If the test shows that the fetus has inherited a chromosome 4 from the affected grandparent, the parents then learn that the fetus's risk is the same as the parent (50-50), but they learn nothing new about the parent's risk. If the test shows that the fetus has inherited a chromosome 4 from the unaffected grandparent, the risk to the fetus is very low (less than 1%) in most cases.

Another option open to parents is in vitro fertilization with pre-implantation screening. In this procedure, embryos are screened to determine which ones carry the HD mutation. Embryos determined not to have the HD gene mutation are then implanted in the woman's uterus.

In terms of emotional and practical consequences, not only for the individual taking the test but for his or her entire family, testing is enormously complex and has been surrounded by considerable controversy. For example, people with a positive test result may risk losing health and life insurance, suffer loss of employment, and other liabilities. People undergoing testing may wish to cover the cost themselves, since coverage by an insurer may lead to loss of health insurance in the event of a positive result, although this may change in the future.

With the participation of health professionals and people from families with HD, scientists have developed testing guidelines. All individuals seeking a genetic test should obtain a copy of these guidelines, either from their testing center or from the organizations listed on the card in the back of this brochure. These organizations have information on sites that perform testing using the established procedures and they strongly recommend that individuals avoid testing that does not adhere to these guidelines.

How Does a Person Decide Whether to be Tested?

The anxiety that comes from living with a 50 percent risk for HD can be overwhelming. How does a young person make important choices about long-term education, marriage, and children? How do older parents of adult children cope with their fears about children and grandchildren? How do people come to terms with the ambiguity and uncertainty of living at risk?

Some individuals choose to undergo the test out of a desire for greater certainty about their genetic status. They believe the test will enable them to make more informed decisions about the future. Others choose not to take the test. They are able to make peace with the uncertainty of being at risk, preferring to forego the emotional consequences of a positive result, as well as possible losses of insurance and employment. There is no right or wrong decision, as each choice is highly individual. The guidelines for genetic testing for HD, discussed in the previous section, were developed to help people with this life-changing choice.

Whatever the results of genetic testing, the at-risk individual and family members can expect powerful and complex emotional responses. The health and happiness of spouses, brothers and sisters, children, parents, and grandparents are affected by a positive test result, as are an individual's friends, work associates, neighbors, and others. Because receiving test results may prove to be devastating, testing guidelines call for continued counseling even after the test is complete and the results are known.

Is There a Treatment for HD?

Physicians may prescribe a number of medications to help control emotional and movement problems associated with HD. It is important to remember, however, that while medicines may help keep these clinical symptoms under control, there is no treatment to stop or reverse the course of the disease.

In August 2008 the U.S. Food and Drug Administration approved tetrabenazine to treat Huntington's chorea, making it the first drug approved for use in the United States to treat the disease. Antipsychotic drugs, such as haloperidol, or other drugs, such as clonazepam, may help to alleviate choreic movements and may also be used to help control hallucinations, delusions, and violent outbursts. Antipsychotic drugs, however, are not prescribed for another form of muscle contraction associated with HD, called dystonia, and may in fact worsen the condition, causing stiffness and rigidity. These medications may also have severe side effects, including sedation, and for that reason should be used in the lowest possible doses.

For depression, physicians may prescribe fluoxetine, sertraline, nortriptyline, or other compounds. Tranquilizers can help control anxiety and lithium may be prescribed to combat pathological excitement and severe mood swings. Medications may also be needed to treat the severe obsessive-compulsive rituals of some individuals with HD.

Most drugs used to treat the symptoms of HD have side effects such as fatigue, restlessness, or hyperexcitability. Sometimes it may be difficult to tell if a particular symptom, such as apathy or incontinence, is a sign of the disease or a reaction to medication.

What Kind of Care Does the Individual with HD Need?

Although a psychologist or psychiatrist, a genetic counselor, and other specialists may be needed at different stages of the illness, usually the first step in diagnosis and in finding treatment is to see a neurologist. While the family doctor may be able to diagnose HD, and may continue to monitor the individual's status, it is better to consult with a neurologist about management of the varied symptoms.

Problems may arise when individuals try to express complex thoughts in words they can no longer pronounce intelligibly. It can be helpful to repeat words back to the person with HD so that he or she knows that some thoughts are understood. Sometimes people mistakenly assume that if individuals do not talk, they also do not understand. Never isolate individuals by not talking, and try to keep their environment as normal as possible. Speech therapy may improve the individual's ability to communicate.

It is extremely important for the person with HD to maintain physical fitness as much as his or her condition and the course of the disease allows. Individuals who exercise and keep active tend to do better than those who do not. A daily regimen of exercise can help the person feel better physically and mentally. Although their coordination may be poor, individuals should continue walking, with assistance if necessary. Those who want to walk independently should be allowed to do so as long as possible, and careful attention should be given to keeping their environment free of hard, sharp objects. This will help ensure maximal independence while minimizing the risk of injury from a fall. Individuals can also wear special padding during walks to help protect against injury from falls. Some people have found that small weights around the ankles can help stability. Wearing sturdy shoes that fit well can help too, especially shoes without laces that can be slipped on or off easily.

Impaired coordination may make it difficult for people with HD to feed themselves and to swallow. As the disease progresses, persons with HD may even choke. In helping individuals to eat, caregivers should allow plenty of time for meals. Food can be cut into small pieces, softened, or pureed to ease swallowing and prevent choking. While some foods may require the addition of thickeners, other foods may need to be thinned. Dairy products, in particular, tend to increase the secretion of mucus, which in turn increases the risk of choking. Some individuals may benefit from swallowing therapy, which is especially helpful if started before serious problems arise. Suction cups for plates, special tableware designed for people with disabilities, and plastic cups with tops can help prevent spilling. The individual's physician can offer additional advice about diet and about how to handle swallowing difficulties or gastrointestinal problems that might arise, such as incontinence or constipation.

Caregivers should pay attention to proper nutrition so that the individual with HD takes in enough calories to maintain his or her body weight. Sometimes people with HD, who may burn as many as 5,000 calories a day without gaining weight, require five meals a day to take in the necessary number of calories. Physicians may recommend vitamins or other nutritional supplements. In a long-term care institution, staff will need to assist with meals in order to ensure that the individual's special caloric and nutritional requirements are met. Some individuals and their families choose to use a feeding tube; others choose not to.

Individuals with HD are at special risk for dehydration and therefore require large quantities of fluids, especially during hot weather. Bendable straws can make drinking easier for the person. In some cases, water may have to be thickened with commercial additives to give it the consistency of syrup or honey.

What Community Resources are Available?

Individuals and families affected by HD can take steps to ensure that they receive the best advice and care possible. Physicians and state and local health service agencies can provide information on community resources and family support groups that may exist. Possible types of help include:

Legal and social aid. HD affects a person's capacity to reason, make judgments, and handle responsibilities. Individuals may need help with legal affairs. Wills and other important documents should be drawn up early to avoid legal problems when the person with HD may no longer be able to represent his or her own interests. Family members should also seek out assistance if they face discrimination regarding insurance, employment, or other matters.

Home care services. Caring for a person with HD at home can be exhausting, but part-time assistance with household chores or physical care of the individual can ease this burden. Domestic help, meal programs, nursing assistance, occupational therapy, or other home services may be available from federal, state, or local health service agencies.

Recreation and work centers. Many people with HD are eager and able to participate in activities outside the home. Therapeutic work and recreation centers give individuals an opportunity to pursue hobbies and interests and to meet new people. Participation in these programs, including occupational, music, and recreational therapy, can reduce the person's dependence on family members and provides home caregivers with a temporary, much needed break.

Group housing. A few communities have group housing facilities that are supervised by a resident attendant and that provide meals, housekeeping services, social activities, and local transportation services for residents. These living arrangements are particularly suited to the needs of individuals who are alone and who, although still independent and capable, risk injury when they undertake routine chores like cooking and cleaning.

Institutional care. The individual's physical and emotional demands on the family may eventually become overwhelming. While many families may prefer to keep relatives with HD at home whenever possible, a long-term care facility may prove to be best. To hospitalize or place a family member in a care facility is a difficult decision; professional counseling can help families with this.

Finding the proper facility can itself prove difficult. Organizations such as the Huntington's Disease Society of America (www.hdsa.org) may be able to refer the family to facilities that have met standards set for the care of individuals with HD. Very few of these exist, however, and even fewer have experience with individuals with juvenile or early-onset HD who require special care because of their age and symptoms.

What Research is Being Done?

Although HD attracted considerable attention from scientists in the early 20th century, there was little sustained research on the disease until the late 1960s when the Committee to Combat Huntington's Disease and the Huntington's Chorea Foundation, later called the Hereditary Disease Foundation, first began to fund research and to campaign for federal funding. In 1977, Congress established the Commission for the Control of Huntington's Disease and Its Consequences, which made a series of important recommendations. Since then, Congress has provided consistent support for federal research, primarily through the National Institute of Neurological Disorders and Stroke, the government's lead agency for biomedical research on disorders of the brain and nervous system. The effort to combat HD proceeds along the following lines of inquiry, each providing important information about the disease:

Basic neurobiology. Now that the HD gene has been located, investigators in the field of neurobiology-which encompasses the anatomy, physiology, and biochemistry of the nervous system-are continuing to study the HD gene with an eye toward understanding how it causes disease in the human body.

Clinical research. Neurologists, psychologists, psychiatrists, and other investigators are improving our understanding of the symptoms and progression of the disease in patients while attempting to develop new therapeutics.

Imaging. Scientific investigations using PET and other technologies are enabling scientists to see what the defective gene does to various structures in the brain and how it affects the body's chemistry and metabolism.

Animal models. Laboratory animals, such as mice, are being bred in the hope of duplicating the clinical features of HD and can soon be expected to help scientists learn more about the symptoms and progression of the disease.

Fetal tissue research. Investigators are implanting fetal tissue in rodents and nonhuman primates with the hope that success in this area will lead to understanding, restoring, or replacing functions typically lost by neuronal degeneration in individuals with HD.

These areas of research are slowly converging and, in the process, are yielding important clues about the gene's relentless destruction of mind and body. The NINDS supports much of this exciting work.

Molecular Genetics

For 10 years, scientists focused on a segment of chromosome 4 and, in 1993, finally isolated the HD gene. The process of isolating the responsible gene—motivated by the desire to find a cure—was more difficult than anticipated. Scientists now believe that identifying the location of the HD gene is the first step on the road to a cure.

Finding the HD gene involved an intense molecular genetics research effort with cooperating investigators from around the globe. In early 1993, the collaborating scientists announced they had isolated the unstable triplet repeat DNA sequence that has the HD gene. Investigators relied on the NINDS-supported Research Roster for Huntington's Disease, based at Indiana University in Indianapolis, to accomplish this work. First started in 1979, the roster contains data on many American families with HD, provides statistical and demographic data to scientists, and serves as a liaison between investigators and specific families. It provided the DNA from many families affected by HD to investigators involved in the search for the gene and was an important component in the identification of HD markers.

For several years, NINDS-supported investigators involved in the search for the HD gene made yearly visits to the largest known kindred with HD—14,000 individuals—who live on Lake Maracaibo in Venezuela. The continuing trips enable scientists to study inheritance patterns of several interrelated families.

The HD Gene and Its Product

Although scientists know that certain brain cells die in HD, the cause of their death is still unknown. Recessive diseases are usually thought to result from a gene that fails to produce adequate amounts of a substance essential to normal function. This is known as a loss-of-function gene. Some dominantly inherited disorders, such as HD, are thought to involve a gene that actively interferes with the normal function of the cell. This is known as a gain-of-function gene.

How does the defective HD gene cause harm? The HD gene encodes a protein—which has been named huntingtin—the function of which is as yet unknown. The repeated CAG sequence in the gene causes an abnormal form of huntingtin to be made, in which the amino acid glutamine is repeated. It is the presence of this abnormal form, and not the absence of the normal form, that causes harm in HD. This explains why the disease is dominant and why two copies of the defective gene—one from both the mother and the father—do not cause a more serious case than inheritance from only one parent.

With the HD gene isolated, NINDS-supported investigators are now turning their attention toward discovering the normal function of huntingtin and how the altered form causes harm. Scientists hope to reproduce, study, and correct these changes in animal models of the disease.

Huntingtin is found everywhere in the body but only outside the cell's nucleus. Mice called "knockout mice" are bred in the laboratory to produce no huntingtin; they fail to develop past a very early embryo stage and quickly die. Huntingtin, scientists now know, is necessary for life. Investigators hope to learn why the abnormal version of the protein damages only certain parts of the brain. One theory is that cells in these parts of the brain may be supersensitive to this abnormal protein.

Cell Death in HD

Although the precise cause of cell death in HD is not yet known, scientists are paying close attention to the process of genetically programmed cell death that occurs deep within the brains of individuals with HD. This process involves a complex series of interlinked events leading to cellular suicide. Related areas of investigation include:

- Excitotoxicity. Overstimulation of cells by natural chemicals found in the brain.

- Defective energy metabolism. A defect in the power plant of the cell, called mitochondria, where energy is produced.

- Oxidative stress. Normal metabolic activity in the brain that produces toxic compounds called free radicals.

- Trophic factors. Natural chemical substances found in the human body that may protect against cell death.

Several HD studies are aimed at understanding losses of nerve cells and receptors in HD. Neurons in the striatum are classified both by their size (large, medium, or small) and appearance (spiny or aspiny). Each type of neuron contains combinations of neurotransmitters. Scientists know that the destructive process of HD affects different subsets of neurons to varying degrees. The hallmark of HD, they are learning, is selective degeneration of medium-sized spiny neurons in the striatum. NINDS-supported studies also suggest that losses of certain types of neurons and receptors are responsible for different symptoms and stages of HD.

What do these changes look like? In spiny neurons, investigators have observed two types of changes, each affecting the nerve cells' dendrites. Dendrites, found on every nerve cell, extend out from the cell body and are responsible for receiving messages from other nerve cells. In the intermediate stages of HD, dendrites grow out of control. New, incomplete branches form and other branches become contorted. In advanced, severe stages of HD, degenerative changes cause sections of dendrites to swell, break off, or disappear altogether. Investigators believe that these alterations may be an attempt by the cell to rebuild nerve cell contacts lost early in the disease. As the new dendrites establish connections, however, they may in fact contribute to nerve cell death. Such studies give compelling, visible evidence of the progressive nature of HD and suggest that new experimental therapies must consider the state of cellular degeneration. Scientists do not yet know exactly how these changes affect subsets of nerve cells outside the striatum.

Animal Models of HD

As more is learned about cellular degeneration in HD, investigators hope to reproduce these changes in animal models and to find a way to correct or halt the process of nerve cell death. Such models serve the scientific community in general by providing a means to test the safety of new classes of drugs in nonhuman primates. NINDS-supported scientists are currently working to develop both nonhuman primate and mouse models to investigate nerve degeneration in HD and to study the effects of excitotoxicity on nerve cells in the brain.

Investigators are working to build genetic models of HD using transgenic mice. To do this, scientists transfer the altered human HD gene into mouse embryos so that the animals will develop the anatomical and biological characteristics of HD. This genetic model of mouse HD will enable in-depth study of the disease and testing of new therapeutic compounds.

Another idea is to insert into mice a section of DNA containing CAG repeats in the abnormal, disease gene range. This mouse equivalent of HD could allow scientists to explore the basis of CAG instability and its role in the disease process.

Fetal Tissue Research

A relatively new field in biomedical research involves the use of brain tissue grafts to study, and potentially treat, neurodegenerative disorders. In this technique, tissue that has degenerated is replaced with implants of fresh, fetal tissue, taken at the very early stages of development. Investigators are interested in applying brain tissue implants to HD research. Extensive animal studies will be required to learn if this technique could be of value in patients with HD.

Clinical Studies

Scientists are pursuing clinical studies that may one day lead to the development of new drugs or other treatments to halt the disease's progression. Examples of NINDS-supported investigations, using both asymptomatic and symptomatic individuals, include:

Genetic studies on age of onset, inheritance patterns, and markers found within families. These studies may shed additional light on how HD is passed from generation to generation.

Studies of cognition, intelligence, and movement. Studies of abnormal eye movements, both horizontal and vertical, and tests of patients' skills in a number of learning, memory, neuropsychological, and motor tasks may serve to identify when the various symptoms of HD appear and to characterize their range and severity.

Clinical trials of drugs. Testing of various drugs may lead to new treatments and at the same time improve our understanding of the disease process in HD. Classes of drugs being tested include those that control symptoms, slow the rate of progression of HD, and block effects of excitotoxins, and those that might correct or replace other metabolic defects contributing to the development and progression of HD.

Imaging

NINDS-supported scientists are using positron emission tomography (PET) to learn how the gene affects the chemical systems of the body. PET visualizes metabolic or chemical abnormalities in the body, and investigators hope to ascertain if PET scans can reveal any abnormalities that signal HD. Investigators conducting HD research are also using PET to characterize neurons that have died and chemicals that are depleted in parts of the brain affected by HD.

Like PET, a form of Magnetic Resonance Imaging (MRI) called functional MRI can measure increases or decreases in certain brain chemicals thought to play a key role in HD. Functional MRI studies are also helping investigators understand how HD kills neurons in different regions of the brain.

Imaging technologies allow investigators to view changes in the volume and structures of the brain and to pinpoint when these changes occur in HD. Scientists know that in brains affected by HD, the basal ganglia, cortex, and ventricles all show atrophy or other alterations.

Chapter 7

Amyotrophic Lateral Sclerosis (ALS)

What is amyotrophic lateral sclerosis?

Amyotrophic Lateral Sclerosis (ALS), sometimes called Lou Gehrig's disease, is a rapidly progressive, invariably fatal neurological disease that attacks the nerve cells (*neurons*) responsible for controlling voluntary muscles (muscle action we are able to control, such as those in the arms, legs, and face). The disease belongs to a group of disorders known as *motor neuron diseases*, which are characterized by the gradual degeneration and death of motor neurons.

Motor neurons are nerve cells located in the brain, brain stem, and spinal cord that serve as controlling units and vital communication links between the nervous system and the voluntary muscles of the body. Messages from motor neurons in the brain (called *upper motor neurons*) are transmitted to motor neurons in the spinal cord (called *lower motor neurons*) and from them to particular muscles. In ALS, both the upper motor neurons and the lower motor neurons degenerate or die, and stop sending messages to muscles. Unable to function, the muscles gradually weaken, waste away (*atrophy*), and have very fine twitches (called *fasciculations*). Eventually, the ability of the brain to start and control voluntary movement is lost.

Text in this chapter is excerpted from "Amyotrophic Lateral Sclerosis (ALS) Fact Sheet," National Institute of Neurological Disorders and Stroke (NINDS), February 23, 2015.

ALS causes weakness with a wide range of disabilities (see "What are the symptoms?"). Eventually, all muscles under voluntary control are affected, and individuals lose their strength and the ability to move their arms, legs, and body. When muscles in the diaphragm and chest wall fail, people lose the ability to breathe without ventilatory support. Most people with ALS die from respiratory failure, usually within 3 to 5 years from the onset of symptoms. However, about 10 percent of those with ALS survive for 10 or more years.

Although the disease usually does not impair a person's mind or intelligence, several recent studies suggest that some persons with ALS may have depression or alterations in cognitive functions involving decision-making and memory.

ALS does not affect a person's ability to see, smell, taste, hear, or recognize touch. Patients usually maintain control of eye muscles and bladder and bowel functions, although in the late stages of the disease most individuals will need help getting to and from the bathroom.

Who gets ALS?

More than 12,000 people in the U.S. have a definite diagnosis of ALS, for a prevalence of 3.9 cases per 100,000 persons in the U.S. general population, according to a report on data from the **National ALS Registry**. ALS is one of the most common neuromuscular diseases worldwide, and people of all races and ethnic backgrounds are affected. ALS is more common among white males, non-Hispanics, and persons aged 60–69 years, but younger and older people also can develop the disease. Men are affected more often than women.

In 90 to 95 percent of all ALS cases, the disease occurs apparently at random with no clearly associated risk factors. Individuals with this sporadic form of the disease do not have a family history of ALS, and their family members are not considered to be at increased risk for developing it.

About 5 to 10 percent of all ALS cases are inherited. The familial form of ALS usually results from a pattern of inheritance that requires only one parent to carry the gene responsible for the disease. Mutations in more than a dozen genes have been found to cause familial ALS.

About one-third of all familial cases (and a small percentage of sporadic cases) result from a defect in a gene known as "chromosome 9 open reading frame 72," or C9orf72. The function of this gene is still unknown. Another 20 percent of familial cases result from mutations in the gene that encodes the enzyme copper-zinc superoxide dismutase 1 (SOD1).

What are the symptoms?

The onset of ALS may be so subtle that the symptoms are overlooked. The earliest symptoms may include fasciculations, cramps, tight and stiff muscles (*spasticity*), muscle weakness affecting an arm or a leg, slurred and nasal speech, or difficulty chewing or swallowing. These general complaints then develop into more obvious weakness or atrophy that may cause a physician to suspect ALS.

The parts of the body showing early symptoms of ALS depend on which muscles in the body are affected. Many individuals first see the effects of the disease in a hand or arm as they experience difficulty with simple tasks requiring manual dexterity such as buttoning a shirt, writing, or turning a key in a lock. In other cases, symptoms initially affect one of the legs, and people experience awkwardness when walking or running or they notice that they are tripping or stumbling more often. When symptoms begin in the arms or legs, it is referred to as "limb onset" ALS. Other individuals first notice speech problems, termed "bulbar onset" ALS.

Regardless of the part of the body first affected by the disease, muscle weakness and atrophy spread to other parts of the body as the disease progresses. Individuals may develop problems with moving, swallowing (*dysphagia*), and speaking or forming words (*dysarthria*). Symptoms of upper motor neuron involvement include spasticity and exaggerated reflexes (*hyperreflexia*) including an overactive gag reflex. An abnormal reflex commonly called Babinski's sign (the large toe extends upward as the sole of the foot is stimulated in a certain way) also indicates upper motor neuron damage. Symptoms of lower motor neuron degeneration include muscle weakness and atrophy, muscle cramps, and fasciculations.

To be diagnosed with ALS, people must have signs and symptoms of both upper and lower motor neuron damage that cannot be attributed to other causes.

Although the sequence of emerging symptoms and the rate of disease progression vary from person to person, eventually individuals will not be able to stand or walk, get in or out of bed on their own, or use their hands and arms. Difficulty swallowing and chewing impair the person's ability to eat normally and increase the risk of choking. Maintaining weight will then become a problem. Because cognitive abilities are relatively intact, people are aware of their progressive loss of function and may become anxious and depressed. A small percentage of individuals may experience problems with memory or decision-making, and there is growing evidence that some may even develop a form of dementia over time. Health care professionals need to explain the course of the disease and describe available treatment options so that people can make informed decisions in advance. In later stages of the disease, individuals have difficulty breathing as the muscles of the respiratory system weaken. They eventually lose the ability to breathe on their own and must depend on ventilatory support for survival. Affected individuals also face an increased risk of pneumonia during later stages of ALS.

How is ALS diagnosed?

No one test can provide a definitive diagnosis of ALS, although the presence of upper and lower motor neuron signs is strongly suggestive. Instead, the diagnosis of ALS is primarily based on the symptoms and signs the physician observes in the patient and a series of tests to rule out other diseases. Physicians obtain the individual's full medical history and usually conduct a neurologic examination at regular intervals to assess whether symptoms such as muscle weakness, atrophy of muscles, hyperreflexia, and spasticity are getting progressively worse.

Since ALS symptoms in the early stages of the disease can be similar to those of a wide variety of other, more treatable diseases or disorders, appropriate tests must be conducted to exclude the possibility of other conditions. One of these tests is *Electromyography* (EMG), a special recording technique that detects electrical activity in muscles. Certain EMG findings can support the diagnosis of ALS. Another common test is a *Nerve Conduction Study* (NCS), which measures electrical energy by assessing the nerve's ability to send a signal. Specific abnormalities in the NCS and EMG may suggest, for example, that the individual has a form of peripheral neuropathy (damage to peripheral nerves) or myopathy (muscle disease) rather than ALS. The physician may order *Magnetic Resonance Imaging* (MRI), a noninvasive procedure that uses a magnetic field and radio waves to take detailed images of the brain and spinal cord. Standard MRI scans are normal in people with ALS. However, they can reveal evidence of other problems that may be causing the symptoms, such as a spinal cord tumor, a herniated disk in the neck that compresses the spinal cord, syringomyelia (a cyst in the spinal cord), or cervical spondylosis (abnormal wear affecting the spine in the neck).

Based on the person's symptoms and findings from the examination and from these tests, the physician may order tests on blood and urine samples to eliminate the possibility of other diseases as well as routine laboratory tests. In some cases, for example, if a physician suspects that the individual may have a myopathy rather than ALS, a muscle biopsy may be performed.

Infectious diseases such as Human Immunodeficiency Virus (HIV), Human T-Cell Leukemia Virus (HTLV), polio, West Nile virus, and Lyme disease can in some cases cause ALS-like symptoms. Neurological disorders such as multiple sclerosis, post-polio syndrome, multifocal motor neuropathy, and spinal muscular atrophy also can mimic certain facets of the disease and should be considered by physicians attempting to make a diagnosis. Fasciculations, the fine rippling movements in the muscle, and muscle cramps also occur in benign conditions.

Because of the prognosis carried by this diagnosis and the variety of diseases or disorders that can resemble ALS in the early stages of the disease, individuals may wish to obtain a second neurological opinion.

What causes ALS?

The cause of ALS is not known, and scientists do not yet know why ALS strikes some people and not others. An important step toward answering this question was made in 1993 when scientists supported by the National Institute of Neurological Disorders and Stroke (NINDS) discovered that mutations in the gene that produces the SOD1 enzyme were associated with some cases of familial ALS. Although it is still not clear how mutations in the SOD1 gene lead to motor neuron degeneration, there is increasing evidence that mutant SOD1 protein can become toxic.

Since then, over a dozen additional genetic mutations have been identified, many through NINDS-supported research, and each of these gene discoveries has provided new insights into possible mechanisms of ALS.

For example, the discovery of certain genetic mutations involved in ALS suggests that changes in the processing of RNA molecules (involved with functions including gene regulation and activity) may lead to ALS-related motor neuron degeneration. Other gene mutations implicate defects in protein recycling. And still others point to possible defects in the structure and shape of motor neurons, as well as increased susceptibility to environmental toxins. Overall, it is becoming increasingly clear that a number of cellular defects can lead to motor neuron degeneration in ALS.

Another research advance was made in 2011 when scientists found that a defect in the C9orf72 gene is not only present in a significant subset of ALS patients but also in some patients who suffer from a type of Frontotemporal Dementia (FTD). This observation provides evidence for genetic ties between these two neurodegenerative disorders. In fact, some researchers are proposing that ALS and some forms of FTD are related disorders with genetic, clinical, and pathological overlap.

In searching for the cause of ALS, researchers are also studying the role of environmental factors such as exposure to toxic or infectious agents, as well as physical trauma or behavioral and occupational factors. For example, studies of populations of military personnel who were deployed to the Gulf region during the 1991 war show that those veterans were more likely to develop ALS compared to military personnel who were not in the region.

Future research may show that many factors, including a genetic predisposition, are involved in the development of ALS.

How is ALS treated?

No cure has yet been found for ALS. However, the Food and Drug Administration (FDA) approved the first drug treatment for the disease—riluzole (Rilutek)—in 1995. Riluzole is believed to reduce damage to motor neurons by decreasing the release of glutamate. Clinical trials with ALS patients showed that riluzole prolongs survival by several months, mainly in those with difficulty swallowing. The drug also extends the time before an individual needs ventilation support. Riluzole does not reverse the damage already done to motor neurons, and persons taking the drug must be monitored for liver damage and other possible side effects. However, this first disease-specific therapy offers hope that the progression of ALS may one day be slowed by new medications or combinations of drugs.

Other treatments for ALS are designed to relieve symptoms and improve the quality of life for individuals with the disorder. This supportive care is best provided by multidisciplinary teams of health care professionals such as physicians; pharmacists; physical, occupational, and speech therapists; nutritionists; and social workers and home care and hospice nurses. Working with patients and caregivers, these teams can design an individualized plan of medical and physical therapy and provide special equipment aimed at keeping patients as mobile and comfortable as possible.

Physicians can prescribe medications to help reduce fatigue, ease muscle cramps, control spasticity, and reduce excess saliva and phlegm. Drugs also are available to help patients with pain, depression, sleep disturbances, and constipation. Pharmacists can give advice on the proper use of medications and monitor a patient's prescriptions to avoid risks of drug interactions.

Physical therapy and special equipment can enhance an individual's independence and safety throughout the course of ALS. Gentle, low-impact aerobic exercise such as walking, swimming, and stationary bicycling can strengthen unaffected muscles, improve cardiovascular health, and help patients fight fatigue and depression. Range of motion and stretching exercises can help prevent painful spasticity and shortening (contracture) of muscles. Physical therapists can recommend exercises that provide these benefits without overworking muscles. Occupational therapists can suggest devices such as ramps, braces, walkers, and wheelchairs that help individuals conserve energy and remain mobile.

People with ALS who have difficulty speaking may benefit from working with a speech therapist. These health professionals can teach individuals adaptive strategies such as techniques to help them speak louder and more clearly. As ALS progresses, speech therapists can help people develop ways for responding to yes-or-no questions with their eyes or by other nonverbal means and can recommend aids such as speech synthesizers and computer-based communication systems. These methods and devices help people communicate when they can no longer speak or produce vocal sounds.

Nutritional support is an important part of the care of people with ALS. Individuals and caregivers can learn from speech therapists and nutritionists how to plan and prepare numerous small meals throughout the day that provide enough calories, fiber, and fluid and how to avoid foods that are difficult to swallow. People may begin using suction devices to remove excess fluids or saliva and prevent choking. When individuals can no longer get enough nourishment from eating, doctors may advise inserting a feeding tube into the stomach. The use of a feeding tube also reduces the risk of choking and pneumonia that can result from inhaling liquids into the lungs. The tube is not painful and does not prevent individuals from eating food orally if they wish.

When the muscles that assist in breathing weaken, use of nocturnal ventilatory assistance (*Intermittent Positive Pressure Ventilation* [IPPV] or *Bilevel Positive Airway Pressure* [BIPAP]) may be used to aid breathing during sleep. Such devices artificially inflate the person's lungs from various external sources that are applied directly to the face or body. Individuals with ALS will have breathing tests on a regular basis to determine when to start Non-Invasive Ventilation (NIV). When muscles are no longer able to maintain normal oxygen and carbon dioxide levels, these devices may be used full-time. The NeuRx Diaphragm Pacing System, which uses implanted electrodes and a battery pack to cause the diaphragm (breathing muscle) to contract, has been approved by the Food and Drug Administration to help certain individuals who have ALS and breathing problems an average benefit of up to 16 months before onset of severe respiratory failure.

Individuals may eventually consider forms of mechanical ventilation (respirators) in which a machine inflates and deflates the lungs. To be effective, this may require a tube that passes from the nose or mouth to the windpipe (trachea) and for long-term use, an operation such as a tracheostomy, in which a plastic breathing tube is inserted directly in the patient's windpipe through an opening in the neck. Patients and their families should consider several factors when deciding whether and when to use one of these options. Ventilation devices differ in their effect on the person's quality of life and in cost. Although ventilation support can ease problems with breathing and prolong survival, it does not affect the progression of ALS. People need to be fully informed about these considerations and the long-term effects of life without movement before they make decisions about ventilation support.

Social workers and home care and hospice nurses help patients, families, and caregivers with the medical, emotional, and financial challenges of coping with ALS, particularly during the final stages of the disease. Respiratory therapists can help caregivers with tasks such as operating and maintaining respirators, and home care nurses are available not only to provide medical care but also to teach caregivers about giving tube feedings and moving patients to avoid painful skin problems and contractures. Home hospice nurses work in consultation with physicians to ensure proper medication and pain control.

What research is being done?

The National Institute of Neurological Disorders and Stroke, part of the National Institutes of Health, is the Federal Government's leading supporter of biomedical research on ALS. The goals of this research are to find the cause or causes of ALS, understand the mechanisms involved in the progression of the disease, and develop effective treatments.

Scientists are seeking to understand the mechanisms that selectively trigger motor neurons to degenerate in ALS, and to find effective approaches to halt the processes leading to cell death. This work includes studies in animals to identify the molecular means by which ALS-causing gene mutations lead to the destruction of neurons. To this end, scientists have developed models of ALS in a variety of animal species, including fruit flies, zebrafish, and rodents. Initially, these genetically modified animal models focused on mutations in the SOD1 gene but more recently, models harboring other ALS-causing mutations also have been developed. Research in these models suggests that depending on the gene mutation, motor neuron death is caused by a variety of cellular defects, including in the processing of RNA molecules and recycling of proteins, as well as impaired energy metabolism, and hyperactivation of motor neurons. Increasing evidence also suggests that various types of glial support cells and inflammation cells of the nervous system play an important role in the disease.

Overall, the work in familial ALS is already leading to a greater understanding of the more common sporadic form of the disease. Because familial ALS is virtually indistinguishable from sporadic ALS clinically, some researchers believe that familial ALS genes may also be involved in sporadic ALS. For example, recent research has shown that the defect in the C9orf72 gene found in familial ALS is also present in a small percentage of sporadic ALS cases. Further, there is evidence that mutant SOD1 is present in spinal cord tissue in some sporadic cases of ALS.

Another active area of research is the development of innovative cell culture systems to serve as "patient-derived" model systems for ALS research. For example, scientists have developed ways of inducing skin cells from individuals with ALS into becoming pluripotent stem cells (cells that are capable of becoming all the different cell types of the body). In the case of ALS, researchers have been able to convert pluripotent stem cells derived from skin into becoming motor neurons and other cell types that may be involved in the disease. NINDS is supporting research on the development of pluripotent cell lines for a number of neurodegenerative diseases, including ALS.

Scientists are also working to develop biomarkers for ALS that could serve as tools for diagnosis, as markers of disease progression, or correlated with therapeutic targets. Such biomarkers can be molecules derived from a bodily fluid (such as spinal fluid), an imaging assay of the brain or spinal cord, or an electrophysiological measure of nerve and muscle ability to process an electrical signal.

Potential therapies for ALS are being investigated in a range of animal models, especially in rodent models. This work involves the testing of drug-like compounds, gene therapy approaches, antibodies and cell-based therapies. In addition, at any given time, a number of exploratory treatments are in clinical testing in ALS patients. Investigators are optimistic that these and other basic, translational, and clinical research studies will eventually lead to new and more effective treatments for ALS.

Chapter 8

Alzheimer's Disease

Introduction

Alzheimer's disease is an irreversible, progressive brain disease that slowly destroys memory and thinking skills, and eventually even the ability to carry out the simplest tasks. In most people with Alzheimer's, symptoms first appear after age 65. Estimates vary, but experts suggest that as many as 5 million Americans age 65 and older may have Alzheimer's disease.

Alzheimer's disease is the most common cause of dementia among older people. Dementia is the loss of cognitive functioning—thinking, remembering, and reasoning—and behavioral abilities, to such an extent that it interferes with a person's daily life and activities. Dementia ranges in severity from the mildest stage, when it is just beginning to affect a person's functioning, to the most severe stage, when the person must depend completely on others for basic activities of daily living.

Alzheimer's disease is named after Dr. Alois Alzheimer. In 1906, Dr. Alzheimer noticed changes in the brain tissue of a woman who had died of an unusual mental illness. Her symptoms included memory loss, language problems, and unpredictable behavior. After she died, he examined her brain and found many abnormal clumps (now called amyloid plaques) and tangled bundles of fibers (now called neurofibrillary tangles). Plaques and tangles in the brain are two of the main features of Alzheimer's disease. The third is the loss of connections between nerve cells (neurons) in the brain.

Text in this chapter is excerpted from "Alzheimer's Disease Fact Sheet," National Institute on Aging (NIA), February 23, 2015.

Changes in the Brain in Alzheimer's Disease

Although we still don't know how the Alzheimer's disease process begins, it seems likely that damage to the brain starts a decade or more before problems become evident. During the preclinical stage of Alzheimer's disease, people are free of symptoms but toxic changes are taking place in the brain. Abnormal deposits of proteins form amyloid plaques and tau tangles throughout the brain, and once-healthy neurons begin to work less efficiently. Over time, neurons lose their ability to function and communicate with each other, and eventually they die.

Before long, the damage spreads to a nearby structure in the brain called the hippocampus, which is essential in forming memories. As more neurons die, affected brain regions begin to shrink. By the final stage of Alzheimer's, damage is widespread, and brain tissue has shrunk significantly.

Very Early Signs and Symptoms

Memory problems are typically one of the first warning signs of cognitive loss, possibly due to the development of Alzheimer's disease. Some people with memory problems have a condition called amnestic mild cognitive impairment (MCI). People with this condition have more memory problems than normal for people their age, but their symptoms are not as severe as those seen in people with Alzheimer's disease. Other recent studies have found links between some movement difficulties and MCI. Researchers also have seen links between MCI

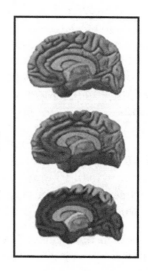

Figure 8.1. *Neurofibrillary Tangles in the Brain*

As Alzheimer's disease progresses, neurofibrillary tangles and amyloid plaques spread throughout the brain.

and some problems with the sense of smell. The ability of people with MCI to perform normal daily activities is not significantly impaired. However, more older people with MCI, compared with those without MCI, go on to develop Alzheimer's.

A decline in other aspects of cognition, such as word-finding, vision/spatial issues, and impaired reasoning or judgment, may also signal the very early stages of Alzheimer's disease. Scientists are looking to see whether brain imaging and biomarker studies, for example, of people with MCI and those with a family history of Alzheimer's, can detect early changes in the brain like those seen in Alzheimer's. Initial studies indicate that early detection using biomarkers and imaging may be possible, but findings will need to be confirmed by other studies before these techniques can be used to help with diagnosis in everyday medical practice.

These and other studies offer hope that someday we may have tools that could help detect Alzheimer's early, track the course of the disease, and monitor response to treatments.

Mild Alzheimer's Disease

As Alzheimer's disease progresses, memory loss worsens, and changes in other cognitive abilities are evident. Problems can include, for example, getting lost, trouble handling money and paying bills (PDF, 159K), repeating questions, taking longer to complete normal daily tasks, using poor judgment, and having some mood and personality changes. People often are diagnosed in this stage.

Moderate Alzheimer's Disease

In this stage, damage occurs in areas of the brain that control language, reasoning, sensory processing, and conscious thought. Memory loss and confusion grow worse, and people begin to have problems recognizing family and friends. They may be unable to learn new things, carry out tasks that involve multiple steps (such as getting dressed), or cope with new situations. They may have hallucinations, delusions, and paranoia, and may behave impulsively.

Severe Alzheimer's Disease

By the final stage, plaques and tangles have spread throughout the brain, and brain tissue has shrunk significantly. People with severe Alzheimer's cannot communicate and are completely dependent on others for their care. Near the end, the person may be in bed most or all of the time as the body shuts down.

What Causes Alzheimer's

Scientists don't yet fully understand what causes Alzheimer's disease, but it has become increasingly clear that it develops because of a complex series of events that take place in the brain over a long period of time. It is likely that the causes include some mix of genetic, environmental, and lifestyle factors. Because people differ in their genetic make-up and lifestyle, the importance of any one of these factors in increasing or decreasing the risk of developing Alzheimer's may differ from person to person.

The Basics of Alzheimer's

Scientists are conducting studies to learn more about plaques, tangles, and other features of Alzheimer's disease. Advances in brain imaging techniques now allow researchers to visualize abnormal levels of beta-amyloid and tau proteins in the living brain. Scientists are also exploring the very earliest steps in the disease process. Findings from these studies will help them understand the causes of Alzheimer's.

One of the great mysteries of Alzheimer's disease is why it largely strikes older adults. Research on how the brain changes normally with age is shedding light on this question. For example, scientists are learning how age-related changes in the brain may harm neurons and contribute to Alzheimer's damage. These age-related changes include atrophy (shrinking) of certain parts of the brain, inflammation, the production of unstable molecules called free radicals, and mitochondrial dysfunction (a breakdown of energy production within a cell).

Genetics

Early-onset Alzheimer's is a rare form of the disease. It occurs in people age 30 to 60 and represents less than 5 percent of all people who have Alzheimer's disease. Most cases of early-onset Alzheimer's are familial Alzheimer's disease, caused by changes in one of three known genes inherited from a parent.

Most people with Alzheimer's disease have "late-onset" Alzheimer's, which usually develops after age 60. Many studies have linked the apolipoprotein E (APOE) gene to late-onset Alzheimer's. This gene has several forms. One of them, APOE ε4, seems to increase a person's risk of getting the disease. However, carrying the APOE ε4 form of the gene does not necessarily mean that a person will develop Alzheimer's disease, and people carrying no APOE ε4 can also develop the disease.

Most experts believe that additional genes may influence the development of late-onset Alzheimer's. Scientists around the world are searching for these genes, and have identified a number of common genes in addition to APOE ε4 that may increase a person's risk for late-onset Alzheimer's.

Environmental/Lifestyle Factors

Research also suggests that a host of factors beyond basic genetics may play a role in the development and course of Alzheimer's disease. There is a great deal of interest, for example, in associations between cognitive decline and vascular and metabolic conditions such as heart disease, stroke, high blood pressure, diabetes, and obesity. Understanding these relationships and testing them in clinical trials will help us understand whether reducing risk factors for these conditions may help with Alzheimer's as well.

Further, a nutritious diet, physical activity, social engagement, and mentally stimulating pursuits can all help people stay healthy as they age. New research suggests the possibility that these and other factors also might help to reduce the risk of cognitive decline and Alzheimer's disease. Clinical trials of specific interventions are underway to test some of these possibilities.

Diagnosing Alzheimer's Disease

Alzheimer's disease can be definitively diagnosed only after death, by linking clinical measures with an examination of brain tissue and pathology in an autopsy. But doctors now have several methods and tools to help them determine fairly accurately whether a person who is having memory problems has "possible Alzheimer's dementia" (dementia may be due to another cause) or "probable Alzheimer's dementia" (no other cause for dementia can be found).

To diagnose Alzheimer's, doctors may:

- Ask questions about overall health, past medical problems, ability to carry out daily activities, and changes in behavior and personality

- Conduct tests of memory, problem solving, attention, counting, and language

- Carry out standard medical tests, such as blood and urine tests, to identify other possible causes of the problem

- Perform brain scans, such as computed tomography (CT) or magnetic resonance imaging (MRI), to distinguish Alzheimer's from other possible causes for symptoms, like stroke or tumor

These tests may be repeated to give doctors information about how the person's memory is changing over time.

Early, accurate diagnosis is beneficial for several reasons. It can tell people whether their symptoms are from Alzheimer's or another cause, such as stroke, tumor, Parkinson's disease, sleep disturbances, side effects of medications, or other conditions that may be treatable and possibly reversible.

Beginning treatment early on in the disease process can help preserve function for some time, even though the underlying disease process cannot be changed. Having an early diagnosis also helps families plan for the future, make living arrangements, take care of financial and legal matters, and develop support networks.

In addition, an early diagnosis can provide greater opportunities for people to get involved in clinical trials. In a typical clinical trial, scientists test a drug or treatment to see if that intervention is effective and for whom it would work best.

Treating Alzheimer's Disease

Alzheimer's disease is complex, and it is unlikely that any one intervention will be found to delay, prevent, or cure it. That's why current approaches in treatment and research focus on several different aspects, including helping people maintain mental function, managing behavioral symptoms, and slowing or delaying the symptoms of disease.

Maintaining Mental Function

Four medications are approved by the U.S. Food and Drug Administration to treat Alzheimer's. Donepezil (Aricept®), rivastigmine (Exelon®), and galantamine (Razadyne®) are used to treat mild to moderate Alzheimer's (donepezil can be used for severe Alzheimer's as well). Memantine (Namenda®) is used to treat moderate to severe Alzheimer's. These drugs work by regulating neurotransmitters (the chemicals that transmit messages between neurons). They may help maintain thinking, memory, and speaking skills, and help with certain behavioral problems. However, these drugs don't change the underlying disease process, are effective for some but not all people, and may help only for a limited time.

Managing Behavioral Symptoms

Common behavioral symptoms of Alzheimer's include sleeplessness, agitation, wandering, anxiety, anger, and depression. Scientists are learning why these symptoms occur and are studying new treatments—drug and non-drug—to manage them. Treating behavioral symptoms often makes people with Alzheimer's more comfortable and makes their care easier for caregivers.

Slowing, Delaying, or Preventing Alzheimer's Disease

Alzheimer's disease research has developed to a point where scientists can look beyond treating symptoms to think about addressing underlying disease processes. In ongoing clinical trials, scientists are looking at many possible interventions, such as immunization therapy, cognitive training, physical activity, antioxidants, and the effects of cardiovascular and diabetes treatments.

Supporting Families and Caregivers

Caring for a person with Alzheimer's disease can have high physical, emotional, and financial costs. The demands of day-to-day care, changing family roles, and difficult decisions about placement in a care facility can be hard to handle. Researchers have learned much about Alzheimer's caregiving, and studies are helping to develop new ways to support caregivers.

Becoming well-informed about the disease is one important long-term strategy. Programs that teach families about the various stages of Alzheimer's and about flexible and practical strategies for dealing with difficult caregiving situations provide vital help to those who care for people with Alzheimer's.

Developing good coping skills and a strong support network of family and friends also are important ways that caregivers can help themselves handle the stresses of caring for a loved one with Alzheimer's disease. For example, staying physically active provides physical and emotional benefits.

Some Alzheimer's caregivers have found that participating in a support group is a critical lifeline. These support groups allow caregivers to find respite, express concerns, share experiences, get tips, and receive emotional comfort. There are a growing number of groups for people in the early stage of Alzheimer's and their families. Support networks can be especially valuable when caregivers face the difficult decision of whether and when to place a loved one in a nursing home or assisted living facility.

Research

Thirty years ago, we knew very little about Alzheimer's disease. Since then, scientists have made important advances. Research supported by NIA and other organizations has expanded knowledge of brain function in healthy older people, identified ways we might lessen normal age-related declines in mental function, and deepened our understanding of the disease. Many scientists and physicians are now working together to untangle the genetic, biological, and environmental factors that, over many years, ultimately result in Alzheimer's. This effort is bringing us closer to better managing and, ultimately, preventing this devastating disease.

Chapter 9

Parkinson's Disease

What Is Parkinson's Disease?

A Brain Disorder

Parkinson's disease is a brain disorder that leads to shaking, stiffness, and difficulty with walking, balance, and coordination. It affects about half a million people in the United States although the numbers may be much higher. The average age of onset is 60 years, and the risk of developing Parkinson's goes up with age.

Parkinson's disease was first described in 1817 by James Parkinson, a British doctor who published a paper on what he called "the shaking palsy." In this paper, he described the major symptoms of the disease that would later bear his name.

Four Main Symptoms

Parkinson's disease belongs to a group of neurological conditions called movement disorders. The four main symptoms of Parkinson's are:

- tremor, or trembling in hands, arms, legs, jaw, or head
- rigidity, or stiffness of the limbs and trunk
- bradykinesia, or slowness of movement
- postural instability, or impaired balance.

Text in this chapter is excerpted from "Parkinson's Disease," National Institutes of Health (NIH), June, 2012.

Parkinson's symptoms usually begin gradually and get worse over time. As the symptoms become more severe, people with the disorder may have difficulty walking, talking, or completing other simple tasks. They also experience non-motor, or movement, symptoms including mental and behavioral changes, sleep problems, depression, memory difficulties, and fatigue.

Parkinson's disease not only affects the brain, but the entire body. While the brain involvement is responsible for the core features, other affected locations contribute to the complicated picture of Parkinson's.

Parkinson's disease is both chronic, meaning it lasts for a long time, and progressive, meaning its symptoms grow worse over time. It is not contagious.

Diagnosis Can Be Difficult

About 60,000 Americans are diagnosed with Parkinson's disease each year. However, it's difficult to know exactly how many have it because many people in the early stages of the disease think their symptoms are due to normal aging and do not seek help from a doctor. Also, diagnosis is sometimes difficult because there are no medical tests that can diagnose the disease with certainty and because other conditions may produce symptoms of Parkinson's.

For example, people with Parkinson's may sometimes be told by their doctors that they have other disorders, and people with diseases similar to Parkinson's may be incorrectly diagnosed as having Parkinson's. A person's good response to the drug levodopa may support the diagnosis. Levodopa is the main therapy for Parkinson's disease.

Who Is at Risk?

Both men and women can have Parkinson's disease. However, the disease affects about 50 percent more men than women.

While the disease is more common in developed countries, studies also have found an increased risk of Parkinson's disease in people who live in rural areas and in those who work in certain professions, suggesting that environmental factors may play a role in the disorder.

Researchers are focusing on additional risk factors for Parkinson's disease. One clear risk factor for Parkinson's is age. The average age of onset is 60 years and the risk rises significantly with advancing age. However, about 5 to 10 percent of people with Parkinson's have "early-onset" disease which begins before the age of 50. Early-onset forms of Parkinson's are often inherited, though not always, and some have been linked to specific gene mutations.

Juvenile Parkinsonism

In very rare cases, parkinsonian symptoms may appear in people before the age of 20. This condition is called juvenile parkinsonism. It is most commonly seen in Japan but has been found in other countries as well. It usually begins with dystonia (sustained muscle contractions causing twisting movements) and bradykinesia (slowness of movement), and the symptoms often improve with levodopa medication. Juvenile parkinsonism often runs in families and is sometimes linked to a mutated gene.

Some Cases Are Inherited

Evidence suggests that, in some cases, Parkinson's disease may be inherited. An estimated 15 to 25 percent of people with Parkinson's have a known relative with the disease. People with one or more close relatives who have Parkinson's have an increased risk of developing the disease themselves, but the total risk is still just 2 to 5 percent unless the family has a known gene mutation for the disease. A gene mutation is a change or alteration in the DNA or genetic material that makes up a gene.

Researchers have discovered several genes that are linked to Parkinson's disease. The first to be identified was alpha-synuclein or SNCA. Inherited cases of Parkinson's disease are caused by mutations in the LRRK2, PARK2 or parkin, PARK7 or DJ-1, PINK1, or SNCA genes, or by mutations in genes that have not yet been identified.

What Causes Parkinson's Disease?

A Shortage of Dopamine

Parkinson's disease occurs when nerve cells, or neurons, in an area of the brain that controls movement become impaired and/or die. Normally, these neurons produce an important brain chemical known as *dopamine*, but when the neurons die or become impaired, they produce less dopamine. This shortage of dopamine causes the movement problems of people with Parkinson's.

Dopamine is a chemical messenger, or *neurotransmitter*. Dopamine is responsible for transmitting signals between the substantia nigra and multiple brain regions. The connection between the substantia nigra and the *corpus striatum* is critical to produce smooth, purposeful movement. Loss of dopamine in this circuit results in abnormal nerve-firing patterns within the brain that cause impaired movement.

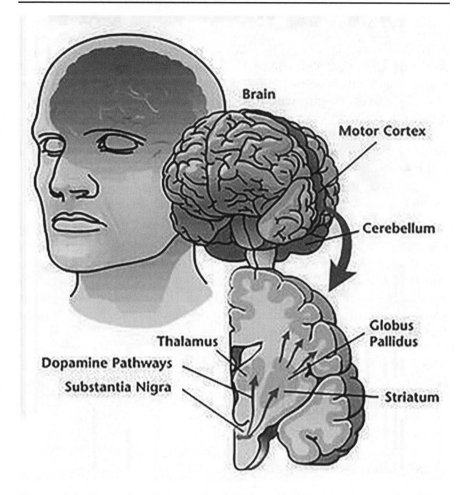

Figure 9.1. *Dopamine Pathway for the Motor System*

Here is the dopamine pathway for the motor system. Dopamine signals travel from the substantia nigra to brain regions including the corpus striatum, the globus pallidus, and the thalamus in order to control movement and balance. In Parkinson's disease, most of the dopamine signals from the substantia nigra are lost.

Loss of Norepinephrine

People with Parkinson's also have loss of the nerve endings that produce the neurotransmitter *norepinephrine*. Norepinephrine, which is closely related to dopamine, is the main chemical messenger of the sympathetic nervous system. The sympathetic nervous system controls many automatic functions of the body, such as heart rate and blood pressure. The loss of norepinephrine might help explain several of the non-movement features of Parkinson's, such as fatigue, irregular blood pressure, decreased gastric motility or movement of food through the digestive tract, and postural hypotension. Postural hypotension is a sudden drop in blood pressure when a person stands up from a sitting or lying-down position. It may cause dizziness, lightheadedness, and in some cases, loss of balance or fainting.

Lewy Bodies in Brain Cells

Many brain cells of people with Parkinson's contain *Lewy bodies*. Lewy bodies are unusual deposits or clumps of the brain protein *alpha-synuclein*, along with other proteins, which are seen upon microscopic examination of the brain. Researchers do not yet know why Lewy bodies form or what role they play in the development of Parkinson's. The clumps may prevent the cell from functioning normally, or they may actually be helpful, perhaps by keeping harmful proteins "locked up" so the cells can function.

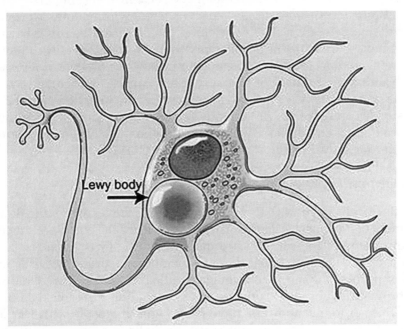

Figure 9.2. *A Lewy Body*

This drawing shows a Lewy body, a hallmark of Parkinson's disease, inside the cell body of a neuron, or nerve cell. Lewy bodies are clumps of the brain protein alpha-synuclein and other proteins.

Genetic Mutations

Although some cases of Parkinson's appear to be hereditary, and a few can be traced to specific genetic mutations, most cases are sporadic. Sporadic means the disease occurs randomly and does not seem to run in families. Many researchers now believe that Parkinson's disease results from a combination of genetic and environmental factors.

Scientists have identified several genetic mutations associated with Parkinson's including mutations in the alpha-synuclein gene. They think that many more genes may be linked to the disorder. Studying the genes responsible for inherited cases of Parkinson's can help researchers understand both inherited and sporadic cases. The same genes and proteins that are altered in inherited cases may also be altered in sporadic cases by environmental toxins or other factors. Researchers also hope that discovering genes will help identify new ways of treating Parkinson's.

Environmental Toxins

Although researchers increasingly recognize the importance of genetics in Parkinson's disease, most believe environmental exposures increase a person's risk of developing the disease. Even in inherited cases, exposure to toxins or other environmental factors may influence when symptoms of the disease appear or how the disease progresses.

There are a number of toxins that can cause parkinsonian symptoms in humans. Researchers are pursuing the question of whether pesticides and other environmental factors not yet identified also may cause Parkinson's disease. Viruses are another possible environmental trigger for Parkinson's.

Mitochondria and Free Radicals

Research suggests that *mitochondria* may play a role in the development of Parkinson's disease. Mitochondria are the energy-producing components of the cell and are major sources of *free radicals*. Free radicals are molecules that damage membranes, proteins, DNA, and other parts of the cell. This damage is called *oxidative stress*. Changes to brain cells caused by oxidative stress, including free radical damage to DNA, proteins, and fats, have been found in people with Parkinson's. Clinical studies now underway test whether agents thought to improve energy metabolism and decrease oxidative stress slow the progression of Parkinson's disease. Recent evidence suggests that mutations in genes linked to Parkinson's disease result in mitochondrial dysfunction.

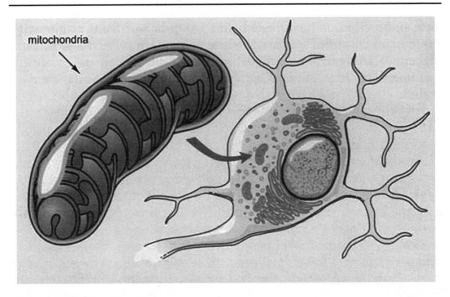

Figure 9.3. *Mitochondria*

Problems with mitochondria, the structures that produce energy for all cells, have been linked to the development of Parkinson's disease.

Buildup of Harmful Proteins

Other research suggests that the cell's protein disposal system may fail in people with Parkinson's, causing proteins like alpha-synuclein to build up to harmful levels and trigger premature cell death. Additional studies have found that clumps of protein that develop inside brain cells of people with Parkinson's may contribute to the death of nerve cells, or neurons. However, the exact role of the protein deposits remains unknown. These studies also found that inflammation, because of protein accumulation, toxins or other factors, may play a role in the disease. However, the exact role of the protein deposits remains unknown. Researchers are exploring the possibility of vaccine development to decrease or prevent the accumulation of alpha-synuclein.

While mitochondrial dysfunction, oxidative stress, inflammation, and many other cellular processes may contribute to Parkinson's disease, scientists still do not know what causes cells that produce dopamine to die.

Genes Linked to Parkinson's

Researchers have discovered several genes that are linked to Parkinson's disease. The first to be identified was alpha-synuclein or SNCA . Studies have found that Lewy bodies from people with the sporadic form of Parkinson's contain clumps of alpha-synuclein protein. This discovery revealed a possible link between hereditary and sporadic forms of the disease. Other genes linked to Parkinson's include PARK2, PARK7, PINK1, and LRRK2. PARK2, PARK7, and PINK1 cause rare, early-onset forms of the disease. Mutations in the LRRK2 gene are common in specific populations, including in people with Parkinson's in North Africa.

Researchers are continuing to study the normal functions and interactions of these genes in order to find clues about how Parkinson's develops. They also have identified a number of other genes and chromosome regions that may play a role in Parkinson's, but the nature of these links is not yet clear. Whole genome wide association studies, or GWAS, of thousands of people with Parkinson's disease are now underway to find gene variants that allow for an increased risk of developing Parkinson's but are not necessarily causes of this disorder by themselves.

A recent international study found that two genes containing mutations known to cause rare hereditary forms of Parkinson's disease are also associated with the more common sporadic form of the disease. This finding came from a GWAS which looked at DNA samples of European people who had Parkinson's disease and from those who did not have the disorder.

Symptoms and Diagnosis

Parkinson's disease does not affect everyone the same way. Symptoms of the disorder and the rate of progression differ among people with the disease. Sometimes people dismiss early symptoms of Parkinson's as the effects of normal aging. There are no medical tests to definitively diagnose the disease, so it can be difficult to diagnose accurately.

Early Symptoms

Early symptoms of Parkinson's disease are subtle and occur gradually. For example, affected people may feel mild tremors or have difficulty getting out of a chair. They may notice that they speak too softly or that their handwriting is slow and looks cramped or small. This very early period may last a long time before the more classic and obvious symptoms appear.

Friends or family members may be the first to notice changes in someone with early Parkinson's. They may see that the person's face lacks expression and animation, a condition known as "masked face," or that the person does not move an arm or leg normally. They also may notice that the person seems stiff, unsteady, or unusually slow.

As the Disease Progresses

As the disease progresses, symptoms may begin to interfere with daily activities. The shaking or tremor may make it difficult to hold utensils steady or read a newspaper. Tremor is usually the symptom that causes people to seek medical help.

People with Parkinson's often develop a so-called *parkinsonian gait* that includes a tendency to lean forward, small quick steps as if hurrying forward (called festination), and reduced swinging of the arms. They also may have trouble initiating or continuing movement, which is known as *freezing*.

Symptoms often begin on one side of the body or even in one limb on one side of the body. As the disease progresses, it eventually affects both sides. However, the symptoms may still be more severe on one side than on the other.

Four Primary Symptoms

The four primary symptoms of Parkinson's are tremor, rigidity, slowness of movement (bradykinesia), and impaired balance (postural instability).

- Tremor often begins in a hand, although sometimes a foot or the jaw is affected first. It is most obvious when the hand is at rest or when a person is under stress. It usually disappears during sleep or improves with a deliberate movement.

- Rigidity, or a resistance to movement, affects most people with Parkinson's. It becomes obvious when another person tries to move the individual's arm, such as during a neurological examination. The arm will move only in ratchet-like or short, jerky movements known as "cogwheel" rigidity.

- Bradykinesia, or the slowing down and loss of spontaneous and automatic movement, is particularly frustrating because it may make simple tasks somewhat difficult. Activities once performed quickly and easily, such as washing or dressing, may take several hours.

- Postural instability, or impaired balance, causes people with Parkinson's to fall easily. They also may develop a stooped posture with a bowed head and droopy shoulders.

Other Symptoms

A number of other symptoms may accompany Parkinson's disease. Some are minor; others are not. Many can be treated with medication or physical therapy. No one can predict which symptoms will affect an individual person, and the intensity of the symptoms varies from person to person. Many people note that prior to experiencing motor problems of stiffness and tremor, they had symptoms of a sleep disorder, constipation, decreased ability to smell, and restless legs.

Other symptoms include:

- depression
- emotional changes
- difficulty swallowing and chewing
- speech changes
- urinary problems or constipation
- skin problems, sleep problems
- dementia or other cognitive problems
- orthostatic hypotension (a sudden drop in blood pressure when standing up from a sitting or lying down position)
- muscle cramps and dystonia (twisting and repetitive movements)
- pain
- fatigue and loss of energy
- sexual dysfunction

A number of disorders can cause symptoms similar to those of Parkinson's disease. People with Parkinson's-like symptoms that result from other causes are sometimes said to have parkinsonism. While these disorders initially may be misdiagnosed as Parkinson's, certain medical tests, as well as response to drug treatment, may help to distinguish them from Parkinson's.

Diagnosis Can Be Difficult

There are currently no blood, or laboratory tests to diagnose sporadic Parkinson's disease. Diagnosis is based on a person's medical history and a neurological examination, but the disease can be difficult to diagnose accurately. Early signs and symptoms of Parkinson's may sometimes be dismissed as the effects of normal aging. A doctor may need to observe the person for some time until it is clear that the symptoms are consistently present. Improvement after initiating medication is another important hallmark of Parkinson's disease.

Doctors may sometimes request brain scans or laboratory tests to rule out other diseases. However, computed tomography (CT) and magnetic resonance imaging (MRI) brain scans of people with Parkinson's usually appear normal. Recently, the FDA (Food and Drug Administration) has approved an imaging technique called DaTscan, which may help to increase accuracy of the diagnosis of Parkinson's disease. Since many other diseases have similar features but require different treatments, it is very important to make an exact diagnosis as soon as possible to ensure proper treatment.

Medications

Although there is no cure for Parkinson's disease, medicines can often provide dramatic relief from the symptoms. However, there are limits to their effectiveness, and scientists are working to find better ways to treat the disease.

Three classes of medications

Medications for Parkinson's fall into three groups.

- The first group includes drugs that increase the level of dopamine in the brain.

- The second group affects other neurotransmitters in the body in order to ease some of the symptoms of the disease.

- The third group includes medications that help control non-motor symptoms (those that do not affect movement) of Parkinson's.

Levodopa Is the Main Therapy

The main therapy for Parkinson's is the drug levodopa, also called L-dopa. It is a simple chemical found naturally in plants and animals.

Nerve cells use levodopa to make dopamine to replenish the brain's dwindling supply. People cannot simply take dopamine pills because dopamine does not easily pass through the blood-brain barrier. The blood-brain barrier is a lining of cells inside blood vessels that controls the transport of oxygen, glucose, and other substances into the brain.

Usually, people take levodopa along with another medication called *carbidopa*. Carbidopa delays the body's conversion of levodopa into dopamine until the levodopa reaches the brain. This prevents or reduces some of the side effects that often accompany levodopa therapy. Carbidopa also reduces the amount of levodopa needed.

Usually Successful in Early Stages

Levodopa successfully reduces the tremors and other symptoms of Parkinson's during the early stages of the disease. It allows most people with Parkinson's to extend the period of time in which they can lead relatively normal, productive lives.

However, not all symptoms respond equally to levodopa. It usually helps most with bradykinesia (slowness of movement) and rigidity. Problems with balance and other non-motor symptoms may not be helped at all.

People with Parkinson's disease often see dramatic improvement in their symptoms after starting levodopa therapy. However, they may need to increase the dose gradually over time to maintain maximum benefit.

Levodopa is often so effective that some people may temporarily forget they have Parkinson's during the early stages of the disease. But levodopa is not a cure. Although it can reduce the symptoms, it does not replace lost nerve cells or stop the gradual loss of brain cells that causes the disease.

Side Effects of Levodopa

Levodopa can have a variety of side effects including nausea, vomiting, low blood pressure, and restlessness. It can also cause drowsiness or sudden sleep onset. Levodopa in excess sometimes causes hallucinations and psychosis.

Dyskinesias, or involuntary movements such as twitching, twisting, and writhing, commonly develop in people who take large doses of levodopa for a long time. The dose of levodopa is often reduced in order to lessen the movements brought on by the drug. However, symptoms of Parkinson's disease often reappear even with lower doses of medication. People with Parkinson's must work closely with their doctor to find a tolerable balance between the drug's benefits and side effects.

Other troubling and distressing problems may occur with levodopa use in people with advanced Parkinson's disease. People may begin to notice more pronounced symptoms before their first dose of medication in the morning, and they may develop muscle spasms or other problems when each dose begins to wear off. The period of effectiveness after each dose may begin to shorten, called the "wearing-off" effect.

Another potential problem is referred to as the "on-off" effect—sudden fluctuations in movement, from normal or dyskinesia to parkinsonian slowness and stiffness and back again. These effects indicate that the person's response to the drug is changing as the disease progresses.

One approach to reducing these side effects is to take levodopa more often and in smaller amounts. People with Parkinson's disease should never stop taking levodopa without telling their doctor because suddenly stopping the drug may have serious side effects, such as being unable to move or having difficulty breathing.

Other Drug Treatments

Fortunately, doctors have other treatment choices for some symptoms and stages of Parkinson's disease. These include:

- direct dopamine agonists
- MAO-B inhibitors
- COMT inhibitors
- Amantadine, an old antiviral drug which can reduce dyskinesia
- anticholinergic drugs.

Direct Dopamine Agonists

Direct dopamine agonists are drugs that mimic the role of dopamine in the brain as opposed to levodopa which requires conversion in the brain to dopamine. They may be used in the early stages of the disease, or later on to give a more prolonged, steady dopaminergic effect in people who experience wearing off or on-off effects. Dopamine agonists are generally less effective than levodopa in controlling rigidity and bradykinesia. They can cause confusion in older adults.

MAO-B Inhibitors

MAO-B inhibitors are drugs that slow down the enzyme mono-amine oxidase B, or MAO-B, which breaks down dopamine in the brain. MAO-B inhibitors cause dopamine to build up in surviving nerve cells, thereby reducing symptoms of Parkinson's.

One MAO-B inhibitor, rasagiline, may be used alone or in combination with other medication to treat Parkinson's disease symptoms.

COMT Inhibitors

COMT, which stands for catechol-O-methyltransferase, is another enzyme that helps to break down dopamine. COMT inhibitors prolong the effects of levodopa by preventing the breakdown of dopamine. They can decrease the duration of "off" periods, and they usually make it possible to reduce the person's dose of levodopa.

Other Drugs

- Amantadine is an old antiviral drug that can help reduce symptoms of Parkinson's and dyskinesias caused by levodopa. It is often used alone in the early stages of the disease, and again in later stages to treat dyskinesias.

- Anticholinergics decrease the activity of the neurotransmitter acetylcholine and help to reduce tremors and muscle rigidity.

When recommending a course of treatment, a doctor will tailor therapy to the person's particular condition. Since no two people react the same way to a given drug, it may take time and patience to get the dose just right. Even then, symptoms may not go away completely.

Medications for Non-Motor Symptoms

Doctors may prescribe a variety of medications to treat the non-motor symptoms of Parkinson's disease, such as depression and anxiety. Hallucinations, delusions, and other psychotic symptoms may be caused by some drugs prescribed for Parkinson's. Therefore, reducing or stopping those medications may reduce these symptoms of psychosis. Various treatment options, including medications, also are available to treat orthostatic hypotension, the sudden drop in blood pressure that occurs upon standing.

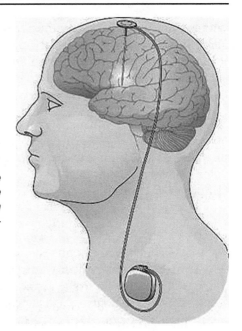

Figure 9.4. *Deep Brain Stimulation*

Deep brain stimulation, or DBS, can be performed on one or both sides of the brain. DBS is used more frequently than surgeries such as pallidotomy or thalamotomy.

Surgical Treatments and Other Therapies

Deep Brain Stimulation

Deep brain stimulation, or DBS, is a surgical procedure used to treat a variety of disabling disorders. It is most commonly used to treat the debilitating symptoms of Parkinson's disease.

Deep brain stimulation uses an electrode surgically implanted into part of the brain. The electrodes are connected by a wire under the skin to a small electrical device called a pulse generator that is implanted in the chest. The pulse generator and electrodes painlessly stimulate the brain in a way that helps to stop many of the symptoms of Parkinson's such as tremor, bradykinesia, and rigidity. DBS is primarily used to stimulate one of three brain regions: the subthalamic nucleus, the globus pallidus, or the thalamus. Researchers are exploring optimal generator settings for DBS, whether DBS of other brain regions will also improve symptoms of Parkinson's disease, and also whether DBS may slow disease progression.

Deep brain stimulation usually reduces the need for levodopa and related drugs, which in turn decreases dyskinesias and other side effects. It also helps to relieve "on-off" fluctuation of symptoms. People who respond well to treatment with levodopa tend to respond well to DBS. Unfortunately, older people who have only a partial response to levodopa may not improve with DBS.

Complementary and Supportive Therapies

A wide variety of complementary and supportive therapies may be used for Parkinson's disease. Among these therapies are standard physical, occupational, and speech therapies, which help with gait and voice disorders, tremors and rigidity, and decline in mental functions. Other supportive therapies include diet and exercise.

Diet

At this time there are no specific vitamins, minerals, or other nutrients that have any proven therapeutic value in Parkinson's disease. Some early reports have suggested that dietary supplements might protect against Parkinson's. Also, a preliminary clinical study of a supplement called coenzyme Q10 suggested that large doses of this substance might slow disease progression in people with early-stage Parkinson's. This supplement is now being tested in a large clinical trial.

Other studies are being conducted to find out if caffeine, antioxidants, nicotine, and other dietary factors may help prevent or treat the disease. While there is currently no proof that any specific dietary factor is beneficial, a normal, healthy diet can promote overall well-being for people with Parkinson's disease, just as it would for anyone else. A high protein meal, however, may limit levodopa's effectiveness because for a time afterwards less levodopa passes through the blood-brain barrier.

Exercise

Exercise can help people with Parkinson's improve their mobility and flexibility. It can also improve their emotional well-being. Exercise may improve the brain's dopamine production or increase levels of beneficial compounds called neurotrophic factors in the brain.

Other Therapies

Other complementary therapies include massage therapy, yoga, tai chi, hypnosis, acupuncture, and the Alexander technique, which improves posture and muscle activity. There have been limited studies suggesting mild benefits from some of these therapies, but they do not slow Parkinson's disease and to date there is no convincing evidence that they help. However, this remains an active area of investigation.

Research

In recent years, research on Parkinson's has advanced to the point that halting the progression of the disease, restoring lost function, and even preventing the disease are all considered realistic goals. While the goal of preventing Parkinson's disease may take years to achieve, researchers are making great progress in understanding and treating it.

Genetics Research

One of the most exciting areas of Parkinson's research is genetics. Studying the genes responsible for inherited cases can help researchers understand both inherited and sporadic cases of the disease. Identifying gene defects can also help researchers:

- understand how Parkinson's occurs

- develop animal models that accurately mimic the death of nerve cells in humans

- identify new approaches to drug therapy

- improve diagnosis.

Researchers funded by the National Institute of Neurological Disorders and Stroke are gathering information and DNA samples from hundreds of families with members who have Parkinson's and are conducting large-scale studies to identify gene variants that are associated with increased risk of developing the disease. They are also comparing gene activity in Parkinson's with gene activity in similar diseases such as progressive supranuclear palsy.

In addition to identifying new genes for Parkinson's disease, researchers are trying to learn about the function of genes known to be associated with the disease, and about how gene mutations cause disease.

Effects of Environmental Toxins

Scientists continue to study environmental toxins such as pesticides and herbicides that can cause Parkinson's symptoms in animals. They have found that exposing rodents to the pesticide rotenone and several other agricultural chemicals can cause cellular and behavioral changes that mimic those seen in Parkinson's.

Role of Lewy Bodies

Other studies focus on how Lewy bodies form and what role they play in Parkinson's disease. Some studies suggest that Lewy bodies are a byproduct of a breakdown that occurs within nerve cells, while others indicate that Lewy bodies are protective, helping neurons "lock away" abnormal molecules that might otherwise be harmful.

Identifying Biomarkers

Biomarkers for Parkinson's—measurable characteristics that can reveal whether the disease is developing or progressing—are another focus of research. Such biomarkers could help doctors detect the disease before symptoms appear and improve diagnosis of the disease. They also would show if medications and other types of therapy have a positive or negative effect on the course of the disease. The National Disorders of Neurological Disorders and Stroke has developed an initiative, the Parkinson's Disease Biomarkers Identification Network (PD-BIN), designed specifically to address these questions and to discover and validate biomarkers for Parkinson's disease.

Transcranial Therapies

Researchers are conducting many studies of new or improved therapies for Parkinson's disease. Studies are testing whether transcranial electrical polarization (TEP) or transcranial magnetic stimulation (TMS) can reduce the symptoms of the disease. In TEP, electrodes placed on the scalp are used to generate an electrical current that modifies signals in the brain's cortex. In TMS, an insulated coil of wire on the scalp is used to generate a brief electrical current.

Drug Discovery

A variety of new drug treatments for Parkinson's disease are in clinical trials. Several MAO-B inhibitors including selegiline, lazabemide, and rasagiline, are being tested to determine if they have neuroprotective effects in people with Parkinson's disease.

The National Institute of Neurological Disorders and Stroke has launched a broad effort to find drugs to slow the progression of Parkinson's disease, called NET-PD or NIH Exploratory Trials in Parkinson's Disease. The first studies tested several compounds; one of these, *creatine*, is now being evaluated in a larger clinical trial. The NET-PD investigators are testing a highly purified form of creatine, a nutritional supplement, to find out if it slows the decline seen in people with Parkinson's. Creatine is a widely used dietary supplement thought to improve exercise performance. Cellular energy is stored in a chemical bond between creatine and a phosphate.

More recently, NET-PD has initiated pilot studies to test pioglitazone, a drug that has been shown to stimulate mitochondrial function. Because mitochondrial function may be less active in Parkinson's disease, this drug may protect vulnerable dopamine neurons by boosting mitochondrial function.

Cell Implantation

Another potential approach to treating Parkinson's disease is to implant cells to replace those lost in the disease. Starting in the 1990s, researchers conducting a controlled clinical trial of fetal tissue implants tried to replace lost dopamine-producing nerve cells with healthy ones from fetal tissue in order to improve movement and the response to medications. While many of the implanted cells survived in the brain and produced dopamine, this therapy was associated with only modest functional improvements, mostly in patients under the age of 60. Some of the people who received the transplants developed disabling dyskinesias that could not be relieved by reducing anti-parkinsonian medications.

Stem Cells

Another type of cell therapy involves stem cells. Some stem cells derived from embryos can develop into any kind of cell in the body, while others, called progenitor cells, are less flexible. Researchers are developing methods to improve the number of dopamine-producing cells that can be grown from embryonic stem cells in culture. Other researchers are also exploring whether stem cells from adult brains might be useful in treating Parkinson's disease.

Recent studies suggest that some adult cells from skin can be reprogrammed to an embryonic-like state, resulting in induced pluripotent stem cells (iPSC) that may someday be used for treatment of Parkinson's. In addition, development and characterization of cells from people with sporadic or inherited Parkinson's may reveal information about cellular mechanisms of disease and identify targets for drug development.

Gene Therapy

A number of early clinical trials are now underway to test whether gene therapy can improve Parkinson's disease. Genes which are found to improve cellular function in models of Parkinson's are inserted into modified viruses. The genetically engineered viruses are then injected into the brains of people with Parkinson's disease. Clinical studies have focused on the therapeutic potential of neurotrophic factors, including GDNF and neurturin, and enzymes that produce dopamine. These trials will test whether the viruses, by lending to the production of the protective gene product, improve symptoms of Parkinson's over time.

The National Institute of Neurological Disorders and Stroke also supports the Morris K. Udall Centers of Excellence for Parkinson's Disease Research program . These Centers, located across the USA, study cellular mechanisms underlying Parkinson's disease, identify and characterize disease-associated genes, and discover and develop potential therapeutic targets. The Centers' multidisciplinary research environment allows scientists to take advantage of new discoveries in the basic, translational and clinical sciences that could lead to clinical advances for Parkinson's disease.

Chapter 10

Cerebral Palsy

What is Cerebral Palsy?

Cerebral palsy refers to a group of neurological disorders that appear in infancy or early childhood and permanently affect body movement and muscle coordination Cerebral palsy (CP) is caused by damage to or abnormalities inside the developing brain that disrupt the brain's ability to control movement and maintain posture and balance. The term *cerebral* refers to the brain; *palsy* refers to the loss or impairment of motor function.

Cerebral palsy affects the motor area of the brain's outer layer (called the cerebral cortex), the part of the brain that directs muscle movement.

In some cases, the cerebral motor cortex hasn't developed normally during fetal growth. In others, the damage is a result of injury to the brain either before, during, or after birth. In either case, the damage is not repairable and the disabilities that result are permanent.

Children with CP exhibit a wide variety of symptoms, including:

- lack of muscle coordination when performing voluntary movements (*ataxia*);

- stiff or tight muscles and exaggerated reflexes (*spasticity*);

- weakness in one or more arm or leg;

Text in this chapter is excerpted from "Cerebral Palsy: Hope Through Research," National Institute of Neurological Disorders and Stroke (NINDS), February 2, 2015.

- walking on the toes, a crouched gait, or a "scissored" gait;
- variations in muscle tone, either too stiff or too floppy;
- excessive drooling or difficulties swallowing or speaking;
- shaking (*tremor*) or random involuntary movements;
- delays in reaching motor skill milestones; and
- difficulty with precise movements such as writing or buttoning a shirt.

The symptoms of CP differ in type and severity from one person to the next, and may even change in an individual over time. Symptoms may vary greatly among individuals, depending on which parts of the brain have been injured. All people with cerebral palsy have problems with movement and posture, and some also have some level of intellectual disability, seizures, and abnormal physical sensations or perceptions, as well as other medical disorders. People with CP also may have impaired vision or hearing, and language, and speech problems.

CP is the leading cause of childhood disabilities, but it doesn't always cause profound disabilities. While one child with severe CP might be unable to walk and need extensive, lifelong care, another child with mild CP might be only slightly awkward and require no special assistance. The disorder isn't progressive, meaning it doesn't get worse over time. However, as the child gets older, certain symptoms may become more or less evident.

A study by the Centers for Disease Control and Prevention shows the average prevalence of cerebral palsy is 3.3 children per 1,000 live births.

There is no cure for cerebral palsy, but supportive treatments, medications, and surgery can help many individuals improve their motor skills and ability to communicate with the world.

What are the early signs?

The signs of cerebral palsy usually appear in the early months of life, although specific diagnosis may be delayed until age two years or later. Infants with CP frequently have *developmental delay*, in which they are slow to reach developmental milestones such as learning to roll over, sit, crawl, or walk. Some infants with CP have abnormal muscle tone. Decreased muscle tone (*hypotonia*) can make them appear relaxed, even floppy. Increased muscle tone (*hypertonia*) can make them seem stiff or rigid. In some cases, an early period of hypotonia will progress to hypertonia after the first 2 to 3 months of life. Children with CP may also have unusual posture or favor one side of the body when they reach, crawl, or move. It is important to note that some children *without* CP also might have some of these signs.

Some early warning signs:

In a Baby Younger Than 6 Months of Age

- His head lags when you pick him up while he's lying on his back
- He feels stiff
- He feels floppy
- When you pick him up, his legs get stiff and they cross or scissor

In a Baby Older Than 6 Months of Age

- She doesn't roll over in either direction
- She cannot bring her hands together
- She has difficulty bringing her hands to her mouth
- She reaches out with only one hand while keeping the other fisted

In a Baby Older Than 10 Months of Age

- He crawls in a lopsided manner, pushing off with one hand and leg while dragging the opposite hand and leg
- He cannot stand holding onto support

What causes cerebral palsy?

Cerebral palsy is caused by abnormal development of part of the brain or by damage to parts of the brain that control movement. This damage can occur before, during, or shortly after birth. The majority of children have *congenital cerebral palsy* CP (that is, they were born with it), although it may not be detected until months or years later. A small number of children have *acquired cerebral palsy*, which means the disorder begins after birth. Some causes of acquired cerebral palsy include brain damage in the first few months or years of life, brain infections such as bacterial meningitis or viral encephalitis, problems with blood flow to the brain, or head injury from a motor vehicle accident, a fall, or child abuse.

In many cases, the cause of cerebral palsy is unknown. Possible causes include genetic abnormalities, congenital brain malformations, maternal infections or fevers, or fetal injury, for example. The following types of brain damage may cause its characteristic symptoms:

Damage to the white matter of the brain (*periventricular leukomalacia, or PVL*). The white matter of the brain is responsible for transmitting signals inside the brain and to the rest of the body. Damage from PVL looks like tiny holes in the white matter of an infant's brain. These gaps in brain tissue interfere with the normal transmission of signals. Researchers have identified a period of selective vulnerability in the developing fetal brain, a period of time between 26 and 34 weeks of *gestation*, in which periventricular white matter is particularly sensitive to insults and injury.

Abnormal development of the brain (*cerebral dysgenesis*). Any interruption of the normal process of brain growth during fetal development can cause brain malformations that interfere with the transmission of brain signals. Mutations in the genes that control brain development during this early period can keep the brain from developing normally. Infections, fevers, trauma, or other conditions that cause unhealthy conditions in the womb also put an unborn baby's nervous system at risk.

Bleeding in the brain (*intracranial hemorrhage*). Bleeding inside the brain from blocked or broken blood vessels is commonly caused by fetal stroke. Some babies suffer a stroke while still in the womb because of blood clots in the *placenta* that block blood flow in the brain. Other types of fetal stroke are caused by malformed or weak blood vessels in the brain or by blood-clotting abnormalities. Maternal high blood pressure (hypertension) is a common medical disorder during pregnancy and is more common in babies with fetal stroke. Maternal infection, especially pelvic inflammatory disease, has also been shown to increase the risk of fetal stroke.

Severe lack of oxygen in the brain. *Asphyxia*, a lack of oxygen in the brain caused by an interruption in breathing or poor oxygen supply, is common for a brief period of time in babies due to the stress of labor and delivery. If the supply of oxygen is cut off or reduced for lengthy periods, an infant can develop a type of brain damage called *hypoxic-ischemic encephalopathy*, which destroys tissue in the cerebral motor cortex and other areas of the brain. This kind of damage can also be caused by severe maternal low blood pressure, rupture of the uterus, detachment of the placenta, or problems involving the umbilical cord, or severe trauma to the head during labor and delivery.

What are the risk factors?

There are some medical conditions or events that can happen during pregnancy and delivery that may increase a baby's risk of being born with cerebral palsy. These risks include:

Low birth weight and premature birth. Premature babies (born less than 37 weeks into pregnancy) and babies weighing less than 5½ pounds at birth have a much higher risk of developing cerebral palsy than full-term, heavier weight babies. Tiny babies born at very early gestational ages are especially at risk.

Multiple births. Twins, triplets, and other multiple births -- even those born at term—are linked to an increased risk of cerebral palsy. The death of a baby's twin or triplet further increases the risk.

Infections during pregnancy. Infections such as toxoplasmosis, rubella (German measles), cytomegalovirus, and herpes, can infect the womb and placenta. Inflammation triggered by infection may then go on to damage the developing nervous system in an unborn baby. Maternal fever during pregnancy or delivery can also set off this kind of inflammatory response.

Blood type incompatibility between mother and child. *Rh incompatibility* is a condition that develops when a mother's Rh blood type (either positive or negative) is different from the blood type of her baby. The mother's system doesn't tolerate the baby's different blood type and her body will begin to make antibodies that will attack and kill her baby's blood cells, which can cause brain damage.

Exposure to toxic substances. Mothers who have been exposed to toxic substances during pregnancy, such as methyl mercury, are at a heightened risk of having a baby with cerebral palsy.

Mothers with thyroid abnormalities, intellectual disability, excess protein in the urine, or seizures. Mothers with any of these conditions are slightly more likely to have a child with CP.

There are also medical conditions during labor and delivery, and immediately after delivery that act as warning signs for an increased risk of CP. However, most of these children will not develop CP. Warning signs include:

Breech presentation. Babies with cerebral palsy are more likely to be in a breech position (feet first) instead of head first at the beginning of labor. Babies who are unusually floppy as fetuses are more likely to be born in the breech position.

Complicated labor and delivery. A baby who has vascular or respiratory problems during labor and delivery may already have suffered brain damage or abnormalities.

Small for gestational age. Babies born smaller than normal for their gestational age are at risk for cerebral palsy because of factors that kept them from growing naturally in the womb.

Low Apgar score. The Apgar score is a numbered rating that reflects a newborn's physical health. Doctors periodically score a baby's heart rate, breathing, muscle tone, reflexes, and skin color during the first minutes after birth. A low score at 10-20 minutes after delivery is often considered an important sign of potential problems such as CP.

Jaundice. More than 50 percent of newborns develop jaundice (a yellowing of the skin or whites of the eyes) after birth when *bilirubin*, a substance normally found in bile, builds up faster than their livers can break it down and pass it from the body. Severe, untreated jaundice can kill brain cells and can cause deafness and CP.

Seizures. An infant who has seizures faces a higher risk of being diagnosed later in childhood with CP.

Can cerebral palsy be prevented?

Cerebral palsy related to genetic abnormalities cannot be prevented, but a few of the risk factors for congenital cerebral palsy can be managed or avoided. For example, *rubella*, or German measles, is preventable if women are vaccinated against the disease before becoming pregnant. Rh incompatibilities can also be managed early in pregnancy. Acquired cerebral palsy, often due to head injury, is often preventable using common safety tactics, such as using car seats for infants and toddlers.

What are the different forms?

The specific forms of cerebral palsy are determined by the extent, type, and location of a child's abnormalities. Doctors classify CP according to the type of movement disorder involved—*spastic* (stiff muscles), *athetoid* (writhing movements), or *ataxic* (poor balance and coordination)—plus any additional symptoms, such weakness (*paresis*) or paralysis (*plegia*). For example, *hemiparesis* (*hemi* = half) indicates that only one side of the body is weakened. *Quadriplegia* (*quad* = four) means all four limbs are afffected.

Spastic **cerebral palsy** is the most common type of the disorder. People have stiff muscles and awkward movements. Forms of spastic cerebral palsy include:

- *Spastic hemiplegia / hemiparesis* typically affects the arm and hand on one side of the body, but it can also include the leg. Children with spastic hemiplegia generally walk later and on tip-toe because of tight heel tendons. The arm and leg of the affected side are frequently shorter and thinner. Some children will develop an abnormal curvature of the spine (*scoliosis*). A child with spastic hemiplegia may also have seizures. Speech will be delayed and, at best, may be competent, but intelligence is usually normal.

- *Spastic diplegia / diparesis* involves muscle stiffness that is predominantly in the legs and less severely affects the arms and face, although the hands may be clumsy. Tendon reflexes in the legs are hyperactive. Toes point up when the bottom of the foot is stimulated. Tightness in certain leg muscles makes the legs move like the arms of a scissor. Children may require a walker or leg braces. Intelligence and language skills are usually normal.

- *Spastic quadriplegia / quadriparesis* is the most severe form of cerebral palsy and is often associated with moderate-to-severe intellectual disability. It is caused by widespread damage to the brain or significant brain malformations. Children will often have severe stiffness in their limbs but a floppy neck. They are rarely able to walk. Speaking and being understood are difficult. Seizures can be frequent and hard to control.

Dyskinetic **cerebral palsy (also includes athetoid, choreoathetoid, and dystonic cerebral palsies)** is characterized by slow and uncontrollable writhing or jerky movements of the hands, feet, arms, or legs. Hyperactivity in the muscles of the face and tongue makes some children grimace or drool. They find it difficult to sit straight or walk. Some children have problems hearing, controlling their breathing, and/or coordinating the muscle movements required for speaking. Intelligence is rarely affected in these forms of cerebral palsy.

Ataxic **cerebral palsy** affects balance and depth perception. Children with ataxic CP will often have poor coordination and walk unsteadily with a wide-based gait. They have difficulty with quick or precise movements, such as writing or buttoning a shirt, or a hard time controlling voluntary movement such as reaching for a book.

Mixed types of cerebral palsy refer to symptoms that don't correspond to any single type of CP but are a mix of types. For example, a child with mixed CP may have some muscles that are too tight and others that are too relaxed, creating a mix of stiffness and floppiness.

What other conditions are associated with cerebral palsy?

Intellectual disability. Approximately 30–50 percent of individuals with CP will be intellectually impaired. Mental impairment is more common among those with spastic quadriplegia than in those with other types of cerebral palsy.

Seizure disorder. As many as half of all children with CP have one or more seizures. Children with both cerebral palsy and epilepsy are more likely to have intellectual disability.

Delayed growth and development. Children with moderate to severe CP, especially those with spastic quadriparesis, often lag behind in growth and development. In babies this lag usually takes the form of too little weight gain. In young children it can appear as abnormal shortness, and in teenagers it may appear as a combination of shortness and lack of sexual development. The muscles and limbs affected by CP tend to be smaller than normal, especially in children with spastic hemiplegia, whose limbs on the affected side of the body may not grow as quickly or as long as those on the normal side.

Spinal deformities and osteoarthritis. Deformities of the spine—curvature (*scoliosis*), humpback (*kyphosis*), and saddle back (*lordosis*)—are associated with CP. Spinal deformities can make sitting, standing, and walking difficult and cause chronic back pain. Pressure on and misalignment of the joints may result in osteoporosis (a breakdown of cartilage in the joints and bone enlargement).

Impaired vision. Many children with CP have strabismus, commonly called "cross eyes," which left untreated can lead to poor vision in one eye and can interfere with the ability to judge distance. Some children with CP have difficulty understanding and organizing visual information. Other children may have defective vision or blindness that blurs the normal field of vision in one or both eyes.

Hearing loss. Impaired hearing is also more frequent among those with CP than in the general population. Some children have partial or complete hearing loss, particularly as the result of jaundice or lack of oxygen to the developing brain.

Speech and language disorders. Speech and language disorders, such as difficulty forming words and speaking clearly, are present in more than a third of persons with CP. Poor speech impairs communication and is often interpreted as a sign of cognitive impairment, which can be very frustrating to children with CP, especially the majority who have average to above average intelligence.

Drooling. Some individuals with CP drool because they have poor control of the muscles of the throat, mouth, and tongue.

Incontinence. A possible complication of CP is incontinence, caused by poor control of the muscles that keep the bladder closed.

Abnormal sensations and perceptions. Some individuals with CP experience pain or have difficulty feeling simple sensations, such as touch.

Learning difficulties. Children with CP may have difficulty processing particular types of spatial and auditory information. Brain damage may affect the development of language and intellectual functioning.

Infections and long-term illnesses. Many adults with CP have a higher risk of heart and lung disease, and pneumonia (often from inhaling bits of food into the lungs), than those without the disorder.

Contractures. Muscles can become painfully fixed into abnormal positions, called contractures, which can increase muscle spasticity and joint deformities in people with CP.

Malnutrition. Swallowing, sucking, or feeding difficulties can make it difficult for many individuals with CP, particularly infants, to get proper nutrition and gain or maintain weight.

Dental problems. Many children with CP are at risk of developing gum disease and cavities because of poor dental hygiene. Certain medications, such as seizure drugs, can exacerbate these problems.

Inactivity. Childhood inactivity is magnified in children with CP due to impairment of the motor centers of the brain that produce and control voluntary movement. While children with CP may exhibit increased energy expenditure during activities of daily living, movement impairments make it difficult for them to participate in sports and other activities at a level of intensity sufficient to develop and maintain strength and fitness. Inactive adults with disability exhibit increased severity of disease and reduced overall health and well-being.

How is cerebral palsy diagnosed?

Most children with cerebral palsy are diagnosed during the first 2 years of life. But if a child's symptoms are mild, it can be difficult for a doctor to make a reliable diagnosis before the age of 4 or 5.

Doctors will order a series of tests to evaluate the child's motor skills. During regular visits, the doctor will monitor the child's development, growth, muscle tone, age-appropriate motor control, hearing and vision, posture, and coordination, in order to rule out other disorders that could cause similar symptoms. Although symptoms may change over time, CP is not progressive. If a child is continuously losing motor skills, the problem more likely is a condition other than CP—such as a genetic or muscle disease, metabolism disorder, or tumors in the nervous system.

Lab tests can identify other conditions that may cause symptoms similar to those associated with CP.

Neuroimaging techniques that allow doctors to look into the brain (such as an MRI scan) can detect abnormalities that indicate a potentially treatable movement disorder. Neuroimaging methods include:

- **Cranial ultrasound** uses high-frequency sound waves to produce pictures of the brains of young babies. It is used for high-risk premature infants because it is the least intrusive of the imaging techniques, although it is not as successful as computed tomography or magnetic resonance imaging at capturing subtle changes in white matter—the type of brain tissue that is damaged in CP.

- **Computed tomography (CT)** uses x-rays to create images that show the structure of the brain and the areas of damage.

- **Magnetic resonance imaging (MRI)** uses a computer, a magnetic field, and radio waves to create an anatomical picture of the brain's tissues and structures. MRI can show the location and type of damage and offers finer levels of details than CT.

Another test, an **electroencephalogram**, uses a series of electrodes that are either taped or temporarily pasted to the scalp to detect electrical activity in the brain. Changes in the normal electrical pattern may help to identify epilepsy.

Some metabolic disorders can masquerade as CP. Most of the childhood metabolic disorders have characteristic brain abnormalities or malformations that will show up on an MRI.

Other types of disorders can also be mistaken for CP or can cause specific types of CP. For example, coagulation disorders (which prevent blood from clotting or lead to excessive clotting) can cause prenatal or perinatal strokes that damage the brain and produce symptoms characteristic of CP, most commonly hemiparetic CP. Referrals to specialists such as a child neurologist, developmental pediatrician, ophthalmologist, or otologist aid in a more accurate diagnosis and help doctors develop a specific treatment plan.

How is cerebral palsy treated?

Cerebral palsy can't be cured, but treatment will often improve a child's capabilities. Many children go on to enjoy near-normal adult lives if their disabilities are properly managed. In general, the earlier treatment begins, the better chance children have of overcoming developmental disabilities or learning new ways to accomplish the tasks that challenge them.

There is no standard therapy that works for every individual with cerebral palsy. Once the diagnosis is made, and the type of CP is determined, a team of health care professionals will work with a child and his or her parents to identify specific impairments and needs, and then develop an appropriate plan to tackle the core disabilities that affect the child's quality of life.

Physical therapy, usually begun in the first few years of life or soon after the diagnosis is made, is a cornerstone of CP treatment. Specific sets of exercises (such as resistive, or strength training programs) and activities can maintain or improve muscle strength, balance, and motor skills, and prevent contractures. Special braces (called orthotic devices) may be used to improve mobility and stretch spastic muscles.

Occupational therapy focuses on optimizing upper body function, improving posture, and making the most of a child's mobility. Occupational therapists help individuals address new ways to meet everyday activities such as dressing, going to school, and participating in day-to-day activities.

Recreation therapy encourages participation in art and cultural programs, sports, and other events that help an individual expand physical and cognitive skills and abilities. Parents of children who participate in recreational therapies usually notice an improvement in their child's speech, self-esteem, and emotional well-being.

Speech and language therapy can improve a child's ability to speak, more clearly, help with swallowing disorders, and learn new ways to communicate—using sign language and/or special communication devices such as a computer with a voice synthesizer, or a special board covered with symbols of everyday objects and activities to which a child can point to indicate his or her wishes.

Treatments for problems with eating and drooling are often necessary when children with CP have difficulty eating and drinking because they have little control over the muscles that move their mouth, jaw, and tongue. They are also at risk for breathing food or fluid into the lungs, as well as for malnutrition, recurrent lung infections, and progressive lung disease.

Drug Treatments

Oral medications such as diazepam, baclofen, dantrolene sodium, and tizanidine are usually used as the first line of treatment to relax stiff, contracted, or overactive muscles. Some drugs have some risk side effects such as drowsiness, changes in blood pressure, and risk of liver damage that require continuous monitoring. Oral medications are most appropriate for children who need only mild reduction in muscle tone or who have widespread spasticity.

- *Botulinum toxin (BT-A)*, injected locally, has become a standard treatment for overactive muscles in children with spastic movement disorders such as CP. BT-A relaxes contracted muscles by keeping nerve cells from over-activating muscle. The relaxing effect of a BT-A injection lasts approximately 3 months. Undesirable side effects are mild and short-lived, consisting of pain upon injection and occasionally mild flu-like symptoms. BT-A injections are most effective when followed by a stretching program including physical therapy and splinting. BT-A injections work best for children who have some control over their motor movements and have a limited number of muscles to treat, none of which is fixed or rigid.

212

- *Intrathecal baclofen* therapy uses an implantable pump to deliver baclofen, a muscle relaxant, into the fluid surrounding the spinal cord. Baclofen decreases the excitability of nerve cells in the spinal cord, which then reduces muscle spasticity throughout the body. The pump can be adjusted if muscle tone is worse at certain times of the day or night. The baclofen pump is most appropriate for individuals with chronic, severe stiffness or uncontrolled muscle movement throughout the body

Surgery **Orthopedic surgery** is often recommended when spasticity and stiffness are severe enough to make walking and moving about difficult or painful. For many people with CP, improving the appearance of how they walk—their gait—is also important. Surgeons can lengthen muscles and tendons that are proportionately too short, which can improve mobility and lessen pain. Tendon surgery may help the symptoms for some children with CP but could also have negative long-term consequences. Orthopedic surgeries may be staggered at times appropriate to a child's age and level of motor development. Surgery can also correct or greatly improve spinal deformities in people with CP. Surgery may not be indicated for all gait abnormalities and the surgeon may request a quantitative gait analysis before surgery.

Surgery to cut nerves. *Selective dorsal rhizotomy* (SDR) is a surgical procedure recommended for cases of severe spasticity when all of the more conservative treatments—physical therapy, oral medications, and intrathecal baclofen—have failed to reduce spasticity or chronic pain. A surgeon locates and selectively severs overactivated nerves at the base of the spinal column. SDR is most commonly used to relax muscles and decrease chronic pain in one or both of the lower or upper limbs. It is also sometimes used to correct an overactive bladder. Potential side effects include sensory loss, numbness, or uncomfortable sensations in limb areas once supplied by the severed nerve.

Assistive Devices

Assistive devices such devices as computers, computer software, voice synthesizers, and picture books can greatly help some individuals with CP improve communications skills. Other devices around the home or workplace make it easier for people with CP to adapt to activities of daily living.

Orthotic devices help to compensate for muscle imbalance and increase independent mobility. Braces and splints use external force to correct muscle abnormalities and improve function such as sitting or walking. Other orthotics help stretch muscles or the positioning of a joint. Braces, wedges, special chairs, and other devices can help people sit more comfortably and make it easier to perform daily functions. Wheelchairs, rolling walkers, and powered scooters can help individuals who are not independently mobile. Vision aids include glasses, magnifiers, and large-print books and computer typeface. Some individuals with CP may need surgery to correct vision problems. Hearing aids and telephone amplifiers may help people hear more clearly.

Complementary and Alternative Therapies

Many children and adolescents with CP use some form of complementary or alternative medicine. Controlled clinical trials involving some of the therapies have been inconclusive or showed no benefit and the therapies have not been accepted in mainstream clinical practice. Although there are anecdotal reports of some benefit in some children with CP, these therapies have not been approved by the U.S. Food and Drug Administration for the treatment of CP. Such therapies include hyperbaric oxygen therapy, special clothing worn during resistance exercise training, certain forms of electrical stimulation, assisting children in completing certain motions several times a day, and specialized learning strategies. Also, dietary supplements, including herbal products, may interact with other products or medications a child with CP may be taking or have unwanted side effects on their own. Families of children with CP should discuss all therapies with their doctor.

Stem cell therapy is being investigated as a treatment for cerebral palsy, but research is in early stages and large-scale clinical trials are needed to learn if stem cell therapy is safe and effective in humans. Stem cells are capable of becoming other cell types in the body. Scientists are hopeful that stem cells may be able to repair damaged nerves and brain tissues. Studies in the U.S. are examining the safety and tolerability of umbilical cord blood stem cell infusion in children with CP.

Are there treatments for other conditions associated with cerebral palsy?

Epilepsy. Many children with intellectual disability and CP also have epilepsy. In general, drugs are prescribed based on the type of seizures an individual experiences, since no one drug controls all types. Some individuals may need a combination of two or more drugs to achieve good seizure control.

214

Incontinence. Medical treatments for incontinence include special exercises, biofeedback, prescription drugs, surgery, or surgically implanted devices to replace or aid muscles.

Osteopenia. Children with CP who are unable to walk risk developing poor bone density (*osteopenia*), which makes them more likely to break bones. In a study of older Americans funded by the National Institutes of Health (NIH), a family of drugs called *bisphosphonates*, which has been approved by the FDA to treat mineral loss in elderly patients, also appeared to increase bone mineral density Doctors may choose to selectively prescribe the drug off-label to children to prevent osteopenia.

Pain. Pain can be a problem for people with CP due to spastic muscles and the stress and strain on parts of the body that are compensating for muscle abnormalities. Some individuals may also have frequent and irregular muscle spasms that can't be predicted or medicated in advance. Diazepam can reduce the pain associated with muscle spasms and gabapentin has been used successfully to decrease the severity and frequency of painful spasms. Botulinum toxin injections have also been shown to decrease spasticity and pain. Intrathecal baclofen has shown good results in reducing pain. Some children and adults have been able to decrease pain by using noninvasive and drug-free interventions such as distraction, relaxation training, biofeedback, and therapeutic massage.

Do adults with cerebral palsy face special health challenges?

Premature aging. The majority of individuals with CP will experience some form of premature aging by the time they reach their 40s because of the extra stress and strain the disease puts upon their bodies. The developmental delays that often accompany CP keep some organ systems from developing to their full capacity and level of performance. As a consequence, organ systems such as the cardiovascular system (the heart, veins, and arteries) and pulmonary system (lungs) have to work harder and they age prematurely.

Functional issues at work. The day-to-day challenges of the workplace are likely to increase as an employed individual with CP reaches middle age. Some individuals will be able to continue working with accommodations such as an adjusted work schedule, assistive equipment, or frequent rest periods.

Depression. Mental health issues can also be of concern as someone with cerebral palsy grows older. The rate of depression is three to four times higher in people with disabilities such as cerebral palsy. It appears to be related not so much to the severity of their disabilities, but to how well they cope with them. The amount of emotional support someone has, how successful they are at coping with disappointment and stress, and whether or not they have an optimistic outlook about the future all have a significant impact on mental health.

Post-impairment syndrome. This syndrome is marked by a combination of pain, fatigue, and weakness due to muscle abnormalities, bone deformities, *overuse syndromes* (sometimes also called repetitive motion injuries), and arthritis. Fatigue is often a challenge, since individuals with CP may use up to three to five times the amount of energy that able-bodied people use when they walk and move about.

Osteoarthritis and degenerative arthritis. Musculoskeletal abnormalities that may not produce discomfort during childhood can cause pain in adulthood. For example, the abnormal relationships between joint surfaces and excessive joint compression can lead to the early development of painful osteoarthritis and degenerative arthritis. Individuals with CP also may have limited strength and restricted patterns of movement, which puts them at risk for overuse syndromes and *nerve entrapments.*

Pain. Individuals with CP may have pain that can be acute (usually comes on quickly and lasts a short while) or chronic, and is experienced most commonly in the hips, knees, ankles, and the upper and lower back. Individuals with spastic CP may have an increased number of painful sites and worse pain than those with other types of cerebral palsy. Preventive treatment aimed at correcting skeletal and muscle abnormalities early in life may help to avoid the progressive accumulation of stress and strain that causes pain. Dislocated hips, which are particularly likely to cause pain, can be surgically repaired.

Other medical conditions. Adults have higher than normal rates of other medical conditions secondary to their cerebral palsy, such as hypertension, incontinence, bladder dysfunction, and swallowing difficulties. Scoliosis is likely to progress after puberty, when bones have matured into their final shape and size. People with CP also have a higher incidence of bone fractures, occurring most frequently during physical therapy sessions.

What research is being done?

The National Institute of Neurological Disorders and Stroke, (NINDS), a part of the National Institutes of Health (NIH), is the nation's leading funder of basic, clinical, and translational research on brain and nervous system disorders. Another NIH agency, the *Eunice Kennedy Shriver* National Institute of Child Health and Human Development (NICHD), also conducts and supports research on cerebral palsy.

Much of what we now know about CP came from research sponsored by the NINDS, including the identification of new causes and risk factors for cerebral palsy, the discovery of drugs to control stiff and spastic muscles and more precise methods to deliver them, refined surgical techniques to correct abnormalities in muscle and bone, and a greater understanding of how and why brain damage at critical stages of fetal development causes CP.

Many scientists think that a significant number of children develop CP because of mishaps early in **brain development**. They are examining how neurons (nerve cells) in the brain specialize and form the right connections with other brain cells, and they are looking for ways to prevent the factors that disrupt the normal processes of brain development.

Genetic defects are sometimes responsible for the brain malformations and abnormalities that cause cerebral palsy. Scientists are searching for the genes responsible for these abnormalities by collecting DNA samples from people with cerebral palsy and their families and using genetic screening techniques to discover linkages between individual genes and specific types of abnormality – primarily those associated with the process in the developing brain in which neurons migrate from where they are born to where they settle into neural circuits (called neural migration).

Scientists are scrutinizing events in newborn babies' brains, such as bleeding, epileptic seizures, and breathing and circulation problems, which can cause the **abnormal release of chemicals** that triggers the kind of damage that causes cerebral palsy. For example, research has shown that bleeding in the brain unleashes dangerously high amounts of glutamate, a chemical that helps neurons communicate. However, too much glutamate overexcites and kills neurons. By learning how brain chemicals that are normally helpful become dangerously toxic, scientists will have opportunities to develop new drugs to block their harmful effects.

Researchers are using **imaging techniques** and neurobehavioral tests to predict those preterm infants who will develop cerebral palsy. If these screening techniques are successful, doctors will be able to identify infants at risk for cerebral palsy before they are born.

Periventricular **white matter damage**—the most common cause of CP—is characterized by death of the white matter around the fluid-filled ventricles in the brain. The periventricular area contains nerve fibers that carry messages from the brain to the body's muscles. NINDS-sponsored researchers are hoping to develop preventative strategies for white matter damage. For example, researchers are examining the role the brain chemicals play on white matter development in the brain. Another NINDS-funded project involves the development of a novel mouse model and cell-based therapies for perinatal white matter injury. Researchers funded by NINDS are studying a chemical found naturally in the body, called erythropoietin to see if it decreases the risk of CP in prematurely born infants.

NIH-funded scientists continue to look at new therapies and novel ways to use existing options to treat individuals with CP, including:

Constraint-induced therapy (CIT) is a promising therapy for CP. CIT typically involves restraining the stronger limb (such as the "good" arm in a person who has been affected by a stroke on one side of the body) in a cast and forcing the weaker arm to perform intensive activities every day over a period of weeks. A clinical study sponsored by the NICHD is examining the use of different dosage levels of daily training using either full-time cast immobilization vs. part-time splint restraint in improving upper body extremity skills in children with weakness on both sides of their body. Study findings will establish evidence-based practice standards to improve lifelong neuromotor capacity in individuals with CP.

Functional electrical stimulation (FES)—the therapeutic use of low-level electrical current to stimulate muscle movement and restore useful movements such as standing or stepping—is an effective way to target and strengthen spastic muscles. Researchers are evaluating how FES-assisted stationary cycling can improve physical conditioning and general lower extremity muscle strength in adolescents. *Robotic therapy* that applies controlled force to the leg during the swing phase of gait is may improve the efficacy of body weight supported treadmill training in children with CP. The results from this NICHD study will lead to an innovative clinical therapy aimed at improving locomotor function in children with CP.

Botulinum toxin (Botox), injected locally, has become a standard treatment in children with spastic movement disorders such as CP. Recent animal studies suggest Botox degrades bone but there are no studies of its skeletal consequences in humans. Other research shows a low intensity vibration treatment can improve bone structure in the lower extremity leg bones of children with CP. In a novel clinical study being conducted by NICHD, researchers are determining the effect of Botox treatment in conjunction with a daily vibration treatment on bone mass and bone structure in children with spastic CP.

Systemic hypothermia—the controlled medical cooling of the body's core temperature—appears to protect the brain and decrease the rate of death and disability from certain disorders and brain injuries. Previous studies have shown that hypothermia is effective in treating neurologic symptoms in term or late preterm babies less than one month old that are attributed to hypoxic-ischemia (HIE, brain injury due to a severe decrease in the oxygen supply to the body), which can cause quadriplegic CP, with or without movement disorder. In an effort to determine the most effective cooling strategies, NICHD-funded researchers are studying different cooling treatments to improve the chance of survival and neurodevelopment outcomes 18-22 months post-treatment in infants with neurologic symptoms attributed to HIE. Other researchers are examining if combined therapy using hypothermia and recombinant erythropoietin (a hormone that promotes the growth of new red blood cells and increases oxygen levels in the blood) is more effective than either therapy alone in treating neurodevelopmental handicaps in an animal model involving lack of oxygen before, during, or just after birth.

As researchers continue to explore new treatments for cerebral palsy and to expand our knowledge of brain development, we can expect significant improvements in the care of children with cerebral palsy and many other disorders that strike in early life.

Chapter 11

Friedreich's Ataxia

What is Friedreich's ataxia?

Friedreich's ataxia (also called FA or FRDA) is a rare inherited disease that causes nervous system damage and movement problems. It usually begins in childhood and leads to impaired muscle coordination (ataxia) that worsens over time. The disorder is named after Nicholaus Friedreich, a German doctor who first described the condition in the 1860s.

In Friedreich's ataxia the spinal cord and peripheral nerves degenerate, becoming thinner. The cerebellum, part of the brain that coordinates balance and movement, also degenerates to a lesser extent. This damage results in awkward, unsteady movements and impaired sensory functions. The disorder also causes problems in the heart and spine, and some people with the condition develop diabetes. The disorder does not affect thinking and reasoning abilities (cognitive functions).

Friedreich's ataxia is caused by a defect (mutation) in a gene labeled FXN. The disorder is recessive, meaning it occurs only in someone who inherits two defective copies of the gene, one from each parent. Although rare, Friedreich's ataxia is the most common form of hereditary ataxia, affecting about 1 in every 50,000 people in the United States. Both male and female children can inherit the disorder.

Text in this chapter is excerpted from "Friedreich's Ataxia Fact Sheet," National Institute of Neurological Disorders and Stroke (NINDS), April 6, 2014.

What are the signs and symptoms?

Symptoms typically begin between the ages of 5 and 15 years, although they sometimes appear in adulthood and on rare occasions as late as age 75. The first symptom to appear is usually gait ataxia, or difficulty walking. The ataxia gradually worsens and slowly spreads to the arms and the trunk. There is often loss of sensation in the extremities, which may spread to other parts of the body. Other features include loss of tendon reflexes, especially in the knees and ankles. Most people with Friedreich's ataxia develop scoliosis (a curving of the spine to one side), which often requires surgical intervention for treatment.

Dysarthria (slowness and slurring of speech) develops and can get progressively worse. Many individuals with later stages of Friedreich's ataxia develop hearing and vision loss.

Other symptoms that may occur include chest pain, shortness of breath, and heart palpitations. These symptoms are the result of various forms of heart disease that often accompany Friedreich's ataxia, such as hypertrophic cardiomyopathy (enlargement of the heart), myocardial fibrosis (formation of fiber-like material in the muscles of the heart), and cardiac failure. Heart rhythm abnormalities such as tachycardia (fast heart rate) and heart block (impaired conduction of cardiac impulses within the heart) are also common.

About 20 percent of people with Friedreich's ataxia develop carbohydrate intolerance and 10 percent develop diabetes. Most individuals with Friedreich's ataxia tire very easily and find that they require more rest and take a longer time to recover from common illnesses such as colds and flu.

The rate of progression varies from person to person. Generally, within 10 to 20 years after the appearance of the first symptoms, the person is confined to a wheelchair, and in later stages of the disease individuals may become completely incapacitated.

Friedreich's ataxia can shorten life expectancy, and heart disease is the most common cause of death. However, some people with less severe features of Friedreich's ataxia live into their sixties, seventies, or older.

How is Friedreich's ataxia diagnosed?

A diagnosis of Friedreich's ataxia requires a careful clinical examination, which includes a medical history and a thorough physical exam, in particular looking for balance difficulty, loss of proprioception (joint sensation), absence of reflexes, and signs of neurological problems. Genetic testing now provides a conclusive diagnosis.

Other tests that may aid in the diagnosis or management of the disorder include:

- electromyogram (EMG), which measures the electrical activity of muscle cells,

- nerve conduction studies, which measure the speed with which nerves transmit impulses,

- electrocardiogram (ECG), which gives a graphic presentation of the electrical activity or beat pattern of the heart,

- echocardiogram, which records the position and motion of the heart muscle,

- blood tests to check for elevated glucose levels and vitamin E levels, and

- magnetic resonance imaging (MRI) or computed tomography (CT) scans, tests which provide brain and spinal cord images that are useful for ruling out other neurological conditions.

How is Friedreich's ataxia inherited?

Friedreich's ataxia is an autosomal recessive disease, meaning individuals only develop symptoms if they inherit two copies of the defective FXN gene, one from their father and one from their mother. A person who has only one abnormal copy of the gene is called a carrier. A carrier will not develop the disease but could pass the gene mutation on to his or her children. If both parents are carriers, their children will have a 1 in 4 chance of having the disease and a 1 in 2 chance of inheriting one abnormal gene that they, in turn, could pass on to their children. About one in 90 Americans of European ancestry carries an abnormal FXN gene.

In 1996, an international research team identified the Friedreich's ataxia gene on chromosome 9. The FXN gene codes for production of a protein called "frataxin." In the normal version of the gene, a sequence of DNA (labeled "GAA") is repeated between 7 and 22 times. In the defective FXN gene, the repeat occurs over and over again—hundreds, even up to a thousand times.

This abnormal pattern, called a triplet repeat expansion, has been implicated as the cause of several dominantly inherited diseases, but Friedreich's ataxia is the only known recessive genetic disorder caused by the problem. Almost all people with Friedreich's ataxia have two copies of this mutant form of FXN, but it is not found in all cases of the disease. About two percent of affected individuals have other defects in the FXN gene that are responsible for causing the disease.

The triplet repeat expansion greatly disrupts the normal production of frataxin. Frataxin is found in the energy-producing parts of the cell called mitochondria. Research suggests that without a normal level of frataxin, certain cells in the body (especially peripheral nerve, spinal cord, brain and heart muscle cells) cannot effectively produce energy and have been hypothesized to have a buildup of toxic byproducts leading to what is called "oxidative stress." It also may lead to increased levels of iron in the mitochondria. When the excess iron reacts with oxygen, free radicals can be produced. Although free radicals are essential molecules in the body's metabolism, they can also destroy cells and harm the body. Research continues on this subject (see section "What research is being done?").

Can Friedreich's ataxia be cured or treated?

As with many degenerative diseases of the nervous system, there is currently no cure or effective treatment for Friedreich's ataxia. However, many of the symptoms and accompanying complications can be treated to help individuals maintain optimal functioning as long as possible. Doctors can prescribe treatments for diabetes, if present; some of the heart problems can be treated with medication as well. Orthopedic problems such as foot deformities and scoliosis can be corrected with braces or surgery. Physical therapy may prolong use of the arms and legs. Advances in understanding the genetics of Friedreich's ataxia are leading to breakthroughs in treatment. Research has moved forward to the point where clinical trials of proposed treatments are presently occurring for Friedreich's ataxia.

What services are useful to Friedreich's ataxia patients and their families?

Genetic testing is essential for proper clinical diagnosis, and can aid in prenatal diagnosis and determining a person's carrier status. Genetic counselors can help explain how Friedreich's ataxia is inherited. Psychological counseling and support groups for people with genetic diseases may also help affected individuals and their families cope with the disease.

A primary care physician can screen people for complications such as heart disease, diabetes and scoliosis, and can refer individuals to specialists such as cardiologists, physical therapists, and speech therapists to help deal with some of the other associated problems.

Support and information for families is also available through a number of private organizations. These groups can offer ways to network and communicate with others affected by Friedreich's ataxia. They can also provide access to patient registries, clinical trials information, and other useful resources.

What research is being done?

Within the Federal government the National Institute of Neurological Disorders and Stroke (NINDS), a component of the National Institutes of Health (NIH), has primary responsibility for sponsoring research on neurological disorders. As part of this mission, the NINDS conducts research on Friedreich's ataxia and other forms of inherited ataxias at its facilities at the NIH and supports additional studies at medical centers throughout the United States. Several nonprofit organizations also provide substantial support research.

Researchers are optimistic that they have begun to understand the causes of the disease, and work has begun to develop effective treatments and prevention strategies for Friedreich's ataxia. Scientists have been able to create various models of the disease in yeast and mice which have facilitated understanding the cause of the disease and are now being used for drug discovery and the development of novel treatments.

Studies have revealed that frataxin is an important mitochondrial protein for proper function of several organs. Yet in people with the disease, the amount of frataxin in affected cells is severely reduced. It is believed that the loss of frataxin makes the nervous system, heart, and pancreas particularly susceptible to damage from free radicals (produced when the excess iron reacts with oxygen). Once certain cells in these tissues are destroyed by free radicals they cannot be replaced. Nerve and muscle cells also have metabolic needs that may make them particularly vulnerable to this damage. Free radicals have been implicated in other degenerative diseases such as Parkinson's and Alzheimer's diseases.

Based upon this information, scientists and physicians have tried to reduce the levels of free radicals, also called oxidants, using treatment with "antioxidants." Initial clinical studies in Europe suggested that antioxidants like coenzyme Q10, vitamin E, and idebenone may offer individuals some limited benefit. However, recent clinical trials in the United States and Europe have not revealed effectiveness of idebenone in people with Friedreich's ataxia, but more powerful modified forms of this agent and other antioxidants are in trials at this time. There is also a clinical trial to examine the efficacy of selectively removing excess iron from the mitochondria.

Scientists also are exploring ways to increase frataxin levels through drug treatments, genetic engineering and protein delivery systems. Several compounds that are directed at increasing levels of frataxin may be brought to clinical trials in the near future.

Armed with what they currently know about frataxin and Friedreich's ataxia, scientists are working to better define fraxatin's role, clarify how defects in iron metabolism may be involved in the disease process, and explore new therapeutic approaches for therapy.

Chapter 12

Batten Disease

What is Batten disease?

Batten disease is a fatal, inherited disorder of the nervous system that typically begins in childhood. Early symptoms of this disorder usually appear between the ages of 5 and 10 years, when parents or physicians may notice a previously normal child has begun to develop vision problems or seizures. In some cases the early signs are subtle, taking the form of personality and behavior changes, slow learning, clumsiness, or stumbling. Over time, affected children suffer mental impairment, worsening seizures, and progressive loss of sight and motor skills. Eventually, children with Batten disease become blind, bedridden, and demented. Batten disease is often fatal by the late teens or twenties.

Batten disease is named after the British pediatrician who first described it in 1903. Also known as Spielmeyer-Vogt-Sjogren-Batten disease, it is the most common form of a group of disorders called the neuronal ceroid lipofuscinoses, or NCLs. Although Batten disease originally referred specifically to the juvenile form of NCL (JNCL), the term Batten disease is increasingly used by pediatricians to describe all forms of NCL.

What are the other forms of NCL?

There are four other main types of NCL, including three forms that begin earlier in childhood and a very rare form that strikes adults.

Text in this chapter is excerpted from "Batten Disease Fact Sheet," National Institute of Neurological Disorders and Stroke (NINDS), February 23, 2015.

The symptoms of these childhood types are similar to those caused by Batten disease, but they become apparent at different ages and progress at different rates.

- Congenital NCL is a very rare and severe form of NCL. Babies have abnormally small heads (microcephaly) and seizures, and die soon after birth.

- Infantile NCL (INCL or Santavuori-Haltia disease) begins between about ages 6 months and 2 years and progresses rapidly. Affected children fail to thrive and have microcephaly. Also typical are short, sharp muscle contractions called myoclonic jerks. These children usually die before age 5, although some have survived in a vegetative state a few years longer.

- Late infantile NCL (LINCL, or Jansky-Bielschowsky disease) begins between ages 2 and 4. The typical early signs are loss of muscle coordination (ataxia) and seizures that do not respond to drugs. This form progresses rapidly and ends in death between ages 8 and 12.

- Adult NCL (also known as Kufs disease, Parry's disease, and ANCL) generally begins before age 40, causes milder symptoms that progress slowly, and does not cause blindness. Although age of death varies among affected individuals, this form does shorten life expectancy.

There are also "variant" forms of late-infantile NCL (vLINCL) that do not precisely conform to classical late-infantile NCL.

How many people have these disorders?

Batten disease and other forms of NCL are relatively rare, occurring in an estimated 2 to 4 of every 100,000 live births in the United States. These disorders appear to be more common in Finland, Sweden, other parts of northern Europe, and Newfoundland, Canada. Although NCLs are classified as rare diseases, they often strike more than one person in families that carry the defective genes.

How are NCLs inherited?

Childhood NCLs are autosomal recessive disorders; that is, they occur only when a child inherits two copies of the defective gene, one from each parent. When both parents carry one defective gene, each of their children faces a one in four chance of developing NCL. At the same time, each child also faces a one in two chance of inheriting just one copy of the defective gene. Individuals who have only one defective gene are known as carriers, meaning they do not develop the disease, but they can pass the gene on to their own children. Because the mutated genes that are involved in certain forms of Batten disease are known, carrier detection is possible in some instances.

Adult NCL may be inherited as an autosomal recessive or, less often, as an autosomal dominant disorder. In autosomal dominant inheritance, all people who inherit a single copy of the disease gene develop the disease. As a result, there are no unaffected carriers of the gene.

What causes these diseases?

Symptoms of Batten disease and other NCLs are linked to a buildup of substances called lipofuscins (lipopigments) in the body's tissues. These lipopigments are made up of fats and proteins. Their name comes from the technical word *lipo*, which is short for "lipid" or fat, and from the term *pigment*, used because they take on a greenish-yellow color when viewed under an ultraviolet light microscope. The lipopigments build up in cells of the brain and the eye as well as in skin, muscle, and many other tissues. The substances are found inside a part of cells called lysosomes. Lysosomes are responsible for getting rid of things that become damaged or are no longer needed and must be cleared from inside the cell. The accumulated lipopigments in Batten disease and the other NCLs form distinctive shapes that can be seen under an electron microscope. Some look like half-moons, others like fingerprints. These deposits are what doctors look for when they examine a skin sample to diagnose Batten disease. The specific appearance of the lipopigment deposits can be useful in guiding further diagnostic tests that may identify the specific gene defect.

To date, eight genes have been linked to the varying forms of NCL. Mutations of other genes in NCL are likely since some individuals do not have mutations in any of the known genes. More than one gene may be associated with a particular form of NCL. The known NCL genes are:

CLN1, also known as *PPT1*, encodes an enzyme called palmitoyl-protein thioesterase 1 that is insufficiently active in Infantile NCL.

CLN2, or *TPP1*, produces an enzyme called tripeptidyl peptidase 1—an acid protease that degrades proteins. The enzyme is insufficiently active in Late Infantile NCL (also referred to as CLN2).

CLN3 mutation is the major cause of Juvenile NCL. The gene codes for a protein called CLN3 or battenin, which is found in the membranes of the cell (most predominantly in lysosomes and in related structures called endosomes). The protein's function is currently unknown.

CLN5, which causes variant Late Infantile NCL (vLINCL, also referred to as CLN5), produces a lysosomal protein called CLN5, whose function has not been identified.

CLN6, which also causes Late Infantile NCL, encodes a protein called CLN6 or linclin. The protein is found in the membranes of the cell (most predominantly in a structure called the endoplasmic reticulum). Its function has not been identified.

MFSD8, seen in variant Late Infantile NCL (also referred to as CLN7), encodes the MFSD8 protein that is a member of a protein family called the *major facilitator superfamily*. This superfamily is involved with transporting substances across the cell membranes. The precise function of MFSD8 has not been identified.

CLN8 causes progressive epilepsy with mental retardation. The gene encodes a protein also called CLN8, which is found in the membranes of the cell—most predominantly in the endoplasmic reticulum. The protein's function has not been identified.

CTSD, involved with Congenital NCL (also referred to as CLN10), encodes cathepsin D, a lysosomal enzyme that breaks apart other proteins. A deficiency of cathepsin D causes the disorder.

How are these disorders diagnosed?

Because vision loss is often an early sign, Batten disease may be first suspected during an eye exam. An eye doctor can detect a loss of cells within the eye that occurs in the childhood forms of NCL. However, because such cell loss occurs in other eye diseases, the disorder cannot be diagnosed by this sign alone. Often an eye specialist or other physician who suspects NCL may refer the child to a neurologist for additional testing.

In order to diagnose NCL, the neurologist needs the individual's medical and family history and information from various laboratory tests. Diagnostic tests used for NCLs include:

- *blood or urine tests*. These tests can detect abnormalities that may indicate Batten disease. For example, elevated levels of a chemical called dolichol are found in the urine of many individuals with NCL. The presence of vacuolated lymphocytes—white blood cells that contain holes or cavities (observed by microscopic analysis of blood smears)—when combined with other findings that indicate NCL, is suggestive for the juvenile form caused by *CLN3* mutations.

- *skin or tissue sampling*. The doctor can examine a small piece of tissue under an electron microscope. The powerful magnification of the microscope helps the doctor spot typical NCL deposits. These deposits are common in skin cells, especially those from sweat glands.

- *electroencephalogram or EEG*. An EEG uses special patches placed on the scalp to record electrical currents inside the brain. This helps doctors see telltale patterns in the brain's electrical activity that suggest an individual has seizures.

- *electrical studies of the eyes*. These tests, which include visual-evoked responses and electroretinograms, can detect various eye problems common in childhood NCLs.

- *diagnostic imaging using computed tomography (CT) or magnetic resonance imaging (MRI)*. Diagnostic imaging can help doctors look for changes in the brain's appearance. CT uses x-rays and a computer to create a sophisticated picture of the brain's tissues and structures, and may reveal brain areas that are decaying, or "atrophic," in persons with NCL. MRI uses a combination of magnetic fields and radio waves, instead of radiation, to create a picture of the brain.

- *measurement of enzyme activity*. Measurement of the activity of palmitoyl-protein thioesterase involved in CLN1, the acid protease involved in CLN2, and, though more rare, cathepsin D activity involved in CLN10, in white blood cells or cultured skin fibroblasts (cells that strengthen skin and give it elasticity) can be used to confirm or rule out these diagnoses.

- *DNA analysis*. If families where the mutation in the gene for CLN3 is known, DNA analysis can be used to confirm the diagnosis or for the prenatal diagnosis of this form of Batten disease. When the mutation is known, DNA analysis can also be used to detect unaffected carriers of this condition for genetic counseling. If a family mutation has not previously been identified or if the common mutations are not present, recent molecular advanced have made it possible to sequence all of the known NCL genes, increasing the chances of finding the responsible mutation(s).

Is there any treatment?

As yet, no specific treatment is known that can halt or reverse the symptoms of Batten disease or other NCLs. However, seizures can sometimes be reduced or controlled with anticonvulsant drugs, and other medical problems can be treated appropriately as they arise. At the same time, physical and occupational therapy may help patients retain function as long as possible.

Some reports have described a slowing of the disease in children with Batten disease who were treated with vitamins C and E and with diets low in vitamin A. However, these treatments did not prevent the fatal outcome of the disease.

Support and encouragement can help patients and families cope with the profound disability and dementia caused by NCLs. Often, support groups enable affected children, adults, and families to share common concerns and experiences.

Meanwhile, scientists pursue medical research that could someday yield an effective treatment.

What research is being done?

The National Institute of Neurological Disorders and Stroke, a part of the National Institutes of Health, is the Federal government's leading supporter of biomedical research on the brain and central nervous system. As part of its mission, the NINDS conducts research and supports studies through grants to major medical institutions across the country. Through the work of several scientific teams, the search for the molecular basis of the NCLs is gathering speed.

Studying the lipopigment deposits that contain fats and proteins, one NINDS-supported scientist, using animal models of NCL, found that a large portion of this built-up material is a protein called *subunit c*. This protein is normally found inside the cell's mitochondria, small structures that produce the energy cells need to do their jobs. Scientists are now working to understand what role this protein may play in NCL, including how this protein accumulates inside diseased cell and whether its accumulation—or the accumulation of other components in the storage material—is harmful to the cell. An important aspect of these studies is looking at how the different gene mutations lead to the lipoprotein deposits, which may involve the same processes.

In addition, research scientists are working with NCL animal models to improve understanding and treatment of these disorders. These include naturally occurring sheep and dog models, and genetically engineered mouse models. Simpler models in lower organisms (such as yeast, zebrafish, and the fruit fly) are useful tools that are being implemented by scientists to study the function of the NCL proteins, most of which remain unknown. Research suggests that many of the NCL genes have conserved functions in the lower organisms; in other words, they work the same way in yeast, fly, or zebrafish cells as they do in humans. Because mice and lower organisms breed or propagate quickly and can be genetically manipulated, their use can speed NCL research.

More recently, advances in human cell research will assist the translation of findings in the model organisms to individuals with NCL disorders. Skin or other cell types taken from those with an NCL disorder can now be manipulated in the laboratory to become "pluripotent," meaning they can made into cells that have the potential to become any cell type—including brain cells. This process—known as cellular reprogramming—is used to establish patient-derived induced pluripotent stem cells (iPS cells).

Although no therapies at currently available for NCL disorders, a number of NINDS-funded science teams are working toward developing therapies and identifying therapy targets for NCL. The approaches undertaken by scientists include:

- gene therapy (for example, in CLN1 and CLN2)

- enzyme replacement therapy (CLN1 and CLN2)

- stem cell therapy

- identification of the normal protein functions that are lost as a result of the gene mutations

- testing candidate drugs that modify known disease abnormalities (for example, immune suppression to eliminate the observed autoimmunity in JNCL/CLN3); and

- screening to identify drugs or other factors that normalize cellular abnormalities in the NCL disease models.

Part Three

Brain Infections

Chapter 13

Cysticercosis

Cysticercosis is an infection caused by the larvae of the parasite *Taenia solium*. This infection occurs after a person swallows tapeworm eggs. The larvae get into tissues such as muscle and brain, and form cysts there (these are called cysticerci). When cysts are found in the brain, the condition is called neurocysticercosis.

People get cysticercosis when they swallow *T. solium* eggs that are passed in the feces of a human with a tapeworm. Tapeworm eggs are spread through food, water, or surfaces contaminated with feces. Humans swallow the eggs when they eat contaminated food or put contaminated fingers in their mouth. Importantly, someone with a tapeworm can infect him or herself with tapeworm eggs (this is called autoinfection), and can infect others in the family.

People do **not** get cysticercosis by eating undercooked pork. Eating undercooked pork can result in intestinal **tapeworm** if the pork contains larval cysts. Pigs become infected by eating tapeworm eggs in the feces of a human infected with a tapeworm.

Both the tapeworm infection, also known as **taeniasis**, and cysticercosis occur globally. The highest rates of infection are found in areas of Latin America, Asia, and Africa that have poor sanitation and free-ranging pigs that have access to human feces. Although uncommon, cysticercosis can occur in people who have never traveled outside of the United States. For example, a person infected with a tapeworm

Text in this chapter is excerpted from "Cysticercosis," Centers for Disease Control and Prevention (CDC), April 2014.

who does not wash his or her hands might accidentally contaminate food with tapeworm eggs while preparing it for others.

In the United States, cysticercosis is considered one of the **Neglected Parasitic Infections** (NPIs), a group of five parasitic diseases that have been targeted by CDC for public health action.

Epidemiology & Risk Factors

Cysticercosis is an infection caused by the larvae of the tapeworm, *Taenia solium*. A person with an adult tapeworm, which lives in the person's gut, sheds eggs in the stool. The infection with the adult tapeworm is called taeniasis. A pig then eats the eggs in the stool. The eggs develop into larvae inside the pig and form cysts (called cysticerci) in the pig's muscles or other tissues. The infection with the cysts is called cysticercosis. Humans who eat undercooked or raw infected pork swallow the cysts in the meat. The larvae then come out of their cysts in the human gut and develop into adult tapeworms, completing the cycle.

People get cysticercosis when they swallow eggs that are excreted in the stool of people with the adult tapeworm. This may happen when people:

- Drink water or eat food contaminated with tapeworm eggs

- Put contaminated fingers in their mouth

Cysticercosis is not spread by eating undercooked meat. However, people get infected with tapeworms (**taeniasis**) by eating undercooked infected pork. People who have tapeworm infections can infect themselves with the eggs and develop cysticercosis (this is called autoinfection). They can also infect other people if they have poor hygiene and contaminate food or water that other people swallow. People who live with someone who has a tapeworm infection in their intestines have a much higher risk of getting cysticercosis than other people.

Human cysticercosis is found worldwide, especially in areas where pig cysticercosis is common. Both taeniasis and cysticercosis are most often found in rural areas of developing countries with poor sanitation, where pigs roam freely and eat human feces. Taeniasis and cysticercosis are rare among persons who live in countries where pigs are not raised and in countries where pigs do not have contact with human feces. Although uncommon, cysticercosis can occur in people who have never traveled outside of the United States if they are exposed to tapeworm eggs.

Biology

Causal Agent

The cestode (tapeworm) *Taenia solium* (pork tapeworm) is the main cause of human cysticercosis. In addition, the larval stage of other Taenia species (e.g., *multiceps, serialis, brauni, taeniaeformis, crassiceps*) can infect humans in various sites of localization including the brain, subcutaneous tissue, eye, or liver.

Life Cycle

Cysticercosis is an infection of both humans and pigs with the larval stages of the parasitic cestode, Taenia solium. This infection is caused by ingestion of eggs shed in the feces of a human tapeworm carrier (1). (See Figure 13.1.)

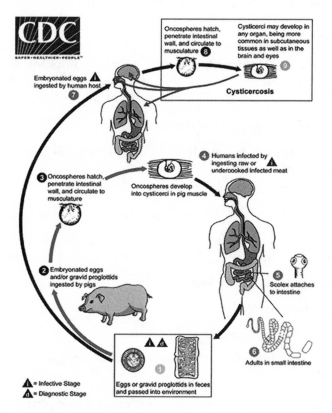

Figure 13.1. *The Cysticercosis Lifecycle*

Pigs and humans become infected by ingesting eggs or gravid proglottids (2), (7). Humans are infected either by ingestion of food contaminated with feces, or by autoinfection. In the latter case, a human infected with adult T. solium can ingest eggs produced by that tapeworm, either through fecal contamination or, possibly, from proglottids carried into the stomach by reverse peristalsis.

Once eggs are ingested, oncospheres hatch in the intestine (3), (8) invade the intestinal wall, and migrate to striated muscles, as well as the brain, liver, and other tissues, where they develop into cysticerci (9). In humans, cysts can cause serious sequellae if they localize in the brain, resulting in neurocysticercosis.

The parasite life cycle is completed, resulting in human tapeworm infection, when humans ingest undercooked pork containing cysticerci (4). Cysts evaginate and attach to the small intestine by their scolex (5). Adult tapeworms develop, (up to 2 to 7 meters in length and produce less than 1,000 proglottids, each with approximately 50,000 eggs) and reside in the small intestine for years (6).

Disease

Cysts, called cysticerci, can develop in the muscles, the eyes, the brain, and/or the spinal cord. Symptoms caused by the cysts depend on the location, size, number, and stage of the cysts.

Cysts in the brain or spinal cord:

- Cause the most serious form of the disease, called neurocysticercosis
- May cause no symptoms
- May cause seizures and/or headaches (these are more common)
- May also cause confusion, difficulty with balance, brain swelling, and excess fluid around the brain (these are less common)
- May cause stroke or death

Cysts in the muscles:

- Generally do not cause symptoms
- May cause lumps under the skin, which can sometimes become tender

The period between initial infection and symptom onset varies from several months to many years. In the United States, infections are detected predominantly in immigrants from Mexico, Guatemala, and other Latin American countries who acquired their infections in their home country.

Clusters and sporadic cases of cysticercosis acquired in the U.S. have been reported. Food handlers with taeniasis are of particular concern in this scenario (see "Prevention and Control" section for more information).

In humans, cysticerci (encysted larvae) often occur in skeletal muscles. However, the manifestations that most frequently lead patients to visit health care providers are caused by cysts in the central nervous system (CNS), known as neurocysticercosis. Less frequently, cysticerci may localize in the eyes, skin, or heart.

Neurocysticercosis may be parenchymal (occurring in the brain substance, the most common location) or extraparenchymal (occurring in the meninges, the ventricles, the basilar cisterns, or the subarachnoid space of the brain or spinal cord).

Clinical manifestations of cysticercosis depend on the number, location, size, and stage (viable, degenerating, or calcified) of the cysticerci and the intensity of the inflammatory response to degenerating cysts. Epilepsy is the most common manifestation, present in 70–90% of symptomatic patients in published case series. Less frequent clinical manifestations include intracranial hypertension, hydrocephalus, chronic meningitis, and cranial nerve abnormalities.

The number of cysticerci in the host can vary from one to more than 1,000. In the absence of massive numbers of cysticerci, the initial host tissue reaction is usually minimal. The developing cysticercus affects the surrounding tissue as a slowly growing mass that may cause pressure atrophy. Most live cysts do not cause an inflammatory reaction, but an acute inflammatory response occurs when the cysts degenerate, which results in the release of parasite antigens. Degeneration of a cyst may occur years after the initial infection. Some calcified cysts may intermittently release antigen, though this process is not fully understood. In the CNS, the inflammatory reaction and resultant edema appear as a contrast-enhancing ring around the cyst on imaging. There may be CSF pleocytosis as well. Necrotic larvae are completely or partially resorbed, but may become calcified, resulting in focal scarring that may provide a focus for seizures.

The distinction between parenchymal and extraparenchymal neurocysticercosis has important prognostic implications. Parenchymal disease with small numbers of cysts carries an excellent long-term prognosis (probably even without anthelminthic therapy) compared to parenchymal disease with > 50 cysts and extraparenchymal disease.

Diagnosis

Diagnosis typically requires both CNS imaging and serological testing. A careful history should be taken, including questions regarding residence or extended travel in developing countries, and consumption of food prepared by someone who has lived in a high-risk area.

Diagnosis often requires both imaging and serological testing because:

- A patient may have clinical disease from a single or very few cysticerci. In this instance, serological results may be negative, but the lesions may be visible on imaging.

- A patient may have cysticerci in locations other than the brain. In this instance, CNS imaging is negative but serological results might be positive, indicating an antibody response to lesions elsewhere (e.g. the spinal cord).

- The location and characteristics of the lesions on imaging, especially on MRI, are essential to determine the best treatment modalities.

Computerized tomography (CT) is superior to magnetic resonance imaging (MRI) for demonstrating small calcifications. However, MRI shows cysts in some locations (cerebral convexity, ventricular ependyma) better than CT, is more sensitive than CT to demonstrate surrounding edema, and may show internal changes indicating the death of cysticerci.

In recent years, the use of CT and MRI has permitted identification of neurocysticercosis cases with a benign course that would not have been detected previously. It is now recognized that most infections are asymptomatic, or mildly symptomatic and benign. Mortality is low in patients with parenchymal cysts or calcification without hydrocephalus. However, untreated cysticercosis with hydrocephalus, large basilar or supratentorial cysts, massive numbers of cysts, intracranial hypertension, or cerebral infarction can be life-threatening.

There are two available serologic tests to detect cysticercosis, the enzyme-linked immunoelectrotransfer blot or EITB, and commercial enzyme-linked immunoassays. The immunoblot is the test preferred by the Centers for Disease Control (CDC), because its sensitivity and specificity have been well characterized in published analyses.

If you think that you may have cysticercosis, please see your health care provider. Your health care provider will ask you about your symptoms, where you have travelled, and what kinds of foods you eat.

If you have been diagnosed with cysticercosis, you and your family members should be tested for intestinal tapeworm infection.

Treatment

The choice of treatment for neurocysticercosis depends on the clinical manifestations and the location, number, size, and stage of cysticerci. Anthelminthic chemotherapy for symptomatic neurocysticercosis is almost never a medical emergency. The focus of initial therapy is control of seizures, edema, intracranial hypertension, or hydrocephalus, when one of these conditions is present. Under certain circumstances, a ventricular shunt or other neurosurgical procedure may be indicated. Rarely, neurocysticercosis—especially large and/or subarachnoid (racemose) lesions—may present with imminent threat of intracranial herniation, a neurosurgical emergency.

Anthelminthic therapy, because it kills viable cysts and provokes an inflammatory response, may actually increase symptoms acutely. Co-administration of corticosteroids that cross the blood brain barrier (e.g. dexamethasone) is used to mitigate these effects. Recent placebo-controlled trials confirm that albendazole treatment in appropriately selected neurocysticercosis patients is effective in decreasing the frequency of generalized seizures in long-term follow-up.

Although the heterogeneity of the clinical picture of neurocysticercosis requires individual tailoring of treatment and management, several general principles apply:

- Anthelminthic therapy is generally indicated for symptomatic patients with multiple, live (noncalcified) cysticerci.

- Anthelminthic treatment will not benefit patients with dead worms (calcified cysts).

- Concomitant administration of steroids (e.g. dexamethasone) is often indicated to suppress the inflammatory response induced by destruction of live cysticerci.

- Conventional anticonvulsant therapy is the mainstay of management of neurocysticercosis-associated seizure disorders.

- Intraventricular cysts should usually be treated by surgical removal (endoscopic if possible). Anthelminthics are relatively contraindicated, because the resulting inflammatory response could precipitate obstructive hydrocephalus.

- Although our understanding of subarachnoid neurocysticercosis is evolving, treatment with both anthelminthics and corticosteroids is usually required. Ventricular shunting is often necessary as well.

Even when anthelminthic therapy is successful, continued use of anticonvulsant and other symptomatic medications may still be needed because the pathology may be irreversible. Decisions regarding discontinuation of anticonvulsant regimens must be made on an individual clinical basis, but data suggest that many patients can be eventually weaned from anticonvulsant therapy.

Drugs

Several studies suggest that **albendazole** (conventional dosage 15 mg/kg/day in 2 divided doses for 15 days) may be superior to **praziquantel** (50 mg/kg/day for 15 days) for the treatment of neurocysticercosis. In comparative clinical trials, albendazole was equivalent or superior to praziquantel in reducing the number of live cysticerci. A recent placebo-controlled, double-blinded trial demonstrated that albendazole treatment (400 mg twice daily plus 6 mg dexamethasone QD for 10 days) significantly decreased generalized seizures over 30 months of follow-up.

More prolonged treatment courses (e.g. 30 days of albendazole, which may be repeated) may be needed for extraparenchymal or extensive disease. Albendazole is more likely to be effective against extraparenchymal forms of the disease because of better penetration than praziquantel into the CSF. Another possible contributing factor to the greater efficacy of albendazole is that serum and CSF metabolite levels appear to be potentiated by concomitant corticosteroids, whereas praziquantel levels are depressed. Albendazole, unlike praziquantel, has been reported to be effective in giant subarachnoid cysticerci (racemose cysts) and in extraocular muscle cysts. Both drugs appear to have a role in therapy, since cases that have not responded to one of the drugs have been reported to respond to the other.

Prevention and Control

To prevent cysticercosis, the following precautions should be taken:

- Wash your hands with soap and warm water after using the toilet, changing diapers, and before handling food

- Teach children the importance of washing hands to prevent infection

- Wash and peel all raw vegetables and fruits before eating
- Use good food and water safety practices while traveling in developing countries such as:

  1. Drink only bottled or boiled (1 minute) water or carbonated (bubbly) drinks in cans or bottles

  2. Filter unsafe water through an "absolute 1 micron or less" filter AND dissolve iodine tablets in the filtered water; "absolute 1 micron" filters can be found in camping and outdoor supply stores

The control and prevention of cysticercosis depends on preventing fecal-oral transmission of eggs from persons with taeniasis. Follow-up of cysticercosis cases reported to the Los Angeles County Health Department from 1988 to 1991 demonstrated at least one active tapeworm carrier among family contacts of 22% of locally acquired cases, and 5% of imported cases. Identification and treatment of tapeworm carriers is an important public health measure that can prevent further cases.

When traveling to areas with poor sanitation, persons should be particularly careful to avoid foods that might be contaminated by human feces. Food handlers should be educated in good handwashing practices. Based on investigations of cases of neurocysticercosis in U.S. citizens who acquired their infections from asymptomatic household employees from Latin America, CDC recommended that such employees should have stool examinations for taeniasis and be treated if found to be infected. CDC does not recommend the routine testing of commercial food handlers, but does support policies aimed at ensuring that food handlers are taught and adhere to good handwashing practices.

Chapter 14

Neurological Complications of AIDS

What is AIDS?

AIDS (acquired immune deficiency syndrome) is a condition that occurs in the most advanced stages of human immunodeficiency virus (HIV) infection. It may take many years for AIDS to develop following the initial HIV infection.

Although AIDS is primarily an immune system disorder, it also affects the nervous system and can lead to a wide range of severe neurological disorders.

How does AIDS affect the nervous system?

The virus does not appear to directly invade nerve cells but it jeopardizes their health and function. The resulting inflammation may damage the brain and spinal cord and cause symptoms such as confusion and forgetfulness, behavioral changes, headaches, progressive weakness, and loss of sensation in the arms and legs. Cognitive motor impairment or damage to the peripheral nerves is also common. Research has shown that the HIV infection can significantly alter the

Text in this chapter is excerpted from "Neurological Complications of AIDS Fact Sheet," National Institute of Neurological Disorders and Stroke (NINDS), February 23, 2015.

size of certain brain structures involved in learning and information processing.

Other nervous system complications that occur as a result of the disease or the drugs used to treat it include pain, seizures, shingles, spinal cord problems, lack of coordination, difficult or painful swallowing, anxiety disorder, depression, fever, vision loss, gait disorders, destruction of brain tissue, and coma. These symptoms may be mild in the early stages of AIDS but can become progressively severe.

In the United States, neurological complications are seen in more than 50 percent of adults with AIDS. Nervous system complications in children may include developmental delays, loss of previously achieved milestones, brain lesions, nerve pain, smaller than normal skull size, slow growth, eye problems, and recurring bacterial infections.

What are some of the neurological complications that are associated with AIDS?

AIDS-related disorders of the nervous system may be caused directly by the HIV virus, by certain cancers and opportunistic infections (illnesses caused by bacteria, fungi, and other viruses that would not otherwise affect people with healthy immune systems), or by toxic effects of the drugs used to treat symptoms. Other neuro-AIDS disorders of unknown origin may be influenced by but are not caused directly by the virus.

AIDS dementia complex (ADC), or HIV-associated dementia (HAD), occurs primarily in persons with more advanced HIV infection. Symptoms include encephalitis (inflammation of the brain), behavioral changes, and a gradual decline in cognitive function, including trouble with concentration, memory, and attention. Persons with ADC also show progressive slowing of motor function and loss of dexterity and coordination. When left untreated, ADC can be fatal. It is rare when anti-retroviral therapy is used. Milder cognitive complaints are common and are termed HIV-associated neurocognitive disorder (HAND). Neuropsychologic testing can reveal subtle deficits even in the absence of symptoms.

Central nervous system (CNS) lymphomas are cancerous tumors that either begin in the brain or result from a cancer that has spread from another site in the body. CNS lymphomas are almost always associated with the Epstein-Barr virus (a common human virus in the herpes family). Symptoms include headache, seizures, vision problems, dizziness, speech disturbance, paralysis, and mental deterioration.

Individuals may develop one or more CNS lymphomas. Prognosis is poor due to advanced and increasing immunodeficiency, but is better with successful HIV therapy.

Cryptococcal meningitis is seen in about 10 percent of untreated individuals with AIDS and in other persons whose immune systems have been severely suppressed by disease or drugs. It is caused by the fungus *Cryptococcus neoformans*, which is commonly found in dirt and bird droppings. The fungus first invades the lungs and spreads to the covering of the brain and spinal cord, causing inflammation. Symptoms include fatigue, fever, headache, nausea, memory loss, confusion, drowsiness, and vomiting. If left untreated, patients with cryptococcal meningitis may lapse into a coma and die.

Cytomegalovirus (CMV) infections can occur concurrently with other infections. Symptoms of CMV encephalitis include weakness in the arms and legs, problems with hearing and balance, altered mental states, dementia, peripheral neuropathy, coma, and retinal disease that may lead to blindness. CMV infection of the spinal cord and nerves can result in weakness in the lower limbs and some paralysis, severe lower back pain, and loss of bladder function. It can also cause pneumonia and gastrointestinal disease. This is rarely seen in HIV-treated individuals since advanced immunity is required for CMV to emerge.

Herpes virus infections are often seen in people with AIDS. The *herpes zoster virus*, which causes chickenpox and shingles, can infect the brain and produce encephalitis and myelitis (inflammation of the spinal cord). It commonly produces shingles, which is an eruption of blisters and intense pain along an area of skin supplied by an infected nerve. In people exposed to herpes zoster, the virus can lay dormant in the nerve tissue for years until it is reactivated as shingles. This reactivation is common in persons with AIDS because of their weakened immune systems. Signs of shingles include painful blisters (like those seen in chickenpox), itching, tingling, and pain in the nerves.

People with AIDS may suffer from several different forms of *neuropathy*, or nerve pain, each strongly associated with a specific stage of active immunodeficiency disease. *Peripheral neuropathy* describes damage to the peripheral nerves, the vast communications network that transmits information between the brain and spinal cord to every other part of the body. Peripheral nerves also send sensory information back to the brain and spinal cord. HIV damages the nerve fibers that help conduct signals and can cause several different forms of neuropathy. *Distal sensory polyneuropathy* causes either a numbing feeling or a mild to painful burning or tingling sensation that normally begins in the legs and feet. These sensations may be particularly strong at night and may spread to the hands. Affected persons have a heightened sensitivity to pain, touch, or other stimuli. Onset usually occurs in the later stages of the HIV infection and may affect the majority of advanced-stage HIV patients.

Neurosyphilis, the result of an insufficiently treated syphilis infection, seems more frequent and more rapidly progressive in people with HIV infection. It may cause slow degeneration of the nerve cells and nerve fibers that carry sensory information to the brain. Symptoms, which may not appear for some decades after the initial infection and vary from person to person, include weakness, diminished reflexes, unsteady gait, progressive degeneration of the joints, loss of coordination, episodes of intense pain and disturbed sensation, personality changes, dementia, deafness, visual impairment, and impaired response to light. The disease is more frequent in men than in women. Onset is common during mid-life.

Progressive multifocal leukoencephalopathy (PML) primarily affects individuals with suppressed immune systems (including nearly 5 percent of people with AIDS). PML is caused by the JC virus, which travels to the brain, infects multiple sites, and destroys the cells that make myelin—the fatty protective covering for many of the body's nerve and brain cells. Symptoms include various types of mental deterioration, vision loss, speech disturbances, ataxia (inability to coordinate movements), paralysis, brain lesions, and, ultimately, coma. Some individuals may also have compromised memory and cognition, and seizures may occur. PML is relentlessly progressive and death usually occurs within 6 months of initial symptoms. However, immune reconstitution with highly active antiretroviral therapy allows survival of more than half of HIV-associated PML cases in the current treatment era.

Editor's Note: For further information on PML, please refer to Chapter 16.

Psychological and neuropsychiatric disorders can occur in different phases of the HIV infection and AIDS and may take various and complex forms. Some illnesses, such as AIDS dementia complex, are caused directly by HIV infection of the brain, while other conditions may be triggered by the drugs used to combat the infection. Individuals may experience anxiety disorder, depressive disorders, increased thoughts of suicide, paranoia, dementia, delirium, cognitive impairment, confusion, hallucinations, behavioral abnormalities, malaise, and acute mania.

Toxoplasma encephalitis, also called cerebral toxoplasmosis, occurs in about 10 percent of untreated AIDS patients. It is caused by the parasite *Toxoplasma gondii*, which is carried by cats, birds, and other animals and can be found in soil contaminated by cat feces and sometimes in raw or undercooked meat. Once the parasite invades the immune system, it remains there; however, the immune system in a healthy person can fight off the parasite, preventing disease. Symptoms include encephalitis, fever, severe headache that does not respond to treatment, weakness on one side of the body, seizures, lethargy, increased confusion, vision problems, dizziness, problems with speaking and walking, vomiting, and personality changes. Not all patients show signs of the infection. Antibiotic therapy, if used early, will generally control the complication.

Vacuolar myelopathy causes the protective myelin sheath to pull away from nerve cells of the spinal cord, forming small holes called vacuoles in nerve fibers. Symptoms include weak and stiff legs and unsteadiness when walking. Walking becomes more difficult as the disease progresses and many patients eventually require a wheelchair. Some people also develop AIDS dementia. Vacuolar myelopathy may affect up to 30 percent of untreated adults with AIDS and its incidence may be even higher in HIV-infected children.

How are these disorders diagnosed?

Based on the results of the individual's medical history and a general physical exam, the physician will conduct a thorough neurological exam to assess various functions: motor and sensory skills, nerve function, hearing and speech, vision, coordination and balance, mental status, and changes in mood or behavior. The physician may order laboratory tests and one or more of the following procedures to help diagnose neurological complications of AIDS.

Brain imaging can reveal signs of brain inflammation, tumors and CNS lymphomas, nerve damage, internal bleeding or hemorrhage, white matter irregularities, and other brain abnormalities. Several painless imaging procedures are used to help diagnose neurological complications of AIDS.

- *Computed tomography* (also called a CT scan) uses x-rays and a computer to produce two-dimensional images of bone and tissue, including inflammation, certain brain tumors and cysts, brain damage from head injury, and other disorders. It provides more details than an x-ray alone.

- *Magnetic resonance* imaging (MRI) uses a computer, radio waves, and a powerful magnetic field to produce either a detailed three-dimensional picture or a two-dimensional "slice" of body structures, including tissues, organs, bones, and nerves. It does not use ionizing radiation (as does an x-ray) and gives physicians a better look at tissue located near bone.

- *Functional MRI* (fMRI) uses the blood's magnetic properties to pinpoint areas of the brain that are active and to note how long they stay active. It can assess brain damage from head injury or degenerative disorders such as Alzheimer's disease and can identify and monitor other neurological disorders, including AIDS dementia complex.

- *Magnetic resonance spectroscopy* (MRS) uses a strong magnetic field to study the biochemical composition and concentration of hydrogen-based molecules, some of which are very specific to nerve cells, in various brain regions. MRS is being used experimentally to identify brain lesions in people with AIDS.

Electromyography, or EMG, is used to diagnose nerve and muscle dysfunction (such as neuropathy and nerve fiber damage caused by the HIV virus) and spinal cord disease. It records spontaneous muscle activity and muscle activity driven by the peripheral nerves.

Biopsy is the removal and examination of tissue from the body. A brain biopsy, which involves the surgical removal of a small piece of the brain or tumor, is used to determine intracranial disorders and tumor type. Unlike most other biopsies, it requires hospitalization. Muscle or nerve biopsies can help diagnose neuromuscular problems, while a brain biopsy can help diagnose a tumor, inflammation, or other irregularity.

Cerebrospinal fluid analysis can detect any bleeding or brain hemorrhage, infections of the brain or spinal cord (such as neurosyphilis), and any harmful buildup of fluid. It can also be used to sample viruses that may be affecting the brain. A sample of the fluid is removed by needle, under local anesthesia, and studied to detect any irregularities.

How are these disorders treated?

No single treatment can cure the neurological complications of AIDS. Some disorders require aggressive therapy while others are treated symptomatically.

Neuropathic pain is often difficult to control. Medicines range from analgesics sold over the counter to antiepileptic drugs, opiates, and some classes of antidepressants. Inflamed tissue can press on nerves, causing pain. Inflammatory and autoimmune conditions leading to neuropathy may be treated with corticosteroids, and procedures such as plasmapheresis (or plasma exchange) can clear the blood of harmful substances that cause inflammation.

Treatment options for AIDS- and HIV-related neuropsychiatric or psychotic disorders include antidepressants and anticonvulsants. Psychostimulants may also improve depressive symptoms and combat lethargy. Antidementia drugs may relieve confusion and slow mental decline, and benzodiazepines may be prescribed to treat anxiety. Psychotherapy may also help some individuals.

Aggressive antiretroviral therapy is used to treat AIDS dementia complex, vacuolar myopathy, progressive multifocal leukoencephalopathy, and cytomegalovirus encephalitis. HAART, or highly active antiretroviral therapy, combines at least three drugs to reduce the amount of virus circulating in the blood and may also delay the start of some infections.

Other neuro-AIDS treatment options include physical therapy and rehabilitation, radiation therapy and/or chemotherapy to kill or shrink cancerous brain tumors that may be caused by the HIV virus, antifungal or antimalarial drugs to combat certain bacterial infections associated with the disorder, and penicillin to treat neurosyphilis.

What research is being done?

Within the Federal government, the National Institute of Neurological Disorders and Stroke (NINDS), one part of the National Institutes of Health (NIH), supports research on the neurological consequences of AIDS. The NINDS works closely with its sister agency, the National Institute of Allergy and Infectious Diseases (NIAID), which has primary responsibility for research related to HIV and AIDS.

Several NINDS-funded projects are studying the role of virally infected brain macrophages (cells that normally work to protect against infection) in causing disease in the central nervous system of adult macaques. The focus of these projects includes gene analyses and the study of key neuroimmune regulatory molecules that are turned on in the brain during the course of viral infection at levels that have been shown to be toxic.

Several animal-based models of HIV (including mouse, rat, and simian models) are used by scientists to study disease mechanisms and the course of AIDS, and NINDS grantees are working to develop new models of HIV. Several projects rely on a mouse model of severe combined immunodeficiency (a group of inherited disorders that are characterized by a lack of or severe defect in cells responsible for protecting the immune system). This model allows researchers to transplant developing human brain tissue from culture into the brains of the mice to monitor and assess neurologic damage caused by HIV infection. Other studies use mice bred to carry symptoms of HIV, and NINDS grantees are using these animals to see if the brain can function as a sanctuary for HIV-infected cells that can migrate to and infect peripheral lymph tissue.

The NINDS also supports research into the mechanisms of neurological illnesses related to immunodeficiency in AIDS patients. Several different investigators are studying the JC virus, which can reproduce in the brains of immunosuppressed patients and cause PML, and one study identified a novel receptor for the JC virus. Other studies of infectious agents include an investigation of the interaction of the fungal agent *Cryptococcus* with the blood vessels of the brain, and an analysis of neurosyphilis in people with AIDS. Scientists are also studying the effect of neurotoxic proteins and antiviral therapies directly on nerve cells as the cause for distal sensory peripheral neuropathy.

Several researchers are studying AIDS dementia and cognitive changes in HIV. NINDS-sponsored scientists are using fMRI and MRS to assess brain function and any behavioral deficits in HIV-affected individuals. Investigators hope to better understand how progressive neuronal cell death contributes to cognitive dysfunction and AIDS dementia. The National NeuroAIDS Tissue Consortium, a project supported jointly by the NINDS and its sister agency, the National Institute of Mental Health, is collecting tissues from people with AIDS who have suffered from dementia and other neurological complications of HIV infection for distribution to researchers around the globe.

The Neurological AIDS Research Consortium was established by the NINDS in 1993 to design and conduct clinical trials on HIV-associated neurologic disease. To date, the Consortium has supported studies of neurological function in advanced AIDS and the treatment of HIV-associated peripheral neuropathy, PML, and CMV infection. Current studies are optimizing therapy for painful neuropathy using methadone and duloxetine. Recent studies evaluated minocycline for dementia treatment and are studying the effects of salvage HAART (using drug therapies to treat HIV strains that have become resistant to drug combination therapy) in the nervous system.

Chapter 15

Meningitis and Encephalitis

What is meningitis? What is encephalitis?

Infections, and less commonly other causes, in the brain and spinal cord can cause dangerous inflammation. This inflammation can produce a wide range of symptoms, including fever, headache, seizures, change in behavior or confusion and, in extreme cases, can cause brain damage, stroke, or even death.

Infection of the meninges, the membranes that surround the brain and spinal cord, is called meningitis and inflammation of the brain itself is called *encephalitis*. *Myelitis* refers to inflammation of the spinal cord. When both the brain and the spinal cord are involved, the condition is called *encephalomyelitis*.

What causes meningitis and encephalitis?

Infectious causes of meningitis and encephalitis include bacteria, viruses, fungi, and parasites. Many of these affect healthy people. For others, environmental and exposure history, recent travel or immunocompromised state (such as HIV, diabetes, steroids, chemotherapy) are important elements. There are also non-infectious causes such as autoimmune causes and medications.

Text in this chapter is excerpted from "Meningitis and Encephalitis Fact Sheet," National Institute of Neurological Disorders and Stroke (NINDS), November 24, 2014.

255

Meningitis

Meningitis is most often caused by a bacterial infection. It also may be caused by a virus, fungal infection, parasite, a reaction to certain medications or medical treatments, a rheumatologic disease such as lupus, some types of cancer, or a traumatic injury to the head or spine.

Bacterial meningitis is a rare but potentially fatal disease. It can be caused by several types of bacteria that first cause an upper respiratory tract infection and then travel through the blood stream to the brain. The disease can also occur when certain bacteria invade the meninges directly. The disease can cause stroke, hearing loss, and permanent brain damage.

Pneumococcal meningitis is the most common form of meningitis and is the most serious form of bacterial meningitis. Some 6,000 cases of pneumococcal meningitis are reported in the United States each year. The disease is caused by the bacterium *Streptococcus pneumoniae*, which also causes pneumonia, blood poisoning (septicemia), and ear and sinus infections. At particular risk are children under age 2 and adults with a weakened or depressed immune system, including the elderly. Persons who have had pneumococcal meningitis often suffer neurological damage ranging from deafness to severe brain damage. There are immunizations available for certain strains of the Pneumococcal bacteria.

Meningococcal meningitis is caused by the bacterium *Neisseria meningitides*. Each year in the United States about 2,600 people get this highly contagious disease. High-risk groups include infants under the age of 1 year, people with suppressed immune systems, travelers to foreign countries where the disease is endemic, and college students (freshmen in particular) who reside in dormitories. Between 10 and 15 percent of cases are fatal, with another 10–15 percent causing brain damage and other serious side effects. If this is diagnosed, people who come in close contact with the affected individual should be given preventative antibiotics.

Haemophilus meningitis was at one time the most common form of bacterial meningitis. Fortunately, the *Haemophilus influenzae b* vaccine has greatly reduced the number of cases in the United States. Those most at risk of getting this disease are children in child-care settings and children who do not have access to the vaccine.

Other forms of bacterial meningitis include *Listeria monocytogenes meningitis*. Certain foods such as unpasteurized dairy or deli meats are sometimes implicated. *Escherichia coli meningitis*, which is most common in elderly adults and newborns and may be transmitted to a baby through the birth canal, and *Mycobacterium tuberculosis meningitis*, a rare disease that occurs when the bacterium that causes tuberculosis attacks the meninges.

Viral, or aseptic, meningitis is usually caused by enteroviruses—common viruses that enter the body through the mouth and travel to the brain and surrounding tissues where they multiply. Enteroviruses are present in mucus, saliva, and feces and can be transmitted through direct contact with an infected person or an infected object or surface. Other viruses that cause meningitis include varicella zoster *(the virus that causes chicken pox and can appear decades later as shingles)*, influenza, mumps, HIV, and *herpes simplex type 2* (genital herpes).

Many fungal infections can affect the brain. The most common form of fungal meningitis is caused by the fungus cryptococcus neoformans (found mainly in dirt and bird droppings). Cryptococcal meningitis mostly occurs in immunocompromised individuals such as in AIDS patients but can also occur in healthy people. Some of these cases can be indolent and smolder for weeks. Although treatable, fungal meningitis often recurs in nearly half of affected persons.

Parasitic causes include cysticercosis, which is common in other parts of the world as well, and cerebral malaria.

There are rare cases of amoebic meningitis, sometimes related to fresh water swimming, which can be rapidly fatal.

Encephalitis

Encephalitis can be caused by the same infections listed above. However, up to 60 percent of cases remain undiagnosed, so this is an active area of research. Several thousand cases of encephalitis are reported each year, but many more may actually occur since the symptoms may be mild to non-existent in most patients.

Most diagnosed cases of encephalitis in the United States are caused by enteroviruses, herpes simplex virus types 1 and 2, rabies virus (this can occur even without a known animal bite, such as for example due to exposure to bats), or arboviruses such as West Nile virus, which are transmitted from infected animals to humans through the bite of an infected tick, mosquito, or other blood-sucking insect. Lyme disease, a bacterial infection spread by tick bite, more typically causes meningitis, and rarely encephalitis.

Herpes simplex encephalitis (HSE) is responsible for about 10 percent of all encephalitis cases, with a frequency of about 2 cases per million persons per year. More than half of untreated cases are fatal. About 30 percent of cases result from the initial infection with the herpes simplex virus; the majority of cases are caused by reactivation of an earlier infection. Most people acquire herpes simplex type 1 (the cause of cold sores or fever blisters) in childhood so it is a ubiquitous exposure.

HSE due to herpes simplex virus type 1 can affect any age group but is most often seen in persons under age 20 or over age 40. This rapidly progressing disease is the single most important cause of fatal sporadic encephalitis in the U.S. Symptoms can include headache and fever for up to 5 days, followed by personality and behavioral changes, seizures, hallucinations, and altered levels of consciousness. Brain damage in adults and in children beyond the neonatal period is usually seen in the frontal (leading to behavioral and personality changes) and temporal lobes (leading to memory and speech problems) and can be severe.

Type 2 virus (genital herpes) is most often transmitted through sexual contact. Many people do not know they are infected and may not have active genital lesions. An infected mother can transmit the disease to her child at birth, and through contact with genital secretions. In newborns, symptoms such as lethargy, irritability, tremors, seizures, and poor feeding generally develop between 4 and 11 days after delivery.

Powassan encephalitis is the only well-documented tick-borne arbovirus in the United States and Canada. Symptoms are noticed 7–10 days following the bite (most people do not notice tick bites) and may include headache, fever, nausea, confusion, partial paralysis, and coma.

Four common forms of mosquito-transmitted viral encephalitis are seen in the United States:

- **Equine encephalitis** affects horses and humans. *Eastern equine encephalitis* also infects birds that live in freshwater swamps of the eastern U.S. seaboard and along the Gulf Coast. In humans, symptoms are seen 4–10 days following transmission and include sudden fever, general flu-like muscle pains, and headache of increasing severity, followed by coma and death in severe cases. About half of infected patients die from the disorder. Fewer than 10 human cases are seen annually in the United States. *Western equine encephalitis* is seen in farming

areas in the western and central plains states. Symptoms begin
5–10 days following infection. Children, particularly those under
12 months of age, are affected more severely than adults and
may have permanent neurologic damage. Death occurs in about
3 percent of cases. *Venezuelan equine encephalitis* is very rare in
this country. Children are at greatest risk of developing severe
complications, while adults generally develop flu-like symptoms.
Epidemics in South and Central America have killed thousands
of persons and left others with permanent, severe neurologic
damage.

- **La Crosse encephalitis** occurs most often in the upper
  mid-western states (Illinois, Wisconsin, Indiana, Ohio,
  Minnesota, and Iowa) but also has been reported in the southeastern and mid-Atlantic regions of the country. Most cases
  are seen in children under age 16. Symptoms such as vomiting,
  headache, fever, and lethargy appear 5–10 days following infection. Severe complications include seizure, coma, and permanent
  neurologic damage. About 100 cases of La Crosse encephalitis
  are reported each year.

- **St. Louis encephalitis** is most prevalent in temperate regions
  of the United States but can occur throughout most of the country. The disease is generally milder in children than in adults,
  with elderly adults at highest risk of severe disease or death.
  Symptoms typically appear 7–10 days following infection and
  include headache and fever. In more severe cases, confusion
  and disorientation, tremors, convulsions (especially in the very
  young), and coma may occur.

- **West Nile encephalitis** was first clinically diagnosed in the
  United States in 1999; 284 people are known to have died of
  the virus the following year. There were 9,862 reported cases of
  human West Nile disease in calendar year 2003, with a total of
  560 deaths from this disorder over 5 years. The disease is usually transmitted by a bite from an infected mosquito, but can
  also occur after transplantation of an infected organ or transfusions of infected blood or blood products. Symptoms are flu-like
  and include fever, headache, and joint pain. Some patients may
  develop a skin rash and swollen lymph glands, while others may
  not show any symptoms. At highest risk are elderly adults and
  people with weakened immune systems.

Who is at risk for encephalitis and meningitis?

Anyone can get encephalitis or meningitis. People with weakened immune systems, including those persons with HIV or those taking immunosuppressant drugs, are at the highest risk of contracting the diseases.

How are these disorders transmitted?

Some forms of bacterial meningitis and encephalitis are contagious and can be spread through contact with saliva, nasal discharge, feces, or respiratory and throat secretions (often spread through kissing, coughing, or sharing drinking glasses, eating utensils, or such personal items as toothbrushes, lipstick, or cigarettes). For example, people sharing a household, at a day care center, or in a classroom with an infected person can become infected. College students living in dormitories—in particular, college freshmen—have a higher risk of contracting meningococcal meningitis than college students overall. Children who do not have access to childhood vaccines are at increased risk of developing certain types of bacterial meningitis.

Because these diseases can occur suddenly, anyone who is suspected of having either meningitis or encephalitis should immediately contact a doctor or go to the hospital.

What are the signs and symptoms?

The hallmark signs of meningitis are sudden fever, severe headache, nausea/vomiting, double vision, drowsiness, sensitivity to bright light, and a stiff neck; encephalitis can be characterized by fever, seizures, change in behavior, confusion and disorientation, and related neurological signs depending on which part of the brain is affected by the encephalitic process, as some of these are quite focal (locally centered) while others are more global.

Meningitis often appears with flu-like symptoms that develop over 1–2 days. Distinctive rashes are typically seen in some forms of the disease. Meningococcal meningitis may be associated with kidney and adrenal gland failure and shock.

Individuals with encephalitis often show mild flu-like symptoms. In more severe cases, patients may experience problems with speech or hearing, double vision, hallucinations, personality changes, loss of consciousness, loss of sensation in some parts of the body, muscle weakness, partial paralysis in the arms and legs, sudden severe dementia, seizures, and memory loss.

Important signs of meningitis or encephalitis to watch for in an infant include fever, lethargy, not waking for feeding, vomiting, body stiffness, unexplained or unusual irritability, and a full or bulging fontanel (the soft spot on the top of the head).

How are meningitis and encephalitis diagnosed?

Following a physical exam and medical history to review activities of the past several days/weeks (such as recent exposure to insects or animals, any contact with ill persons, recent travel, or preexisting medical conditions and medications list), the doctor may order various diagnostic tests to confirm the presence of infection and inflammation. Early diagnosis is vital, as symptoms can appear suddenly and escalate to brain damage, hearing and/or speech loss, blindness, or even death.

A *neurological examination* involves a series of tests designed to assess motor and sensory function, nerve function, hearing and speech, vision, coordination and balance, mental status, and changes in mood or behavior. Doctors may test the function of the nervous system through tests of strength and sensation, with the aid of items including a tuning fork, small light, reflex hammer, and pins.

Laboratory screening of blood, urine, and body secretions can help detect and identify brain and/or spinal cord infection and determine the presence of antibodies and foreign proteins. Such tests can also rule out metabolic conditions that have similar symptoms. For example, a *throat culture* may be taken to check for viral or bacterial organisms that cause meningitis or encephalitis. In this procedure, the back of the throat is wiped with a sterile cotton swab, which is then placed on a culture medium. Viruses and bacteria are then allowed to grow on the medium. Samples are usually taken in the physician's office or in a laboratory setting and sent out for analysis to state laboratories or to the U.S. Centers for Disease Control and Prevention. Results are usually available in 2 to 3 days.

Analysis of the cerebrospinal fluid that surrounds and protects the brain and spinal cord can detect infections in the brain and/or spinal cord, acute and chronic inflammation, and other diseases. In a procedure known as a spinal tap (or lumbar puncture), a small amount of cerebrospinal fluid is removed by a special needle that is inserted into the lower back. The skin is anesthetized with a local anesthetic prior to the sampling. The fluid, which is completely clear in healthy people, is tested to detect the presence of bacteria or blood, as well as to measure glucose levels (a low glucose level can be seen in bacterial or fungal meningitis) and white blood cells (elevated white blood cell counts are also a sign of infection). The procedure is done in a hospital and takes about 45 minutes. The individual will most often be placed on antibiotics and an antiviral drug while awaiting the final microbiology results as delay in treatment can be life-threatening.

Brain imaging can reveal signs of brain inflammation, internal bleeding or hemorrhage, or other brain abnormalities. Two painless, noninvasive imaging procedures are routinely used to diagnose meningitis and encephalitis.

- *Computed tomography*, also known as a CT scan, combines x-rays and computer technology to produce rapid, clear, two-dimensional images of organs, bones, and tissues. Occasionally a contrast dye is injected into the bloodstream to highlight the different tissues in the brain and to detect signs of encephalitis or inflammation of the meninges. CT scans can also detect bone and blood vessel irregularities, certain brain tumors and cysts, herniated discs, spinal stenosis (narrowing of the spinal canal), blood clots or intracranial bleeding in patients with stroke, brain damage from a head injury, and other disorders. If the individual has abnormal results on a neurological examination, often a CT scan is performed to look for brain swelling, hemorrhage, or abscess which if present, could make a spinal tap unsafe.

- *Magnetic resonance imaging* (MRI) uses computer-generated radio waves and a strong magnet to produce detailed images of body structures, including tissues, organs, bones, and nerves. There is no radiation involved in this test and it gives a much better picture of the actual brain tissue. This may not be available in the emergency setting so a CT scan is usually performed first in very ill individuals. The pictures, which are clearer than those produced by CT, can help identify brain and spinal cord inflammation, infection, tumors, eye disease, and blood vessel irregularities that may lead to stroke. A contrast dye may be injected prior to the test to reveal more detail.

Electroencephalography, or EEG, can identify abnormal brain waves by monitoring electrical activity in the brain through the skull. Among its many functions, EEG is used to help diagnose seizures or patterns that may suggest specific viral infections such as herpes virus. This painless, risk-free test can be performed in a doctor's office or at a hospital or testing facility.

How are these infections treated?

Persons who are suspected of having meningitis or encephalitis should receive immediate, aggressive medical treatment. Both diseases can progress quickly and have the potential to cause severe, irreversible neurological damage.

Meningitis

Early treatment of bacterial meningitis is important to its outcome, with antibiotics that can cross the protective blood-brain lining. Appropriate antibiotic treatment for most types of meningitis can reduce the risk of dying from the disease to below 15 percent.

Infected sinuses may need to be drained. Corticosteroids such as prednisone may be ordered to relieve brain pressure and swelling and to prevent hearing loss that is common in patients with *Haemophilus influenza* meningitis. Lyme disease is treated with intravenous antibiotics.

Unlike bacteria, viruses cannot be killed by antibiotics; generally there is no specific treatment for viruses except for the herpes virus, which can be treated with the antiviral drug acyclovir. The physician may prescribe anticonvulsants such as dilantin or phenytoin to prevent seizures and corticosteroids to reduce brain inflammation. If inflammation is severe, pain medicine and sedatives may be prescribed to make the person more comfortable.

Acute disseminated encephalomyelitis is treated with steroids. Fungal meningitis is treated with intravenous antifungal medications.

Encephalitis

Antiviral drugs used to treat viral encephalitis include acyclovir and ganciclovir.

Anticonvulsants may be prescribed to stop or prevent seizures. Corticosteroids can reduce brain swelling. Individuals with breathing difficulties may require artificial respiration.

Individuals should receive evaluation for comprehensive rehabilitation that might include cognitive rehabilitation, physical, speech, and occupational therapy once the acute illness is under control.

Can meningitis and encephalitis be prevented?

Avoid sharing food, utensils, glasses, and other objects with a person who may be exposed to or have the infection. Wash hands often with soap and rinse under running water.

Effective vaccines are available to prevent pneumonia, H. influenza, pneumococcal meningitis, and infection with other bacteria that can cause meningococcal meningitis.

People who live, work, or go to school with someone who has been diagnosed with bacterial meningitis may be asked to take antibiotics for a few days as a preventive measure.

To lessen the risk of being bitten by an infected mosquito or other insect, people should limit outdoor activities at night, wear long-sleeved clothing when outdoors, use insect repellents that are most effective for that particular region of the country, and rid lawn and outdoor areas of free-standing pools of water, in which mosquitoes breed. Do not over-apply repellants, particularly on young children and especially infants, as chemicals such as DEET may be absorbed through the skin.

What is the prognosis for these infections?

Outcome generally depends on the particular infectious agent involved, the severity of the illness, and how quickly treatment is given. In most cases, people with very mild encephalitis or meningitis can make a full recovery, although the process may be slow.

Individuals who experience only headache, fever, and stiff neck may recover in 2–4 weeks. Those with bacterial meningitis typically show some relief 48–72 hours following initial treatment but are more likely to experience complications caused by the disease. In more serious cases, these diseases can cause hearing and/or speech loss, blindness, permanent brain and nerve damage, behavioral changes, cognitive disabilities, lack of muscle control, seizures, and memory loss. These patients may need long-term therapy, medication, and supportive care. The recovery from encephalitis is variable depending on the cause and extent of brain inflammation.

What research is being done?

The National Institute of Neurological Disorders and Stroke (NINDS), a component of the National Institutes of Health (NIH) within the U.S. Department of Health and Human Services, conducts and supports a wide range of research on neurological disorders, including meningitis and encephalitis. Current research efforts include gaining a better understanding of how the central nervous system responds to inflammation and the role of T cells (blood cells involved in immune system response) in suppressing infection in the brain. Scientists hope to better understand the molecular mechanisms involved in the protection and disruption of the blood-brain barrier, which could lead to the development of new treatments for several neuroinflammatory diseases such as meningitis and encephalitis. Other scientists hope to define, at a molecular level, how certain viruses overcome the body's defense mechanism and interact with target host cells. A possible therapeutic approach under investigation involves testing neuroprotective compounds that block the damage that accumulates after the infection and inflammation of meningitis and encephalitis and can lead to potential complications including loss of cognitive function and dementia.

Chapter 16

Progressive Multifocal Leukoencephalopathy (PML)

What is Progressive Multifocal Leukoencephalopathy?

Progressive multifocal leukoencephalopathy (PML) is a disease of the white matter of the brain, caused by a virus infection that targets cells that make myelin—the material that insulates nerve cells (neurons). Polyomavirus JC (often called JC virus) is carried by a majority of people and is harmless except among those with lowered immune defenses.

Who gets PML?

The disease is rare and occurs in patients undergoing chronic corticosteroid or immunosuppressive therapy for organ transplant, or individuals with cancer (such as Hodgkin's disease or lymphoma). Individuals with autoimmune conditions such as multiple sclerosis, rheumatoid arthritis, and systemic lupus erythematosis—some of whom are treated with biological therapies that allow JC virus reactivation—are at risk for PML as well. PML is most common among individuals with HIV-1 infection.

Text in this chapter is excerpted from "Progressive Multifocal Leukoencephalopathy," National Institute of Neurological Disorders and Stroke (NINDS), February 14, 2014.

Studies estimate that prior to effective antiretroviral therapy, as many as 5 percent of persons infected with HIV-1 eventually develop PML that is an AIDS-defining illness. However, current HIV therapy using antiretroviral drugs (ART), which effectively restores immune system function, allows as many as half of all HIV-PML patients to survive, although they may sometimes have an inflammatory reaction in the regions of the brain affected by PML.

What are the symptoms?

The symptoms of PML are diverse, since they are related to the location and amount of damage in the brain, and may evolve over the course of several weeks to months. The most prominent symptoms are clumsiness; progressive weakness; and visual, speech, and sometimes personality changes.

The progression of deficits leads to life-threatening disability and (frequently) death. A diagnosis of PML can be made following brain biopsy or by combining observations of a progressive course of the disease, consistent white matter lesions visible on a magnetic resonance imaging (MRI) scan, and the detection of the JC virus in spinal fluid.

Is there any treatment?

Currently, the best available therapy is reversal of the immune-deficient state, since there are no effective drugs that block virus infection without toxicity. Reversal may be achieved by using plasma exchange to accelerate the removal of the therapeutic agents that put patients at risk for PML. In the case of HIV-associated PML, immediately beginning anti-retroviral therapy will benefit most individuals. Several new drugs that laboratory tests found effective against infection are being used in PML patients with special permission of the U.S. Food and Drug Administration. Hexadecyloxypropyl-Cidofovir (CMX001) is currently being studied as a treatment option for JVC because of its ability to suppress JVC by inhibiting viral DNA replication.

What is the prognosis?

In general, PML has a mortality rate of 30–50 percent in the first few months following diagnosis but depends on the severity of the underlying disease and treatment received. Those who survive PML can be left with severe neurological disabilities.

Chapter 17

Vasculitis Syndromes of the Central and Peripheral Nervous Systems

What is vasculitis?

Vasculitis is an inflammation of blood vessels, which includes the veins, arteries, and capillaries. Depending on the type, vasculitis can affect blood vessels of any type, size, or location. Inflammation occurs with infection or is thought to be due to a faulty immune system response. Dysfunction may occur due to the inflammation itself or over time as the blood vessel walls swell, harden, thicken, and develop scar tissue. This narrows the passage through which blood can flow. As the condition progresses, it can slow or completely stop the normal flow of blood.

How does vasculitis affect the nervous system?

Vasculitis can cause problems in any organ system, including the central (CNS) and peripheral (PNS) nervous systems. Vasculitic disorders, or syndromes, of the CNS and PNS are characterized by the

---

Text in this chapter is excerpted from "Vasculitis Syndromes of the Central and Peripheral Nervous Systems Fact Sheet," National Institute of Neurological Disorders and Stroke (NINDS), February 23, 2015.

presence of inflammatory cells in and around blood vessels, and secondary narrowing or blockage of the blood vessels that nourish the brain, spinal cord, or peripheral nerves. Any type or size of blood vessel may be involved—arteries, arterioles, veins, venules, or capillaries.

What are the symptoms?

A vasculitis syndrome may begin suddenly or develop over time. Symptoms include:

- headaches, especially a headache that doesn't go away
- fever
- malaise (feeling out-of-sorts)
- rapid weight loss
- confusion or forgetfulness leading to dementia
- aches and pains in the joints and muscles
- pain while chewing or swallowing
- paralysis or numbness, usually in the arms or legs
- visual disturbances, such as double vision, blurred vision, or blindness
- seizures, convulsions
- stroke or transient ischemic attack (TIA, sometimes also called a "mini-stroke")
- unusual rashes or skin discoloration
- problems with the kidneys or other organs

How are these syndromes diagnosed?

A doctor who suspects CNS or PNS vasculitis will gather a comprehensive medical history of the individual, perform a physical examination, order laboratory tests (primarily blood tests), and recommend any other tests that seem appropriate. Electromyography and nerve conduction studies identify blocks and loss of nerve supply to muscle due to vasculitic nerve damage.

Diagnostic imaging of the brain blood vessels such as magnetic resonance or computed tomography angiograms can sometimes identify narrowing in the larger blood vessels. Direct injection of a contrast dye into brain blood vessels may be needed to look for narrowings consistent with vasculitis in medium-sized brain arteries.

However, the diagnosis of vasculitis often requires evidence that there is ongoing inflammation. Inflammatory cells may be found in the spinal fluid. Often there is a need to conduct a tissue biopsy to examine blood vessels under a microscope. In some cases a brain biopsy may be necessary to evaluate the compromised tissue. A definitive diagnosis is important because the treatment usually requires powerful immune-suppressive drugs. In addition, it is important to make sure that an infection is not causing the inflammation.

What are some of these syndromes called and how are they treated?

The diagnosis of a CNS or PNS vasculitis disorder will depend upon the number of blood vessels involved, their size, and their location in the CNS or PNS as well as the types of organs involved. Although these disorders are rare, there are many of them. Some of the better understood syndromes are:

Temporal arteritis (also called giant cell arteritis or cranial arteritis)

Temporal arteritis is a common chronic inflammatory disease of large blood vessels occurring primarily in people 50 and older. It most often involves narrowing and sometimes blockage of the arteries that bring blood to the brain. Doctors will diagnose temporal arteritis if at least three of the following symptoms are present:

- new, severe headache
- visual disturbances
- pain in the jaw or tongue when chewing or swallowing
- tenderness in the temporal arteries (the arteries that run across the temples on either side of the head) or the scalp

Fever, weight loss, and neck or muscle pain can occur, usually in the early phase of the disease. Individuals may also have arthritis; carpal tunnel syndrome; fatigue; and weakness, paralysis, or numbness in isolated muscles. The disease is usually limited to one to two years and is rarely fatal.

Abrupt but reversible blindness is the most dramatic complication of temporal arteritis. About one in ten individuals with temporal arteritis will develop blindness in one eye, preceded by visual disturbances. Once one eye is affected, three out of four individuals will go on to lose vision in the other eye, most in two weeks or less.

The main goal of treatment for temporal arteritis is to prevent blindness. Most individuals respond well to steroid drugs, such as prednisone and methylprednisolone, but they must be given promptly and carefully monitored. Long-term use of steroids can cause harmful side effects, such as collapsing vertebrae, muscle pain, diabetes, cataracts, and infection.

Primary angiitis of the CNS (granulomatous angiitis)

The symptoms of this rare disorder develop slowly. Symptoms include headache and encephalopathy-like symptoms such as dementia and tremor. Stroke, TIA, and seizures can occur. Definitive diagnosis may require brain biopsy. Treatment includes steroid and immunosuppressive drugs, such as prednisolone and cyclophosphamide. It is fatal if left untreated.

Takayasu's disease

This disease affects large arteries such as the aorta, which brings blood to the arms, legs, and head. It primarily strikes individuals of Asian descent and predominantly affects females under the age of 40. The main symptoms are fainting and visual disturbances and it may also cause stroke. Although the disorder is serious, the prognosis is positive: more than 90 percent of those diagnosed with Takayasu's disease survive beyond a decade after diagnosis. Steroid drugs are used in the early phase of the disease, but some individuals become steroid-resistant and have to switch to cyclophosphamide or low-dose methotrexate.

Periarteritis nodosa

The onset of this rare and serious disease is generally between the ages of 40 and 50, but it can occur at any age. Men are three times more likely to develop the disease than women. Symptoms can mimic those of many other diseases, but the most common initial complaints are fever, abdominal pain, numbness or pain in the legs and limbs, weakness, and unexplained weight loss. As the disease progresses, the kidneys may fail and high blood pressure may develop rapidly. Certain drugs (for example, those in the sulfa family), vaccines, bacterial infections, and viral infections have been associated with the onset of the disease. Damage to the PNS with neuropathy is more common than damage to the CNS, but if the disease does involve the CNS, damage to brain and spinal cord tissue can occur.

The disease is treated aggressively with high doses of steroids and immunosuppressive drugs such as cyclophosphamide. Eighty percent of individuals who receive appropriate treatment are alive five years later. Untreated disease is often fatal, ending in heart failure, kidney failure, or failure of other vital organs.

Are there additional vasculitis disorders that can cause neurological symptoms?

Other vasculitis syndromes include Kawasaki disease, which can cause stroke or encephalopathy in children; Churg-Strauss syndrome; Wegener's granulomatosis; systemic lupus erythematosus; scleroderma; rheumatoid arthritis; Sjogren's syndrome; and Behcet's disease.

What research is being done to better understand these syndromes?

The National Institute of Neurological Disorders and Stroke (NINDS), a component of the National Institutes of Health (NIH), and other NIH institutes conduct research relating to vasculitis syndromes in laboratories at the NIH and also support vasculitis research through grants to major medical institutions across the country.

The NINDS supports The Vasculitis Clinical Research Consortium (VCRC), a network of academic medical centers, patient support organizations, and clinical research resources dedicated to conducting clinical research and improving the care of individuals with vasculitis, including Wegener's granulomatosis, microscopic polyangiitis, Churg-Strauss syndrome, polyarteritis nodosa, Takayasu's arteritis, and temporal arteritis. The medical centers are located at Boston University School of Medicine, Cleveland Clinic Foundation, The Johns Hopkins Vasculitis Center, and Mayo Clinic College of Medicine. The Consortium's internet site provides information about clinical research and clinical trial opportunities and helps individuals connect with expert doctors and patient support groups.

Part Four

Acquired and Traumatic Brain Injuries

Chapter 18

Concussion and Mild TBI

Definition of Mild Traumatic Brain Injury (MTBI)

The term mild traumatic brain injury (MTBI) is used interchangeably with the term concussion. An MTBI or concussion is defined as a complex pathophysiologic process affecting the brain, induced by traumatic biomechanical forces secondary to direct or indirect forces to the head. MTBI is caused by a blow or jolt to the head that disrupts the function of the brain. This disturbance of brain function is typically associated with normal structural neuroimaging findings (i.e., CT scan, MRI). MTBI results in a constellation of physical, cognitive, emotional and/or sleep-related symptoms and may or may not involve a loss of consciousness (LOC). Duration of symptoms is highly variable and may last from several minutes to days, weeks, months, or even longer in some cases.[1,2]

Physicians can play a key role in helping to prevent mild traumatic brain injury (MTBI or concussion) and in appropriately identifying, diagnosing, and managing it when it does occur. Physicians can also improve patient outcomes when MTBI is suspected or diagnosed by implementing early management and appropriate referral. MTBI symptoms may appear mild, but can lead to significant, life-long impairment affecting an individual's ability to function physically, cognitively, and psychologically. Appropriate diagnosis, referral, and

---

Text in this chapter is excerpted from "Facts for Physicians about Mild Traumatic Brain Injury (MTBI)," Centers for Disease Control and Prevention (CDC).

patient and family/caregiver education are critical for helping patients with MTBI achieve optimal recovery and to reduce or avoid significant sequelae.

Magnitude of MTBI

- An estimated 75%–90% of the 1.4 million traumatic brain injury (TBI)-related deaths, hospitalizations, and emergency department visits that occur each year are concussions or other forms of MTBI.[3-6]

- Approximately 1.6–3.8 million sports and recreation-related TBIs occur in the United States each year.[7] Most of these are MTBIs that are not treated in a hospital or emergency department.

- Blasts are an important cause of MTBI among military personnel in war zones.[8]

- Direct medical costs and indirect costs such as lost productivity from MTBI totaled an estimated $12 billion in the United States in 2000.[9]

- Individuals with a history of concussion are at an increased risk of sustaining a subsequent concussion.[10]

- Duration of symptoms is highly variable and may last from several minutes to days, weeks, months, or even longer in some cases. Research shows that recovery time may be longer for children and adolescents.[11,12]

- Symptoms or deficits that continue beyond three months may be a sign of post-concussion syndrome.[13]

Leading causes of MTBI (seen in emergency departments)[16]

- Falls
- Motor vehicle trauma
- Unintentionally struck by/against events
- Assaults and
- Sports

Groups at highest risk for MTBI[16]

- Infants and children (ages 0 to 4)
- Children and young adults (ages 5 to 24) and
- Older adults (ages 75 or older)

- With proper diagnosis and management, most patients with MTBI recover fully.[14,15]

Neuropathophysiology of MTBI

Unlike more severe TBIs, the disturbance of brain function from MTBI is related more to dysfunction of brain metabolism rather than to structural injury or damage. The current understanding of the underlying pathology of MTBI involves a paradigm shift away from a focus on anatomic damage to an emphasis on neuronal dysfunction involving a complex cascade of ionic, metabolic and physiologic events. Clinical signs and symptoms of MTBI such as poor memory, speed of processing, fatigue, and dizziness result from this underlying neurometabolic cascade.[17]

Signs and Symptoms

Signs and symptoms of MTBI generally fall into four categories: physical, cognitive, emotional, and sleep.

Table 18.1. Categories of Signs and Symptoms

Physical	Cognitive	Emotional	Sleep
• Headache • Nausea • Vomiting • Balance problems • Dizziness • Visual problems • Fatigue • Sensitivity to light • Sensitivity to noise • Numbness/ Tingling • Dazed or stunned	• Feeling mentally "foggy" • Feeling slowed down • Difficulty concentrating • Difficulty remembering • Forgetful of recent information or conversations • Confused about recent events • Answers questions slowly • Repeats questions	• Irritability • Sadness • More emotional • Nervousness	• Drowsiness • Sleeping less than usual • Trouble falling asleep

Diagnosis

Diagnosing MTBIs can be challenging as symptoms of MTBI are common to those of other medical conditions (such as post-traumatic stress disorder [PTSD], depression, and headache syndromes), and the onset and/or recognition of symptoms may occur days or weeks after the initial injury.[14,18]

A systematic assessment of the injury and its manifestations is essential to proper management and reduced morbidity. The Acute Concussion Evaluation (ACE) form was developed to provide physicians with an evidence-based protocol to conduct an initial evaluation and diagnosis of patients (both children and adults) with known or suspected MTBI. The research evidence documenting the importance of these components in the evaluation of an MTBI is provided in the reference list. The ACE can also be used serially to track symptom recovery over time. It provides a systematic protocol for assessing the key components for diagnosing an MTBI and serves as the basis for management and referral recommendations provided by the ACE Care Plan (two versions). These tools were developed to provide physicians with a more individualized assessment of MTBI and to help guide the management and recovery, as well as the referral of patients with such injuries.

Editor's Note: For more information on ACE form please contact your physician or visit http://www.cdc.gov/headsup/pdfs/providers/ace-a.pdf

MTBI is an important concern among military personnel returning from war zones. Symptoms of MTBI may be missed or may not be noticed until after they have returned home. The identification and management of MTBI in these patients may also be complicated by the presence of PTSD.

The ACE contains three major components that require evaluation:

- Characteristics of the injury;
- Types and severity of the symptoms; and
- Risk factors that can lead to a protracted period of recovery.

The ACE should be administered to patients for whom concussion is clearly indicated (e.g., loss of consciousness or change in mental status, confusion or amnesia) and to those for whom concussion should be suspected (e.g., other traumatic injuries are observed or reported; forcible blow to the head with functional changes).

For example, concussions are often not recognized among children with orthopedic injuries. Physicians should consider screening for possible concussion among patients with various other types of injuries such as:

- High-speed activities (motor vehicle crashes, bicycle riding, skateboarding)

- Sports and recreation activities

- Falls (including those among older adults), especially from a significant distance (e.g., off a ladder, from a tree)

- Suspected child maltreatment (e.g., shaking, hitting, throwing)

- Exposure to blasts (includes military personnel returning from war zones)

- Injuries to the external parts of the head and/or scalp (e.g., lacerations)

The following summarizes the information contained on the ACE and outlines steps for diagnosing a patient with a known or suspected MTBI.

A. Injury Characteristics

1. **Injury Description**. Ask the patient (and/or parent, if child) about how the injury occurred, type of force, and location on the head or body where the force (blow) was received. Different biomechanics of injury may result in varied symptom patterns. For example, an injury that occurs to the posterior aspect of the head may result in visual changes, balance problems, and fatigue. The force to the head may be indirect, such as with an individual being struck in the body resulting in the head accelerating forward and then backward quickly (e.g., whiplash).

2. **Cause**. The cause of the injury may also help to estimate the force of the hit or blow the patient sustained. The greater the force associated with the injury, the more likely the patient will present with more severe symptoms. Conversely, significant symptoms associated with a relatively light force might indicate an increased vulnerability to MTBI (especially among patients with a history of multiple MTBIs or preexisting

history of migraine) or the presence of other physical or psychological factors contributing to symptom exacerbation.

3. **Amnesia (Retrograde).** Determine whether amnesia (memory loss) has occurred for events before the injury and attempt to determine the length of time of memory dysfunction. Research indicates that even seconds of amnesia may predict more serious injury.[19]

4. **Amnesia (Anterograde).** Determine whether amnesia has occurred for events after the injury and attempt to determine the length of time of memory dysfunction. Anterograde amnesia is also referred to as post-traumatic amnesia (PTA).

5. **Loss of Consciousness (LOC).** Inquire whether LOC occurred or was observed and the length of time the patient lost consciousness. (Note: Research indicates that up to 90% of concussions do not involve LOC.)[19,20]

6. **Early Signs Observed by Others.** Ask those who know the patient (parent, spouse, friend, etc) about specific signs of the MTBI that they may have observed. These signs are typically observed early after the injury. Record their presence or absence with a checkmark.

7. **Seizures.** Inquire whether seizures were observed (although this is uncommon).

B. Symptom Check List

Record the presence and severity of physical, cognitive, emotional, and sleep symptoms and the early signs since the injury.

1. **Signs and Symptoms.** Use the ACE to record symptoms reported by the patient (and/or parent, if child) in each of the four symptom areas (physical, cognitive, emotional, and sleep). Determine if each symptom is present. If not present, circle "0" for No. If symptom is present (within the past 24 hours), circle "1" for Yes. Since symptoms can be present prior to the injury (e.g., inattention, headaches), it is important to assess any changes from usual symptom presentation.19,21 Sum the total number of symptoms for each of the four symptom areas and for the Total Symptom Score. Any Total Symptom Score greater than "0" indicates a positive symptom profile. (Note: any presentation of lingering and/or persistent symptoms

associated with MTBI indicates incomplete recovery and prudent management is indicated, especially pertaining to activities such as work, school, and sports.)

2. **Exertion.** Inquire whether any symptoms worsen with exertion, that is, with physical activity (e.g., running, climbing stairs, bike riding) and/or cognitive activity (e.g., academic studies, multi-tasking at work, reading or other tasks requiring focused concentration). Physicians should be aware that symptoms will typically worsen or re-emerge with exertion, indicating incomplete recovery, which may also be protracted with over-exertion.

3. **Overall "Difference" Rating.** Obtain an overall rating from the patient (and/or parent, if child) regarding their overall perceived change from their pre-injury self. This rating is helpful in summarizing the overall impact of the symptoms. Use the 7 point scale with "0" reflecting no change from normal, to "6" reflecting a major change.

C. Signs of Deteriorating Neurological Function

It is important to assess whether the patient with an MTBI exhibits any signs or reports any symptoms that would indicate deteriorating neurological functioning. Patients should be carefully observed over the first 24–48 hours for the serious signs listed below.[22] If any of these signs are reported, they should be referred to an emergency department for an immediate medical evaluation.

- Headaches that worsen
- Seizures
- Focal neurologic signs
- Looks very drowsy or can't be awakened
- Repeated vomiting
- Slurred speech
- Can't recognize people or places
- Increasing confusion or irritability
- Weakness or numbness in arms or legs
- Neck pain

- Unusual behavior change

- Significant irritability

- Any loss of consciousness greater than 30 seconds or longer. *(Brief loss of consciousness (under 30 seconds) should be taken seriously and the patient should be carefully monitored.)*

D. Identify Risk Factors that may Complicate the Recovery Process

Each of the factors below has been identified through empirical research to be associated with a longer period of recovery from an MTBI. Identifying any of these factors is helpful for understanding the nature and extent of the patient's injury and for monitoring their recovery.

1. **Concussion (or MTBI) History.** Assess the number and date(s) of prior concussions and the duration of symptoms for each injury. The effects of multiple MTBIs may be cumulative, especially if there is minimal duration of time between injuries and less biomechanical force results in subsequent MTBI (which may indicate incomplete recovery from the initial trauma).[10,21-26]

2. **Headache History.** Assess prior personal and/or family history of diagnosis and treatment for headaches. Headaches (migraines in particular) can result in protracted recovery from MTBI.[27-29]

3. **Developmental History.** Assess for a history of learning disabilities, Attention-Deficit/Hyperactivity Disorder or other developmental disorders. Recovery may take longer in patients with these conditions.[30]

4. **Psychiatric History.** Assess for history of depression/mood disorder, anxiety, and/or sleep disorder.[31-33]

E. Establishing the Diagnosis

Following the above assessment, the diagnosis of concussion or MTBI using the following ICD–9–CM codes may be applicable:

- **850.0 (Concussion, with no loss of consciousness)**–Positive injury description with evidence of a direct or indirect forcible blow to the head, plus evidence of active symptoms and/or signs of any type and number related to the trauma; no evidence of LOC, skull fracture, internal bleed (i.e., intracranial injury).

- **850.1 (Concussion, with brief loss of consciousness < 1 hour)**–Positive injury description with evidence of a direct or indirect forcible blow to the head, plus evidence of active symptoms and/or signs of any type and number related to the trauma; positive evidence of LOC; no skull fracture, internal bleed.

- **850.9 (Concussion, unspecified)**–Positive injury description with evidence of a direct or indirect forcible blow to the head, plus evidence of active symptoms and/or signs of any type and number related to the trauma; unclear or unknown injury details and unclear evidence of LOC; no skull fracture, internal bleed.

If there is evidence of prolonged LOC (>1 hour), skull fracture, and/or intracranial injury, the diagnosis of 854 should be considered (consult the ICD–9–CM manual for detailed codes). Use of ICD–9–CM **959.01 Head injury, unspecified** is not recommended for concussion/MTBI, as it excludes the above concussion diagnoses and is non-specific.

Clinical Management

The first step to improving outcomes for patients with MTBI is to determine a plan of action for follow-up. Based on the findings of an evaluation, such as that provided by the ACE, the physician may decide to:

1. **Monitor the Patient in the Office.** Office monitoring is particularly appropriate if the number and severity of symptoms are steadily decreasing over time and/or fully resolve within 3 to 5 days. However, if symptoms have not fully abated in this time period, or remain steady or worsen, referral to an MTBI specialist may be warranted.

2. **Make a Referral to an MTBI Specialist.** Referral to a specialist who cares for patients with MTBI is appropriate if symptom reduction is not evident within 3 to 5 days post injury, or sooner, and if the type or severity of symptoms is of concern. Referral to a specialist can be particularly valuable to further evaluate the patient's complex presentation and to help manage certain aspects of their condition (e.g., return to sports, school, and work). (Information about specific TBI specialists in a particular area is often available through state or national brain injury associations.)

Infants, Toddlers and Preschool Children

Very young children (i.e. infants, toddlers, and preschoolers) frequently sustain bumps and bruises to their heads from a host of mechanisms including falls (down stairs or from heights such as counter tops or beds), direct impacts (e.g. getting hit in the head with a ball), motor vehicle crashes, tricycle/bike accidents or child abuse.

Sometimes these events can be significant enough to result in a concussion.

Deciding whether a child who has hit his or her head needs an immediate assessment to determine whether he or she has had a concussion can be difficult, as young children may have the same symptoms of a concussion as older children, but do not express them in the same way. For example, young children cannot explain a feeling of nausea or amnesia or even describe where they hurt. Physicians should therefore keep this in mind when they ask parents about the presence of the symptoms listed below and have a low threshold for referring a child for immediate evaluation. Primary care physicians (PCPs) should ask caregivers about all "bumps on the head" and should consider referring a child with a "bump on the head" to the emergency department if they suspect a concussion but are unsure about the symptoms.

Acute signs and symptoms of a concussion:

- Vomiting
- Headache
- Crying and inability to be consoled
- Restlessness or irritability
- Seizures
- Dizziness or confusion
- Change in personality

Follow-up in Young Children who have Sustained Concussions

All children with concussion or suspected concussion should be followed closely by their PCP. A follow-up visit with the PCP after the event can offer the opportunity for families to ask questions and for the PCP to assess the child for ongoing symptoms.

Although diagnosing post-concussion syndrome in young children is difficult, it is important to assess for these symptoms in order to determine whether children need further evaluation. The follow-up visit can also provide an important opportunity for discussion of age-appropriate injury prevention which is important to minimize the possibility of subsequent concussions. Infants and young children less than 3 years of age who have had a concussion can have their development tracked by their county's developmental program for young children; this is particularly important for children who have sustained a complicated concussion (i.e., with contusions or hemorrhage apparent on imaging), those who have had multiple concussions and/or those with underlying neurologic disease.

Persistent signs and symptoms to assess for during follow-up:

- Excessive crying
- Persistent headache
- Poor attention
- Change in sleep patterns
- Change in nursing or eating habitsPersistent headache
- Becoming upset easily or increased temper tantrums
- Sad or lethargic mood
- Lack of interest in favorite toys

Children who display these symptoms for more than several weeks after a concussion may require further assessment and/or evaluation by a neuropsychologist, neurologist, or other specialist.

Abusive TBI

Young children may also sustain mild to severe TBIs from abuse.

- Approximately 1,400 cases of abusive TBI (including concussions) occur in the U.S. each year.[35]
- Injuries resulting from abusive TBI and other types of child maltreatment are often unrecognized or under reported.[35]
- Recognition of abusive TBI in young children is critical. If children are returned to a violent home, they are at very high risk of being hurt again or killed.
- In any young child with injury to the head, it is imperative to assess whether the history provided for the injury is developmentally appropriate for a child that age. If not, it is important to consider child abuse in the differential diagnosis.

- In some cases of abuse, caretakers do not report a history of any trauma either because (a) they do not know that there has been trauma because it is being inflicted by someone else without their knowledge or (b) because they don't want to tell. As a result, if an infant or young child presents with the signs and symptoms listed above, it is important to consider the possibility of abusive TBI even in the absence of a history of trauma.

3. **Refer the Patient for Diagnostic Testing.** During the acute phase, diagnostic tests may include neuroimaging (such as a CT or MRI scan) or neuropsychological testing.[34] Neuropsychological tests, which involve performance of specific cognitive tasks, can be helpful for confirming self-reported symptoms and tracking recovery. They assess a range of abilities such as memory, concentration, information processing, executive function, and reaction time.[34] Brief (approx. 25 minutes) and recently validated computerized test batteries and/or abbreviated traditional (paper and pencil) test batteries may be most practical and informative during this early phase.

Neuropsychological tests may also be helpful for determining the appropriate timing for return to safe sports participation, school, or work. Any indication or suspicion of neurologic deterioration should prompt strong consideration for referral to emergency medical evaluation and/or neuroimaging to rule out intracranial bleed or other structural pathology.

For patients with persisting symptoms, more extensive neuropsychological and neurobehavioral test batteries can be useful for identifying specific deficits and needed supports for return to daily activities, school, or work.

Management Approaches

It is critical for the physician to guide the patient in their recovery with an active management plan based on their current symptom presentation. Careful management can facilitate recovery and prevent further injury. The two ACE Care Plans are based on current research and clinical experience and were developed to help physicians actively manage patients with known or suspected MTBI.

Rest and Careful Management of Physical and Cognitive Exertion are the Keys to Recovery

Patients must not return to high risk activities (e.g., sports, physical education (PE), high speed activity (riding a bicycle or carnival rides), if *any* post-concussion symptoms are present or if results from cognitive testing show persistent deficits. When symptoms are no longer reported or experienced, a patient may slowly, gradually, and carefully return to their daily activities (both physical and cognitive). Children and adolescents will need the help of their parents, teachers, coaches, athletic trainers, etc. to monitor and assist with their recovery. Management planning should involve all aspects of the patient's life including home life, school, work, and social-recreational activities.

Returning to Daily Home / Community Activities

Increased rest and limited exertion are important to facilitate the patient's recovery. Physicians should be cautious about allowing patients to return to driving, especially if the patient has problems with attention, processing speed, or reaction time. Patients should also be advised to get adequate sleep at night and to take daytime naps or rest breaks when significant fatigue is experienced. Symptoms typically worsen or re-emerge with exertion. Let any return of a patient's symptoms be the guide to the level of exertion or activity that is safe.

Patients should limit both physical and cognitive exertion accordingly.

- Physical activity includes PE, sports practices, weight-training, running, exercising, heavy lifting, etc.
- Cognitive activity includes heavy concentration or focus, memory, reasoning, reading or writing (e.g., homework, classwork, job-related mental activity).

As symptoms decrease, or as cognitive test results show improvement, patients may return to their regular activities gradually. However, the patient's overall status should continue to be monitored closely.

Returning to School

Symptomatic students may require active supports and accommodations in school, which may be gradually decreased as their functioning improves. Inform the student's teacher(s), the school nurse, psychologist/counselor, and administrator of the student's injury, symptoms, and cognitive deficits. Students with temporary yet prolonged symptoms (i.e. longer than several weeks) or permanent disability may benefit from referral for special accommodations and services, such as those provided under a Section 504 Plan.

Section 504 Plans:

Section 504 Plans are implemented when students have a disability (temporary or permanent) that affects their performance in any manner. Services and accommodations for students may include environmental, curriculum, methodology, organizational, behavioral, and presentation strategies.

School personnel should be advised to monitor the student for the following signs:

- Increased problems paying attention/concentrating
- Increased problems remembering/learning new information
- Longer time required to complete tasks
- Increased symptoms (e.g., headache, fatigue) during schoolwork
- Greater irritability, less tolerance for stressors

Until a full recovery is achieved, students may need the following supports:

- Time off from school
- Shortened day
- Shortened classes (i.e., rest breaks during classes)
- Rest breaks during the day
- Allowances for extended time to complete coursework/assignments and tests
- Reduced homework/classwork load (it is best to specify for teachers the percent of workload that the student can reasonably handle, e.g., 50% homework load)
- No significant classroom or standardized testing at this time

Physicians and school personnel should monitor the student's symptoms with cognitive exertion (mental effort such as concentration, studying) to evaluate the need and length of time supports should be provided.

Returning to Play (Sports and Recreation)

Guiding the recovery of individuals of any age with MTBI who participate in competitive or recreational activities requires careful management to avoid re-injury or prolonged recovery. Athletes engaged in collision sports require special management and evaluation to ensure full recovery prior to their return to play.

An individual should never return to competitive sporting or recreational activities while experiencing any lingering or persisting MTBI symptoms. This includes PE class, sports practices and games, and other high-risk/high-exertion activities such as running, bike riding, skateboarding, climbing trees, jumping from heights, playful wrestling, etc. The individual should be completely symptom free at rest and with physical exertion (e.g., sprints, non-contact aerobic activity) and cognitive exertion (e.g., studying, schoolwork) prior to return to sports or recreational activities.

Along with parent and teacher observation for continuing signs or symptoms of concussion, objective data in the form of formal neuropsychological testing may provide valuable information to assist with return to play decisions in younger athletes, as their symptom reporting may be more limited and less reliable. Formal neuropsychological testing of competitive athletes may also help physicians with return to play decisions, as athletes may minimize their symptoms to facilitate return to play.[1]

It is important to inform the athlete's coach, PE teacher, and/or athletic trainer that the athlete should not return to play until they are symptom-free and their cognitive function has returned to normal, both at rest and with exertion.

Return to play should occur gradually. Individuals should be monitored for symptoms and cognitive function carefully during each stage of increased exertion. Patients should only progress to the next level of exertion if they are asymptomatic at the current level. In competitive sports, a specific return to play protocol outlining gradual increase in activity has been established by the Concussion in Sport Group:[1]

- Rest

- Aerobic exercise (e.g., stationary bicycle)

- Sport-specific training (e.g., running, skating)

- Non-contact drills (includes cutting and other lateral movements)
- Full contact controlled training
- Full contact game play

Returning to Work

Return-to-work planning should be based upon careful evaluation of symptoms and neurocognitive status. To help expedite recovery from MTBI, patients may initially need to reduce both physical and cognitive exertion. Rest is key. Restricting work during initial stages of recovery may be indicated to help facilitate recovery. Repeated evaluation of both symptoms and cognitive status is recommended to help guide management considerations.

Until a full recovery is achieved, patients may need the following supports:

Schedule Considerations

- Shortened work day (e.g. 8am–12pm)
- Allow for breaks when symptoms increase
- Reduced task assignments and responsibilities

Safety Considerations

- No driving
- No heavy lifting/No working with machinery
- No heights due to risk of dizziness, balance problems

Primary Prevention

As part of preventive care, physicians can provide information to patients, families, and caregivers about behaviors and activities that increase the risk of MTBI/concussion. Recommendations for preventing MTBI include those listed below.

To reduce the risk of sustaining a concussion or a more serious TBI, patients should be advised to:

- Wear a seat belt every time they drive or ride in a motor vehicle.
- Buckle their child in the car using a child safety seat, booster seat, or seat belt (according to the child's height, weight, and age).
  - Children should start using a booster seat when they outgrow their child safety seats (usually when they weigh about 40 pounds). They should continue to ride in a booster seat until the lap/shoulder belts in the car fit properly, typically when they are approximately 4'9" tall.[36]
- Never drive while under the influence of alcohol or drugs.
- Wear a helmet and make sure their children wear helmets that are fitted and maintained properly when:
  - Riding a bike, motorcycle, snowmobile, scooter, or all-terrain vehicle;
  - Playing a contact sport, such as football, ice hockey, lacrosse, or boxing;
  - Using in-line skates or riding a skateboard;
  - Batting and running bases in baseball or softball;
  - Riding a horse; or
  - Skiing, sledding, or snowboarding.
- Ensure that during athletic games and practices that they and/ or their children:
  - Use the right protective equipment (should be fitted and maintained properly in order to provide the expected protection);
  - Follow the safety rules and those for the sport;
  - Practice good sportsmanship; and
  - Do not return to play with a known or suspected concussion until evaluated and given permission by an appropriate health care professional.
- Make living areas safer for seniors by:
  - Removing tripping hazards such as throw rugs and clutter in walkways;
  - Using nonslip mats in the bathtub and on shower floors;
  - Installing grab bars next to the toilet and in the tub or shower;
  - Installing handrails on both sides of stairways;

- Improving lighting throughout the home; and

- Maintaining a regular physical activity program, if their health care provider agrees, to improve lower body strength and balance.[37-40]

- Make living areas safer for children by:

  - Installing window guards to keep young children from falling out of open windows;

  - Using safety gates at the top and bottom of stairs when young children are around;

  - Keeping stairs clear of clutter;

  - Securing rugs and using rubber mats in bathtubs; and

  - Not allowing children to play on fire escapes or on other unsafe platforms.

- Make sure playground surfaces are made of shock-absorbing material, such as hardwood mulch or sand, and are maintained to an appropriate depth.[41,42]

Improving Communication with Patients with MTBI

Patients with MTBI, particularly during the early post-injury phase, may have difficulties communicating with a physician. Obtaining an accurate report from the patient about the injury and its symptoms with tools such as the ACE is critical to proper management. The following provides a summary of types of communication problems related to expression and comprehension that individuals with MTBI may experience, and what physicians can do to improve communication with their patients.

Problem Area	Problem Description	What Physicians Can Do
Expression	• May have trouble thinking of specific words (word finding problems) or expressing the specifics of their symptoms or functional difficulties	• Allow patients time to express themselves • Ask questions about specific symptoms and problems (i.e., are you having headaches?)

Comprehension	**Spoken:**	
	• May become confused if too much information is presented at once or too quickly • May need extra time to understand what others are saying • May have trouble following complex multi-step directions • May take longer than expected to respond to a question	• Speak slowly and clearly • Use short sentences • Repeat complex sentences when necessary • Allow time for patients to comprehend • Provide both spoken and written instructions and directions
	Written: • May read slowly • May have trouble reading material in complex formats or with small print • May have trouble filling out forms	• Allow patients extra time to read and complete forms • Provide written material in simple formats and large print when possible • Have someone read the items and fill out the forms for patients who are having trouble

In addition to the communications problems listed above, it is also important to note that patients may be sensitive to environmental stimuli. In particular, they may become disoriented or confused when exposed to:

• Bright lights;

• Complex visual stimuli such as busy carpet patterns; and/or

• Noise, including from radio or TV.

To address this, physicians should consider offering patients access to a quiet, low-stimulation waiting area if needed.

References

1. Aubry M, et al. Summary and agreement statement of the first International Conference on Concussion in Sport, Vienna 2001. Clinical Journal of Sports Medicine 2002 Jan;12(1):6-11.

2. McCrory P, et al. Summary and agreement statement of the second International Conference on Concussion in Sport, Prague 2004. British Journal of Sports Medicine 2005;39:196-204.

3. Centers for Disease Control and Prevention (CDC), National Center for Injury Prevention and Control. Report to Congress on mild traumatic brain injury in the United States: steps to prevent a serious public health problem. Atlanta (GA): Centers for Disease Control and Prevention; 2003.

4. Kraus JF, Nourjah P. The epidemiology of mild, uncomplicated brain injury. Journal of Trauma 1988;28(12):1637-43.

5. Luerssen TG, Klauber MR, Marshall LF. Outcome from head injury related to patient's age: A longitudinal prospective study of adult and pediatric head injury. Journal of Neurosurgery 1988;68(3):409-16.

6. Lescohier I, DiScala C. Blunt trauma in children: causes and outcomes of head versus intracranial injury. Pediatrics 1993;91(4):721-5.

7. Langlois JA, Rutland-Brown W, Wald M. The epidemiology and impact of traumatic brain injury: a brief overview. Journal of Head Trauma Rehabilitation 2006;21(5):375-8.

8. Warden D. Military TBI During the Iraq and Afghanistan Wars. Journal of Head Trauma and Rehabilitation 2006;21(5):398-402.

9. Finkelstein E, Corso P, Miller T and associates. The Incidence and Economic Burden of Injuries in the United States. New York (NY): Oxford University Press; 2006.

10. Guskiewicz K, et al. Cumulative effects associated with recurrent concussion in collegiate football players: the NCAA Concussion Study. JAMA 2003;290(19):2549-55.

11. Field M, Collins M, Lovell M, Maroon J. Does age play a role in recovery from sports-related concussion? A comparison of high school and collegiate athletes. The Journal of Pediatrics 2003;142(5):546-53.

12. Pellman EJ, Lovell MR, Viano DC, Casson IR. Concussion in professional football: recovery of NFL and high school athletes assessed by computerized neuropsychological testing--Part 12. Neurosurgery 2006;58(2):263-74;discussion 263-74.

13. Kashluba S, Casey JE, Paniak C. Evaluating the utility of ICD-10 diagnostic criteria for postconcussion syndrome following mild traumatic brain injury. Journal of the International Neuropsychological Society 2006;12(1):111-8.

14. Kushner DS. Mild traumatic brain injury: toward understanding manifestations and treatment. Archives of Internal Medicine 1998;158(15):1617-24.

15. Alexander MP. Mild traumatic brain injury: pathophysiology, natural history, and clinical management. Neurology 1995;45:1253-60.

16. Bazarian J, et al. Mild traumatic brain injury in the United States, 1998-2000. Brain Injury 2005;19(2):85-91.

17. Giza C, Hovda D. The neurometabolic cascade of concussion. Journal of Athletic Training 2001;36(3):228-235.

18. Centers for Disease Control and Prevention, Advisory Group, Mild Traumatic Brain Injury Tool Kit. Meeting summary [unpublished]. Atlanta, GA: CDC. 2001.

19. Collins MW, Iverson G, Lovell MR, McKeag DB, Norwig J, Maroon J. On-field predictors of neuropsychological and symptom deficit following sports-related concussion. Clinical Journal of Sport Medicine 2003;13(4):222-9.

20. Schultz MR, et al. Incidence and risk factors for concussion in high school athletes, North Carolina, 1996-1999. American Journal of Epidemiology 2004;160(10):937-944.

21. Collins MW, Lovell MR, Iverson G, Cantu R, Maroon J, Field M. Cumulative effects of concussion in high school athletes. Neurosurgery 2002;51:1175-181.

22. Fung M, Willer B, Moreland D, Leddy J. A proposal for an evidence-based emergency department discharge form for mild traumatic brain injury. Brain Injury 2006;20(9):889-94.

23. Lovell MR, Collins MW, Bradley J. Return to play following sports related concussion. Clinics in Sports Medicine 2004;23(3):421-443.

24. Iverson G, Gaetz M, Lovell MR, Collins MW. Cumulative effects of concussion in amateur athletes. Brain Injury 2004;18(5):433-43.

25. Collins MW, Field M, Lovell MR, Iverson GL, Johnston K, Maroon J, Fu F. Relationship between post-concussion headache and neuropsychological test performance in high school athletes. American Journal of Sports Medicine 2003;31:168-173.

26. Bellanger HG, Vanderploeg RD. The neuropsychological impact of sports-related concussion: a meta-analysis. Journal of the International Neuropsychological Society 2005;11(4):345-57.

27. Mihalik J, Stump J, Collins MW, Lovell MR, Field M, Maroon J. Posttraumatic migraine characteristics in athletes following sports-related concussion. Journal of Neurosurgery 2005;102(5):850-5.

28. Collins MW, Field M, Lovell MR, Iverson G, Johnston KM, Maroon J, Fu FH. Headache following sports-related concussion: To play or not to play. American Journal of Sports Medicine 2003;31(2):168-173.

29. deKruijk J, Leffers P, Menheere P, Meerhoff S, Rutten J, Twijnstra A. Prediction of post-traumatic complaints after mild traumatic brain injury: Early symptoms and biochemical markers. Journal of Neurology, Neurosurgery, and Psychiatry 2002;73(6):727-32.

30. Collins MW, et al. Relationship between concussion and neuropsychological performance in college football players. JAMA 1999;282(10):964-970.

31. Moore EL, Terryberry-Spohr L, Hope DA. Mild traumatic brain injury and anxiety sequelae: a review of the literature. Brain Injury 2006;20(2):117-32.

32. Mooney G, Speed J, Sheppard S. Factors related to recovery after mild traumatic brain injury. Brain Injury 2005;19(12):975-87.

33. Mather FJ, Tate RL, Hannan TJ. Post-traumatic stress disorder in children following road traffic accidents: A comparison of those with and without mild traumatic brain injury. Brain Injury;17(12):1077-87.

34. Bazarian J, Blyth B, Cimpello L. Bench to beside: evidence for brain injury after concussion—looking beyond the computed tomography scan. Academic Emergency Medicine 2006;13(2):199-214.

35. Newton AW, Vandeven AM. Unexplained infant and child death: a review of Sudden Infant Death Syndrome, Sudden Unexplained Infant Death, and child maltreatment fatalities including shaken baby syndrome. Current Opinion in Pediatrics 2006;18:196-200.

36. Centers for Disease Control and Prevention. Warning on interaction between air bags and rear-facing child restraints. MMWR 1993;42(No.14):20-2.

37. Judge JO, Lindsey C, Underwood M, Winsemius D. Balance improvements in older women: effects of exercise training. Physical Therapy 1993;73(4):254-65.

38. Lord SR, Caplan GA, Ward JA. Balance, reaction time, and muscle strength in exercising older women: a pilot study. Archives of Physical Medicine and Rehabilitation 1993;74(8):837-9.

39. Campbell AJ, Robertson MC, Gardner MM, Norton RN, Buchner DM. Falls prevention over 2 years: a randomized controlled trial in women 80 years and older. Age and Aging 1999;28:513-18.

40. Graafmans WC, Ooms ME, Hofstee HMA, Bezemer PD, Bouter LM, Lips P. Falls in the elderly: a prospective study of risk factors and risk profiles. American Journal of Epidemiology 1996;143:1129-36.

41. Mack MG, Sacks JJ, Thompson D. Testing the impact attenuation of loose fill playground surfaces. Injury Prevention 2000;6:141-4.

42. Consumer Product Safety Commission (US). Handbook on Public Playground Safety. Washington, DC; 1997.

References for the Acute Concussion Evaluation (ACE)

1. Collins MW, Iverson G, Lovell MR, McKeag DB, Norwig J, Maroon J. On-field predictors of neuropsychological and symptom deficit following sports-related concussion. Clinical Journal of Sport Medicine 2003;13(4):222-9.

2. Lovell MR, Collins MW. Neuropsychological assessment of the college football player. Journal of Head Trauma Rehabilitation 1998;13(2):9-26.

3. Schultz MR, et al. Incidence and risk factors for concussion in high school athletes, North Carolina, 1996-1999. American Journal of Epidemiology 2004;160(10):937-944.

4. Guskiewicz K, et al. Cumulative effects associated with recurrent concusion in collegiate football players: the NCAA Concussion Study. JAMA 2003;290(19):2549-55.

5. Collins MW, Lovell MR, Iverson G, Cantu R, Maroon J, Field M. Cumulative effects of concussion in high school athletes. Neurosurgery 2002;51:1175-181.

6. Lovell MR, Collins MW, Bradley J. Return to play following sports related concussion. Clinics in Sports Medicine 2004;23(3):421-443.

7. Iverson G, Gaetz M, Lovell MR, Collins MW. Cumulative effects of concussion in amateur athletes. Brain Injury 2004;18(5):433-43.

8. Collins MW, Field M, Lovell MR, Iverson GL, Johnston K, Maroon J, Fu F. Relationship between post-concussion headache and neuropsychological test performance in high school athletes. American Journal of Sports Medicine 2003;31:168-173.

9. Bellanger HG, Vanderploeg RD. The neuropsychological impact of sports-related concussion: A meta-analysis. Journal of the International Neuropsychological Society 2005;11(4):345-57.

10. Mihalik J, Stump J, Collins MW, Lovell MR, Field M, Maroon J. Posttraumatic migraine characteristics in athletes following sports-related concussion. Journal of Neurosurgery 2005;102(5):850-5.

11. Collins MW, Field M, Lovell MR, Iverson G, Johnston KM, Maroon J, Fu FH. Headache following sports-related concussion: To play or not to play. American Journal of Sports Medicine 2003;31(2):168-173.

12. deKruijk J, Leffers P, Menheere P, Meerhoff S, Rutten J, Twijnstra A. Prediction of post-traumatic complaints after mild traumatic brain injury: Early symptoms and biochemical markers. Journal of Neurology, Neurosurgery, and Psychiatry 2002;73(6):727-32.

13. Collins MW, et al. Relationship between concussion and neuropsychological performance in college football players. JAMA 1999;282(10):964-970.

14. Moore E, Terryberry-Spohr L, Hope D. Mild traumatic brain injury and anxiety sequelae: A review of the literature. Brain Injury 2006;20(2):117-32.

15. Mooney G, Speed J, Sheppard S. Factors related to recovery after mild traumatic brain injury. Brain Injury 2005;19(12):975-87.

16. Mather FJ, Tate RL, Hannan TJ. Post-traumatic stress disorder in children following road traffic accidents: a comparison of those with and without mild traumatic brain injury. Brain Injury 2003;17(12):1077-87.

17. Fung M, Willer B, Moreland D, Leddy J. A proposal for an evidence-based emergency department discharge form for mild traumatic brain injury. Brain Injury 2006;20(9):889-94.

Chapter 19

Traumatic Brain Injury

Introduction

Traumatic brain injury (TBI) is a major public health problem, especially among male adolescents and young adults ages 15 to 24, and among elderly people of both sexes 75 years and older. Children aged 5 and younger are also at high risk for TBI.

Perhaps the most famous TBI patient in the history of medicine was Phineas Gage. In 1848, Gage was a 25–year-old railway construction foreman working on the Rutland and Burlington Railroad in Vermont. In the 19th century, little was understood about the brain and even less was known about how to treat an injury to it. Most serious injuries to the brain resulted in death due to bleeding or infection. Gage was working with explosive powder and a packing rod, called a tamping iron, when a spark caused an explosion that propelled the 3-foot long, pointed rod through his head. It penetrated his skull at the top of his head, passed through his brain, and exited the skull by his temple. Amazingly, he survived the accident with the help of physician John Harlow who treated Gage for 73 days. Before the accident Gage was a quiet, mild-mannered man; after his injuries he became an obscene, obstinate, self-absorbed man. He continued to suffer personality and behavioral problems until his death in 1861.

Text in this chapter is excerpted from "Traumatic Brain Injury: Hope through Research," National Institute of Neurological Disorders and Stroke (NINDS), February 23, 2015.

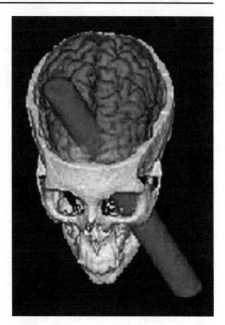

Figure 18.1. *Computer Generated Graphic showing Phineas Gage Accident.*

This computer-generated graphic shows how, in 1848, a 3-foot long, pointed rod penetrated the skull of Phineas Gage, a railway construction foreman. The rod entered at the top of his head, passed through his brain, and exited his skull by his temple. Gage survived the accident but suffered lasting personality and behavioral problems.

Today, we understand a great deal more about the healthy brain and its response to trauma, although science still has much to learn about how to reverse damage resulting from head injuries.

TBI costs the country more than $56 billion a year, and more than 5 million Americans alive today have had a TBI resulting in a permanent need for help in performing daily activities. Survivors of TBI are often left with significant cognitive, behavioral, and communicative disabilities, and some patients develop long-term medical complications, such as epilepsy.

Other statistics dramatically tell the story of head injury in the United States. Each year:

- approximately 1.4 million people experience a TBI

- approximately 50,000 people die from head injury

- approximately 1 million head-injured people are treated in hospital emergency rooms and

- approximately 230,000 people are hospitalized for TBI and survive

What is a Traumatic Brain Injury?

TBI, a form of acquired brain injury, occurs when a sudden trauma causes damage to the brain. The damage can be focal—confined to one area of the brain—or diffuse–involving more than one area of the brain. TBI can result from a closed *head injury* or a *penetrating head injury*. A closed injury occurs when the head suddenly and violently hits an object but the object does not break through the skull. A penetrating injury occurs when an object pierces the skull and enters brain tissue.

What Are the Signs and Symptoms of TBI?

Symptoms of a TBI can be mild, moderate, or severe, depending on the extent of the damage to the brain. Some symptoms are evident immediately, while others do not surface until several days or weeks after the injury. A person with a mild TBI may remain conscious or may experience a loss of consciousness for a few seconds or minutes. The person may also feel dazed or not like himself for several days or weeks after the initial injury. Other symptoms of mild TBI include headache, confusion, lightheadedness, dizziness, blurred vision or tired eyes, ringing in the ears, bad taste in the mouth, fatigue or lethargy, a change in sleep patterns, behavioral or mood changes, and trouble with memory, concentration, attention, or thinking.

A person with a moderate or severe TBI may show these same symptoms, but may also have a headache that gets worse or does not go away, repeated vomiting or nausea, convulsions or *seizures*, inability to awaken from sleep, dilation of one or both pupils of the eyes, slurred speech, weakness or numbness in the extremities, loss of coordination, and/or increased confusion, restlessness, or agitation. Small children with moderate to severe TBI may show some of these signs as well as signs specific to young children, such as persistent crying, inability to be consoled, and/or refusal to nurse or eat. Anyone with signs of moderate or severe TBI should receive medical attention as soon as possible.

What Are the Causes of and Risk Factors for TBI?

Half of all TBIs are due to transportation accidents involving automobiles, motorcycles, bicycles, and pedestrians. These accidents are the major cause of TBI in people under age 75. For those 75 and older, falls cause the majority of TBIs. Approximately 20 percent of TBIs are due to violence, such as firearm assaults and child abuse, and about 3 percent are due to sports injuries. Fully half of TBI incidents involve alcohol use.

The cause of the TBI plays a role in determining the patient's outcome. For example, approximately 91 percent of firearm TBIs (two-thirds of which may be suicidal in intent) result in death, while only 11 percent of TBIs from falls result in death.

What Are the Different Types of TBI?

Concussion is the most minor and the most common type of TBI. Technically, a concussion is a short loss of consciousness in response to a head injury, but in common language the term has come to mean any minor injury to the head or brain.

Other injuries are more severe. As the first line of defense, the skull is particularly vulnerable to injury. Skull fractures occur when the bone of the skull cracks or breaks. A *depressed skull fracture* occurs when pieces of the broken skull press into the tissue of the brain. A *penetrating skull fracture* occurs when something pierces the skull, such as a bullet, leaving a distinct and localized injury to brain tissue.

Skull fractures can cause bruising of brain tissue called a *contusion*. A contusion is a distinct area of swollen brain tissue mixed with blood released from broken blood vessels. A contusion can also occur in response to shaking of the brain back and forth within the confines of the skull, an injury called *contrecoup*. This injury often occurs in car accidents after high-speed stops and in *shaken baby syndrome*, a severe form of head injury that occurs when a baby is shaken forcibly enough to cause the brain to bounce against the skull. In addition, contrecoup can cause *diffuse axonal injury*, also called *shearing*, which involves damage to individual nerve cells (*neurons*) and loss of connections among neurons. This can lead to a breakdown of overall communication among neurons in the brain.

Damage to a major blood vessel in the head can cause a *hematoma*, or heavy bleeding into or around the brain. Three types of hematomas can cause brain damage. An *epidural hematoma* involves bleeding into the area between the skull and the dura. With a *subdural hematoma*, bleeding is confined to the area between the dura and the *arachnoid membrane*. Bleeding within the brain itself is called *intracerebral hematoma*.

Another insult to the brain that can cause injury is *anoxia*. Anoxia is a condition in which there is an absence of oxygen supply to an organ's tissues, even if there is adequate blood flow to the tissue. *Hypoxia* refers to a decrease in oxygen supply rather than a complete absence of oxygen. Without oxygen, the cells of the brain die within several minutes. This type of injury is often seen in near-drowning victims, in heart attack patients, or in people who suffer significant blood loss from other injuries that decrease blood flow to the brain.

What Medical Care Should a TBI Patient Receive?

Medical care usually begins when paramedics or emergency medical technicians arrive on the scene of an accident or when a TBI patient arrives at the emergency department of a hospital. Because little can be done to reverse the initial brain damage caused by trauma, medical personnel try to stabilize the patient and focus on preventing further injury. Primary concerns include insuring proper oxygen supply to the brain and the rest of the body, maintaining adequate blood flow, and controlling blood pressure. Emergency medical personnel may have to open the patient's airway or perform other procedures to make sure the patient is breathing. They may also perform CPR to help the heart pump blood to the body, and they may treat other injuries to control or stop bleeding. Because many head-injured patients may also have spinal cord injuries, medical professionals take great care in moving and transporting the patient. Ideally, the patient is placed on a backboard and in a neck restraint. These devices immobilize the patient and prevent further injury to the head and spinal cord.

As soon as medical personnel have stabilized the head-injured patient, they assess the patient's condition by measuring vital signs and reflexes and by performing a neurological examination. They check the patient's temperature, blood pressure, pulse, breathing rate, and pupil size in response to light. They assess the patient's level of consciousness and neurological functioning using the *Glasgow Coma Scale*, a standardized, 15-point test that uses three measures—eye opening, best verbal response, and best motor response—to determine the severity of the patient's brain injury.

The results of the three tests are added up to determine the patient's overall condition. A total score of 3 to 8 indicates a severe head injury, 9 to 12 indicates a moderate head injury, and 13 to 15 indicates a mild head injury.

Imaging tests help in determining the diagnosis and prognosis of a TBI patient. Patients with mild to moderate injuries may receive skull and neck X-rays to check for bone fractures or spinal instability. The patient should remain immobilized in a neck and back restraint until medical personnel are certain that there is no risk of spinal cord injury. For moderate to severe cases, the gold standard imaging test is a *computed tomography (CT)* scan. The CT scan creates a series of cross-sectional X-ray images of the head and brain and can show bone

Table 19.1. Glasgow Coma Scale

	The eye opening part of the Glasgow Coma Scale has four scores
4	indicates that the patient can open his eyes spontaneously
3	is given if the patient can open his eyes on verbal command
2	indicates that the patient opens his eyes only in response to painful stimuli
1	is given if the patient does not open his eyes in response to any stimulus

	The best verbal response part of the test has five scores
5	is given if the patient is oriented and can speak coherently
4	indicates that the patient is disoriented but can speak coherently
3	means the patient uses inappropriate words or incoherent language
2	is given if the patient makes incomprehensible sounds
1	indicates that the patient gives no verbal response at all

	The best motor response test has six scores
6	Score 6 means the patient can move his arms and legs in response to verbal commands.
5–2	A score between 5 and 2 is given if the patient shows movement in response to a variety of stimuli, including pain.
1	Score 1 indicates that the patient shows no movement in response to stimuli.

fractures as well as the presence of hemorrhage, hematomas, contusions, brain tissue swelling, and tumors. *Magnetic resonance imaging (MRI)* may be used after the initial assessment and treatment of the TBI patient. MRI uses magnetic fields to detect subtle changes in brain tissue content and can show more detail than X-rays or CT. Unfortunately, MRI is not ideal for routine emergency imaging of TBI patients because it is time-consuming and is not available in all hospitals.

Approximately half of severely head-injured patients will need surgery to remove or repair hematomas or contusions. Patients may also need surgery to treat injuries in other parts of the body. These patients usually go to the intensive care unit after surgery.

Sometimes when the brain is injured swelling occurs and fluids accumulate within the brain space. It is normal for bodily injuries to cause swelling and disruptions in fluid balance. But when an injury occurs inside the skull-encased brain, there is no place for swollen tissues to expand and no adjoining tissues to absorb excess fluid. This increased pressure is called *intracranial pressure (ICP)*.

Medical personnel measure patient's ICP using a probe or catheter. The instrument is inserted through the skull to the subarachnoid level and is connected to a monitor that registers the patient's ICP. If a patient has high ICP, he or she may undergo a *ventriculostomy*, a procedure that drains *cerebrospinal fluid (CSF)* from the brain to bring the pressure down. Drugs that can be used to decrease ICP include mannitol or barbiturates, although the safety and effectiveness of the latter are unknown.

How Does a TBI Affect Consciousness?

A TBI can cause problems with arousal, consciousness, awareness, alertness, and responsiveness. Generally, there are five abnormal states of consciousness that can result from a TBI: stupor, coma, persistent vegetative state, locked-in syndrome, and brain death.

Stupor is a state in which the patient is unresponsive but can be aroused briefly by a strong stimulus, such as sharp pain. *Coma* is a state in which the patient is totally unconscious, unresponsive, unaware, and unarousable. Patients in a coma do not respond to external stimuli, such as pain or light, and do not have sleep-wake cycles. Coma results from widespread and diffuse trauma to the brain, including the cerebral hemispheres of the upper brain and the lower brain or brainstem. Coma generally is of short duration, lasting a few days to a few weeks. After this time, some patients gradually come out of the coma, some progress to a vegetative state, and others die.

Patients in a vegetative state are unconscious and unaware of their surroundings, but they continue to have a sleep-wake cycle and can have periods of alertness. Unlike coma, where the patient's eyes are closed, patients in a vegetative state often open their eyes and may move, groan, or show reflex responses. A vegetative state can result from diffuse injury to the cerebral hemispheres of the brain without damage to the lower brain and brainstem. Anoxia, or lack of oxygen to the brain, which is a common complication of cardiac arrest, can also bring about a vegetative state.

Many patients emerge from a vegetative state within a few weeks, but those who do not recover within 30 days are said to be in a *persistent vegetative state (PVS)*. The chances of recovery depend on the extent of injury to the brain and the patient's age, with younger patients having a better chance of recovery than older patients. Generally adults have a 50 percent chance and children a 60 percent chance of recovering consciousness from a PVS within the first 6 months. After a year, the chances that a PVS patient will regain consciousness are very low and most patients who do recover consciousness experience significant disability. The longer a patient is in a PVS, the more severe the resulting disabilities will be. Rehabilitation can contribute to recovery, but many patients never progress to the point of being able to take care of themselves.

Locked-in syndrome is a condition in which a patient is aware and awake, but cannot move or communicate due to complete paralysis of the body.

> **Advances in imaging and other technologies have led to devices that help differentiate among the variety of unconscious states.**

Unlike PVS, in which the upper portions of the brain are damaged and the lower portions are spared, locked-in syndrome is caused by damage to specific portions of the lower brain and brainstem with no damage to the upper brain. Most locked-in syndrome patients can communicate through movements and blinking of their eyes, which are not affected by the paralysis. Some patients may have the ability to move certain facial muscles as well. The majority of locked-in syndrome patients do not regain motor control, but several devices are available to help patients communicate.

With the development over the last half-century of assistive devices that can artificially maintain blood flow and breathing, the term *brain death* has come into use. Brain death is the lack of measurable brain function due to diffuse damage to the cerebral hemispheres and the brainstem, with loss of any integrated activity among distinct areas of the brain. Brain death is irreversible. Removal of assistive devices will result in immediate cardiac arrest and cessation of breathing.

Advances in imaging and other technologies have led to devices that help differentiate among the variety of unconscious states. For example, an imaging test that shows activity in the brainstem but little or no activity in the upper brain would lead a physician to a diagnosis of vegetative state and exclude diagnoses of brain death and locked-in syndrome. On the other hand, an imaging test that shows activity in the upper brain with little activity in the brainstem would confirm a diagnosis of locked-in syndrome, while invalidating a diagnosis of brain death or vegetative state. The use of CT and MRI is standard in TBI treatment, but other imaging and diagnostic techniques that may be used to confirm a particular diagnosis include cerebral angiography, electroencephalography (EEG), transcranial Doppler ultrasound, and single photon emission computed tomography (SPECT).

What Immediate Post-Injury Complications Can Occur From a TBI?

Sometimes, health complications occur in the period immediately following a TBI. These complications are not types of TBI, but are distinct medical problems that arise as a result of the injury. Although complications are rare, the risk increases with the severity of the trauma. Complications of TBI include immediate seizures, hydrocephalus or post-traumatic ventricular enlargement, CSF leaks, infections, vascular injuries, cranial nerve injuries, pain, bed sores, multiple organ system failure in unconscious patients, and polytrauma (trauma to other parts of the body in addition to the brain).

About 25 percent of patients with brain contusions or hematomas and about 50 percent of patients with penetrating head injuries will develop *immediate seizures*, seizures that occur within the first 24 hours of the injury. These immediate seizures increase the risk of *early seizures*—defined as seizures occurring within 1 week after injury—but do not seem to be linked to the development of post-traumatic epilepsy (recurrent seizures occurring more than 1 week after the initial trauma). Generally, medical professionals use anticonvulsant medications to treat seizures in TBI patients only if the seizures persist.

Hydrocephalus or post-traumatic ventricular enlargement occurs when CSF accumulates in the brain resulting in dilation of the cerebral ventricles (cavities in the brain filled with CSF) and an increase in ICP. This condition can develop during the acute stage of TBI or may not appear until later. Generally it occurs within the first year of the injury and is characterized by worsening neurological outcome, impaired consciousness, behavioral changes, ataxia (lack of coordination or balance), incontinence, or signs of elevated ICP. The condition may develop as a result of *meningitis*, subarachnoid hemorrhage, intracranial hematoma, or other injuries. Treatment includes shunting and draining of CSF as well as any other appropriate treatment for the root cause of the condition.

Skull fractures can tear the membranes that cover the brain, leading to CSF leaks. A tear between the dura and the arachnoid membranes, called a *CSF fistula*, can cause CSF to leak out of the subarachnoid space into the subdural space; this is called a *subdural hygroma*. CSF can also leak from the nose and the ear. These tears that let CSF out of the brain cavity can also allow air and bacteria into the cavity, possibly causing infections such as meningitis. *Pneumocephalus* occurs when air enters the intracranial cavity and becomes trapped in the subarachnoid space.

Infections within the intracranial cavity are a dangerous complication of TBI. They may occur outside of the dura, below the dura, below the arachnoid (meningitis), or within the space of the brain itself (abscess). Most of these injuries develop within a few weeks of the initial trauma and result from skull fractures or penetrating injuries. Standard treatment involves antibiotics and sometimes surgery to remove the infected tissue. Meningitis may be especially dangerous, with the potential to spread to the rest of the brain and nervous system.

Any damage to the head or brain usually results in some damage to the vascular system, which provides blood to the cells of the brain. The body's immune system can repair damage to small blood vessels, but damage to larger vessels can result in serious complications. Damage to one of the major arteries leading to the brain can cause a stroke, either through bleeding from the artery (*hemorrhagic stroke*) or through the formation of a clot at the site of injury, called a *thrombus or thrombosis*, blocking blood flow to the brain (*ischemic stroke*). Blood clots also can develop in other parts of the head. Symptoms such as headache, vomiting, seizures, paralysis on one side of the body, and semi-consciousness developing within several days of a head injury may be caused by a blood clot that forms in the tissue of one of the sinuses, or cavities, adjacent to the brain. Thrombotic-ischemic strokes are treated with anticoagulants, while surgery is the preferred treatment for hemorrhagic stroke. Other types of vascular injuries include *vasospasm* and the formation of *aneurysms*.

Skull fractures, especially at the base of the skull, can cause cranial nerve injuries that result in *compressive cranial neuropathies*. All but three of the 12 cranial nerves project out from the brainstem to the head and face. The seventh cranial nerve, called the facial nerve, is the most commonly injured cranial nerve in TBI and damage to it can result in paralysis of facial muscles.

Pain is a common symptom of TBI and can be a significant complication for conscious patients in the period immediately following a TBI. Headache is the most common form of pain experienced by TBI patients, but other forms of pain can also be problematic. Serious complications for patients who are unconscious, in a coma, or in a vegetative state include bed or pressure sores of the skin, recurrent bladder infections, pneumonia or other life-threatening infections, and progressive multiple organ failure.

General Trauma

Most TBI patients have injuries to other parts of the body in addition to the head and brain. Physicians call this polytrauma. These injuries require immediate and specialized care and can complicate treatment of and recovery from the TBI. Other medical complications that may accompany a TBI include pulmonary (lung) dysfunction; cardiovascular (heart) dysfunction from blunt chest trauma; gastrointestinal dysfunction; fluid and hormonal imbalances; and other isolated complications, such as fractures, nerve injuries, *deep vein thrombosis*, excessive blood clotting, and infections.

Trauma victims often develop *hypermetabolism* or an increased metabolic rate, which leads to an increase in the amount of heat the body produces. The body redirects into heat the energy needed to keep organ systems functioning, causing muscle wasting and the starvation of other tissues. Complications related to pulmonary dysfunction can include neurogenic pulmonary edema (excess fluid in lung tissue), aspiration pneumonia (pneumonia caused by foreign matter in the lungs), and fat and blood clots in the blood vessels of the lungs.

Fluid and hormonal imbalances can complicate the treatment of hypermetabolism and high ICP. Hormonal problems can result from dysfunction of the pituitary, the thyroid, and other glands throughout the body. Two common hormonal complications of TBI are *syndrome of inappropriate secretion of antidiuretic hormone (SIADH)* and *hypothyroidism*.

Blunt trauma to the chest can also cause cardiovascular problems, including damage to blood vessels and internal bleeding, and problems with heart rate and blood flow. Blunt trauma to the abdomen can cause damage to or dysfunction of the stomach, large or small intestines, and pancreas. A serious and common complication of TBI is *erosive gastritis*, or inflammation and degeneration of stomach tissue. This syndrome can cause bacterial growth in the stomach, increasing the risk of aspiration pneumonia. Standard care of TBI patients includes administration of prophylactic gastric acid inhibitors to prevent the buildup of stomach acids and bacteria.

What Disabilities Can Result From a TBI?

Disabilities resulting from a TBI depend upon the severity of the injury, the location of the injury, and the age and general health of the patient. Some common disabilities include problems with cognition (thinking, memory, and reasoning), sensory processing (sight, hearing, touch, taste, and smell), communication (expression and understanding), and behavior or mental health (depression, anxiety, personality changes, aggression, acting out, and social inappropriateness).

Within days to weeks of the head injury approximately 40 percent of TBI patients develop a host of troubling symptoms collectively called *post-concussion syndrome (PCS)*. A patient need not have suffered a concussion or loss of consciousness to develop the syndrome and many patients with mild TBI suffer from PCS. Symptoms include headache, dizziness, vertigo (a sensation of spinning around or of objects spinning around the patient), memory problems, trouble concentrating, sleeping problems, restlessness, irritability, apathy, depression, and anxiety. These symptoms may last for a few weeks after the head injury. The syndrome is more prevalent in patients who had psychiatric symptoms, such as depression or anxiety, before the injury. Treatment for PCS may include medicines for pain and psychiatric conditions, and psychotherapy and occupational therapy to develop coping skills.

Cognition is a term used to describe the processes of thinking, reasoning, problem solving, information processing, and memory. Most patients with severe TBI, if they recover consciousness, suffer from cognitive disabilities, including the loss of many higher level mental skills. The most common cognitive impairment among severely head-injured patients is memory loss, characterized by some loss of specific memories and the partial inability to form or store new ones. Some of these patients may experience *post-traumatic amnesia (PTA)*, either anterograde or retrograde. Anterograde PTA is impaired memory of events that happened after the TBI, while retrograde PTA is impaired memory of events that happened before the TBI.

Many patients with mild to moderate head injuries who experience cognitive deficits become easily confused or distracted and have problems with concentration and attention. They also have problems with higher level, so-called executive functions, such as planning, organizing, abstract reasoning, problem solving, and making judgments, which may make it difficult to resume pre-injury work-related activities. Recovery from cognitive deficits is greatest within the first 6 months after the injury and more gradual after that.

> The most common cognitive impairment among severely head-injured patients is memory loss, characterized by some loss of specific memories and the partial inability to form or store new ones.

Patients with moderate to severe TBI have more problems with cognitive deficits than patients with mild TBI, but a history of several mild TBIs may have an additive effect, causing cognitive deficits equal to a moderate or severe injury.

Many TBI patients have sensory problems, especially problems with vision. Patients may not be able to register what they are seeing or may be slow to recognize objects. Also, TBI patients often have difficulty with hand-eye coordination. Because of this, TBI patients may be prone to bumping into or dropping objects, or may seem generally unsteady. TBI patients may have difficulty driving a car, working complex machinery, or playing sports. Other sensory deficits may include problems with hearing, smell, taste, or touch. Some TBI patients develop tinnitus, a ringing or roaring in the ears. A person with damage to the part of the brain that processes taste or smell may develop a persistent bitter taste in the mouth or perceive a persistent noxious smell. Damage to the part of the brain that controls the sense of touch may cause a TBI patient to develop persistent skin tingling, itching, or pain. Although rare, these conditions are hard to treat.

Language and communication problems are common disabilities in TBI patients. Some may experience *aphasia*, defined as difficulty with understanding and producing spoken and written language; others may have difficulty with the more subtle aspects of communication, such as body language and emotional, non-verbal signals.

In *non-fluent aphasia*, also called Broca's aphasia or motor aphasia, TBI patients often have trouble recalling words and speaking in complete sentences. They may speak in broken phrases and pause frequently. Most patients are aware of these deficits and may become extremely frustrated. Patients with *fluent aphasia*, also called Wernicke's aphasia or sensory aphasia, display little meaning in their speech, even though they speak in complete sentences and use correct grammar. Instead, they speak in flowing gibberish, drawing out their sentences with non-essential and invented words. Many patients with fluent aphasia are unaware that they make little sense and become angry with others for not understanding them. Patients with *global aphasia* have extensive damage to the portions of the brain responsible for language and often suffer severe communication disabilities.

TBI patients may have problems with spoken language if the part of the brain that controls speech muscles is damaged. In this disorder, called *dysarthria*, the patient can think of the appropriate language, but cannot easily speak the words because they are unable to use the muscles needed to form the words and produce the sounds. Speech is often slow, slurred, and garbled. Some may have problems with intonation or inflection, called *prosodic dysfunction*. An important aspect of speech, inflection conveys emotional meaning and is necessary for certain aspects of language, such as irony.

These language deficits can lead to miscommunication, confusion, and frustration for the patient as well as those interacting with him or her.

Most TBI patients have emotional or behavioral problems that fit under the broad category of psychiatric health. Family members of TBI patients often find that personality changes and behavioral problems are the most difficult disabilities to handle. Psychiatric problems that may surface include depression, apathy, anxiety, irritability, anger, paranoia, confusion, frustration, agitation, insomnia or other sleep problems, and mood swings. Problem behaviors may include aggression and violence, impulsivity, disinhibition, acting out, noncompliance, social inappropriateness, emotional outbursts, childish behavior, impaired self-control, impaired self-awareness, inability to take responsibility or accept criticism, egocentrism, inappropriate sexual activity, and alcohol or drug abuse/addiction. Some patients' personality problems may be so severe that they are diagnosed with borderline personality disorder, a psychiatric condition characterized by many of the problems mentioned above. Sometimes TBI patients suffer from developmental stagnation, meaning that they fail to mature emotionally, socially, or psychologically after the trauma. This is a serious problem for children and young adults who suffer from a TBI. Attitudes and behaviors that are appropriate for a child or teenager become inappropriate in adulthood. Many TBI patients who show psychiatric or behavioral problems can be helped with medication and psychotherapy.

Are There Other Long-Term Problems Associated With a TBI?

There are other long term problems that can develop after TBI. These include Parkinson's disease and other motor problems, Alzheimer's disease, *dementia pugilistica*, and post-traumatic dementia.

Alzheimer's disease (AD)–AD is a progressive, neurodegenerative disease characterized by dementia, memory loss, and deteriorating cognitive abilities. Recent research suggests an association between head injury in early adulthood and the development of AD later in life; the more severe the head injury, the greater the risk of developing AD. Some evidence indicates that a head injury may interact with other factors to trigger the disease and may hasten the onset of the disease in individuals already at risk. For example, people who have a particular form of the protein apolipoprotein E (apoE4) and suffer a head injury fall into this increased risk category. (ApoE4 is a naturally occurring protein that helps transport cholesterol through the bloodstream.)

Parkinson's disease and other motor problems—Movement disorders as a result of TBI are rare but can occur. Parkinson's disease may develop years after TBI as a result of damage to the basal ganglia. Symptoms of Parkinson's disease include tremor or trembling, rigidity or stiffness, slow movement (bradykinesia), inability to move (akinesia), shuffling walk, and stooped posture. Despite many scientific advances in recent years, Parkinson's disease remains a chronic and progressive disorder, meaning that it is incurable and will progress in severity until the end of life. Other movement disorders that may develop after TBI include tremor, ataxia (uncoordinated muscle movements), and myoclonus (shock-like contractions of muscles).

Dementia pugilistica–Also called chronic traumatic encephalopathy, dementia pugilistica primarily affects career boxers. The most common symptoms of the condition are dementia and parkinsonism caused by repetitive blows to the head over a long period of time. Symptoms begin anywhere between 6 and 40 years after the start of a boxing career, with an average onset of about 16 years.

Post-traumatic dementia–The symptoms of post-traumatic dementia are very similar to those of dementia pugilistica, except that post-traumatic dementia is also characterized by long-term memory problems and is caused by a single, severe TBI that results in a coma.

What Kinds of Rehabilitation Should a TBI Patient Receive?

Rehabilitation is an important part of the recovery process for a TBI patient. During the acute stage, moderately to severely injured patients may receive treatment and care in an intensive care unit of a hospital. Once stable, the patient may be transferred to a subacute unit of the medical center or to an independent rehabilitation hospital. At this point, patients follow many diverse paths toward recovery because there are a wide variety of options for rehabilitation.

Testing by a trained neuropsychologist can assess the individual's cognitive, language, behavioral, motor, and executive functions and provide information regarding the need for rehabilitative services.

In 1998, the NIH held a *Consensus Development Conference on Rehabilitation of Persons with Traumatic Brain Injury*. The Consensus Development Panel recommended that TBI patients receive an individualized rehabilitation program based upon the patient's strengths and capacities and that rehabilitation services should be modified over time to adapt to the patient's changing needs. The panel also recommended that moderately to severely injured patients receive rehabilitation treatment that draws on the skills of many specialists. This involves individually tailored treatment programs in the areas of physical therapy, occupational therapy, speech/language therapy, physiatry (physical medicine), psychology/psychiatry, and social support. Medical personnel who provide this care include rehabilitation specialists, such as rehabilitation nurses, psychologists, speech/language pathologists, physical and occupational therapists, physiatrists (physical medicine specialists), social workers, and a team coordinator or administrator.

The overall goal of rehabilitation after a TBI is to improve the patient's ability to function at home and in society. Therapists help the patient adapt to disabilities or change the patient's living space, called environmental modification, to make everyday activities easier.

Some patients may need medication for psychiatric and physical problems resulting from the TBI. Great care must be taken in prescribing medications because TBI patients are more susceptible to side effects and may react adversely to some pharmacological agents. It is important for the family to provide social support for the patient by being involved in the rehabilitation program. Family members may also benefit from psychotherapy.

It is important for TBI patients and their families to select the most appropriate setting for rehabilitation. There are several options, including home-based rehabilitation, hospital outpatient rehabilitation, inpatient rehabilitation centers, comprehensive day programs at rehabilitation centers, supportive living programs, independent living centers, club-house programs, school based programs for children, and others. The TBI patient, the family, and the rehabilitation team members should work together to find the best place for the patient to recover.

How Can TBI be Prevented?

Unlike most neurological disorders, head injuries can be prevented. The Centers for Disease Control and Prevention (CDC) have issued the following safety tips for reducing the risk of suffering a TBI.

- Wear a seatbelt every time you drive or ride in a car.

- Buckle your child into a child safety seat, booster seat, or seatbelt (depending on the child's age) every time the child rides in a car.

- Wear a helmet and make sure your children wear helmets when

  - riding a bike or motorcycle

  - playing a contact sport such as football or ice hockey

  - using in-line skates or riding a skateboard

  - batting and running bases in baseball or softball

  - riding a horse

  - skiing or snowboarding

- Keep firearms and bullets stored in a locked cabinet when not in use.

- Avoid falls by

  - using a step-stool with a grab bar to reach objects on high shelves

  - installing handrails on stairways

  - installing window guards to keep young children from falling out of open windows

  - using safety gates at the top and bottom of stairs when young children are around

- Make sure the surface on your child's playground is made of shock-absorbing material (e.g., hardwood mulch, sand).

What Research is the NINDS conducting?

The National Institute of Neurological Disorders and Stroke (NINDS) conducts and supports research to better understand CNS injury and the biological mechanisms underlying damage to the brain, to develop strategies and interventions to limit the primary and secondary brain damage that occurs within days of a head trauma, and to devise therapies to treat brain injury and help in long-term recovery of function.

On a microscopic scale, the brain is made up of billions of cells that interconnect and communicate.

The neuron is the main functional cell of the brain and nervous system, consisting of a cell body (soma), a tail or long nerve fiber (axon), and projections of the cell body called dendrites. The axons travel in tracts or clusters throughout the brain, providing extensive interconnections between brain areas.

One of the most pervasive types of injury following even a minor trauma is damage to the nerve cell's axon through shearing; this is referred to as diffuse axonal injury. This damage causes a series of reactions that eventually lead to swelling of the axon and disconnection from the cell body of the neuron. In addition, the part of the neuron that communicates with other neurons degenerates and releases toxic levels of chemical messengers called *neurotransmitters* into the synapse or space between neurons, damaging neighboring neurons through a secondary neuroexcitatory cascade. Therefore, neurons that were unharmed from the primary trauma suffer damage from this secondary insult. Many of these cells cannot survive the toxicity of the chemical onslaught and initiate programmed cell death, or *apoptosis*. This process usually takes place within the first 24 to 48 hours after the initial injury, but can be prolonged.

One area of research that shows promise is the study of the role of calcium ion influx into the damaged neuron as a cause of cell death and general brain tissue swelling. Calcium enters nerve cells through damaged channels in the axon's membrane. The excess calcium inside the cell causes the axon to swell and also activates chemicals, called proteases, that break down proteins. One family of proteases, the calpains, are especially damaging to nerve cells because they break down proteins that maintain the structure of the axon. Excess calcium within the cell is also destructive to the cell's mitochondria, structures that produce the cell's energy. Mitochondria soak up excess calcium until they swell and stop functioning. If enough mitochondria are damaged, the nerve cell degenerates. Calcium influx has other damaging effects: it activates destructive enzymes, such as caspases that damage the DNA in the cell and trigger programmed cell death, and it damages sodium channels in the cell membrane, allowing sodium ions to flood the cell as well. Sodium influx exacerbates swelling of the cell body and axon.

NINDS researchers have shown, in both cell and animal studies, that giving specialized chemicals can reduce cell death caused by calcium ion influx. Other researchers have shown that the use of cyclosporin A, which blocks mitochondrial membrane permeability, protects axons from calcium influx. Another avenue of therapeutic intervention is the use of hypothermia (an induced state of low body temperature) to slow the progression of cell death and axon swelling.

In the healthy brain, the chemical glutamate functions as a neurotransmitter, but an excess amount of glutamate in the brain causes neurons to quickly overload from too much excitation, releasing toxic chemicals. These substances poison the chemical environment of surrounding cells, initiating degeneration and programmed cell death. Studies have shown that a group of enzymes called matrix metalloproteinases contribute to the toxicity by breaking down proteins that maintain the structure and order of the extracellular environment. Other research shows that glutamate reacts with calcium and sodium ion channels on the cell membrane, leading to an influx of calcium and sodium ions into the cell. Investigators are looking for ways to decrease the toxic effects of glutamate and other excitatory neurotransmitters.

The brain attempts to repair itself after a trauma, and is more successful after mild to moderate injury than after severe injury. Scientists have shown that after diffuse axonal injury neurons can spontaneously adapt and recover by sprouting some of the remaining healthy fibers of the neuron into the spaces once occupied by the degenerated axon. These fibers can develop in such a way that the neuron can resume communication with neighboring neurons. This is a very delicate process and can be disrupted by any of a number of factors, such as *neuroexcitation*, hypoxia (low oxygen levels), and hypotension (low blood flow). Following trauma, excessive neuroexcitation, that is the electrical activation of nerve cells or fibers, especially disrupts this natural recovery process and can cause sprouting fibers to lose direction and connect with the wrong terminals.

Scientists suspect that these misconnections may contribute to some long-term disabilities, such as pain, spasticity, seizures, and memory problems. NINDS researchers are trying to learn more about the brain's natural recovery process and what factors or triggers control it. They hope that through manipulation of these triggers they can increase repair while decreasing misconnections.

NINDS investigators are also looking at larger, tissue-specific changes within the brain after a TBI. Researchers have shown that trauma to the frontal lobes of the brain can damage specific chemical messenger systems, specifically the dopaminergic system, the collection of neurons in the brain that uses the neurotransmitter dopamine. Dopamine is an important chemical messenger—for example, degeneration of dopamine-producing neurons is the primary cause of Parkinson's disease. NINDS researchers are studying how the dopaminergic system responds after a TBI and its relationship to neurodegeneration and Parkinson's disease.

The use of stem cells to repair or replace damaged brain tissue is a new and exciting avenue of research. A *neural stem cell* is a special kind of cell that can multiply and give rise to other more specialized cell types. These cells are found in adult neural tissue and normally develop into several different cell types found within the central nervous system. NINDS researchers are investigating the ability of stem cells to develop into neurotransmitter-producing neurons, specifically dopamine-producing cells. Researchers are also looking at the power of stem cells to develop into *oligodendrocytes*, a type of brain cell that produces myelin, the fatty sheath that surrounds and insulates axons. One study in mice has shown that bone marrow stem cells can develop into neurons, demonstrating that neural stem cells are not the only type of stem cell that could be beneficial in the treatment of brain and nervous system disorders. At the moment, stem cell research for TBI is in its infancy, but future research may lead to advances for treatment and rehabilitation.

In addition to the basic research described above, NINDS scientists also conduct broader based clinical research involving patients. One area of study focuses on the *plasticity* of the brain after injury. In the strictest sense, plasticity means the ability to be formed or molded. When speaking of the brain, plasticity means the ability of the brain to adapt to deficits and injury. NINDS researchers are investigating the extent of brain plasticity after injury and developing therapies to enhance plasticity as a means of restoring function.

The plasticity of the brain and the rewiring of neural connections make it possible for one part of the brain to take up the functions of a disabled part. Scientists have long known that the immature brain is generally more plastic than the mature brain, and that the brains of children are better able to adapt and recover from injury than the brains of adults. NINDS researchers are investigating the mechanisms underlying this difference and theorize that children have an overabundance of hard-wired neural networks, many of which naturally decrease through a process called *pruning*. When an injury destroys an important neural network in children, another less useful neural network that would have eventually died takes over the responsibilities of the damaged network. Some researchers are looking at the role of plasticity in memory, while others are using imaging technologies, such as functional MRI, to map regions of the brain and record evidence of plasticity.

In the strictest sense, plasticity means the ability to be formed or molded. When speaking of the brain, plasticity means the ability of the brain to adapt to deficits and injury.

Another important area of research involves the development of improved rehabilitation programs for those who have disabilities from a TBI. The Congressional Children's Health Act of 2000 authorized the NINDS to conduct and support research related to TBI with the goal of designing therapies to restore normal functioning in cognition and behavior.

Chapter 20

Cerebral Aneurysm

What is a cerebral aneurysm?

A cerebral aneurysm (also known as an intracranial or intracerebral aneurysm) is a weak or thin spot on a blood vessel in the brain that balloons out and fills with blood. The bulging aneurysm can put pressure on a nerve or surrounding brain tissue. It may also leak or rupture, spilling blood into the surrounding tissue (called a hemorrhage). Some cerebral aneurysms, particularly those that are very small, do not bleed or cause other problems. Cerebral aneurysms can occur anywhere in the brain, but most are located along a loop of arteries that run between the underside of the brain and the base of the skull.

What causes a cerebral aneurysm?

Cerebral aneurysms can be congenital, resulting from an inborn abnormality in an artery wall. Cerebral aneurysms are also more common in people with certain genetic diseases, such as connective tissue disorders and polycystic kidney disease, and certain circulatory disorders, such as arteriovenous malformations (snarled tangles of arteries and veins in the brain that disrupt blood flow).

Other causes include trauma or injury to the head, high blood pressure, infection, tumors, atherosclerosis (a blood vessel disease in which fats build up on the inside of artery walls) and other diseases of the

Text in this chapter is excerpted from "Cerebral Aneurysms Fact Sheet," National Institute of Neurological Disorders and Stroke (NINDS), February 23, 2015.

vascular system, cigarette smoking, and drug abuse. Some investigators have speculated that oral contraceptives may increase the risk of developing aneurysms.

Aneurysms that result from an infection in the arterial wall are called mycotic aneurysms. Cancer-related aneurysms are often associated with tumors of the head and neck. Drug abuse, particularly the habitual use of cocaine, can inflame blood vessels and lead to the development of brain aneurysms.

How are aneurysms classified?

There are three types of *cerebral* aneurysm. A saccular aneurysm is a rounded or pouch-like sac of blood that is attached by a neck or stem to an artery or a branch of a blood vessel. Also known as a berry aneurysm (because it resembles a berry hanging from a vine), this most common form of cerebral aneurysm is typically found on arteries at the base of the brain. Saccular aneurysms occur most often in adults. A *lateral aneurysm* appears as a bulge on one wall of the blood vessel, while a *fusiform* aneurysm is formed by the widening along all walls of the vessel.

Aneurysms are also classified by size. Small aneurysms are less than 11 millimeters in diameter (about the size of a large pencil eraser), larger aneurysms are 11-25 millimeters (about the width of a dime), and giant aneurysms are greater than 25 millimeters in diameter (more than the width of a quarter).

Who is at risk?

Brain aneurysms can occur in anyone, at any age. They are more common in adults than in children and slightly more common in women than in men. People with certain inherited disorders are also at higher risk.

All cerebral aneurysms have the potential to rupture and cause bleeding within the brain. The incidence of reported ruptured aneurysm is about 10 in every 100,000 persons per year (about 30,000 individuals per year in the U.S.), most commonly in people between ages 30 and 60 years. Possible risk factors for rupture include hypertension, alcohol abuse, drug abuse (particularly cocaine), and smoking. In addition, the condition and size of the aneurysm affects the risk of rupture.

What are the dangers?

Aneurysms may burst and bleed into the brain, causing serious complications, including hemorrhagic stroke, permanent nerve damage, or death. Once it has burst, the aneurysm may burst again and bleed into the brain, and additional aneurysms may also occur. More commonly, rupture may cause a subarachnoid hemorrhage—bleeding into the space between the skull bone and the brain. A delayed but serious complication of subarachnoid hemorrhage is hydrocephalus, in which the excessive buildup of cerebrospinal fluid in the skull dilates fluid pathways called ventricles that can swell and press on the brain tissue. Another delayed post-rupture complication is vasospasm, in which other blood vessels in the brain contract and limit blood flow to vital areas of the brain. This reduced blood flow can cause stroke or tissue damage.

What are the symptoms?

Most cerebral aneurysms do not show symptoms until they either become very large or burst. Small, unchanging aneurysms generally will not produce symptoms, whereas a larger aneurysm that is steadily growing may press on tissues and nerves. Symptoms may include pain above and behind the eye; numbness, weakness, or paralysis on one side of the face; dilated pupils; and vision changes. When an aneurysm hemorrhages, an individual may experience a sudden and extremely severe headache, double vision, nausea, vomiting, stiff neck, and/or loss of consciousness. Individuals usually describe the headache as "the worst headache of my life" and it is generally different in severity and intensity from other headaches people may experience. "Sentinel" or warning headaches may result from an aneurysm that leaks for days to weeks prior to rupture. Only a minority of individuals have a sentinel headache prior to aneurysm rupture.

Other signs that a cerebral aneurysm has burst include nausea and vomiting associated with a severe headache, a drooping eyelid, sensitivity to light, and change in mental status or level of awareness. Some individuals may have seizures. Individuals may lose consciousness briefly or go into prolonged coma. People experiencing this "worst headache," especially when it is combined with any other symptoms, should seek immediate medical attention.

How are cerebral aneurysms diagnosed?

Most cerebral aneurysms go unnoticed until they rupture or are detected by brain imaging that may have been obtained for another condition. Several diagnostic methods are available to provide information about the aneurysm and the best form of treatment. The tests are usually obtained after a subarachnoid hemorrhage, to confirm the diagnosis of an aneurysm.

Angiography is a dye test used to analyze the arteries or veins. An *intracerebral angiogram* can detect the degree of narrowing or obstruction of an artery or blood vessel in the brain, head, or neck, and can identify changes in an artery or vein such as a weak spot like an aneurysm. It is used to diagnose stroke and to precisely determine the location, size, and shape of a brain tumor, aneurysm, or blood vessel that has bled. This test is usually performed in a hospital angiography suite. Following the injection of a local anesthetic, a flexible catheter is inserted into an artery and threaded through the body to the affected artery. A small amount of contrast dye (one that is highlighted on x-rays) is released into the bloodstream and allowed to travel into the head and neck. A series of x-rays is taken and changes, if present, are noted.

Computed tomography (CT) of the head is a fast, painless, non-invasive diagnostic tool that can reveal the presence of a cerebral aneurysm and determine, for those aneurysms that have burst, if blood has leaked into the brain. This is often the first diagnostic procedure ordered by a physician following suspected rupture. X-rays of the head are processed by a computer as two-dimensional cross-sectional images, or "slices," of the brain and skull. Occasionally a contrast dye is injected into the bloodstream prior to scanning. This process, called CT angiography, produces sharper, more detailed images of blood flow in the brain arteries. CT is usually conducted at a testing facility or hospital outpatient setting.

Magnetic resonance imaging (MRI) uses computer-generated radio waves and a powerful magnetic field to produce detailed images of the brain and other body structures. *Magnetic resonance angiography (MRA)* produces more detailed images of blood vessels. The images may be seen as either three-dimensional pictures or two-dimensional cross-slices of the brain and vessels. These painless, noninvasive procedures can show the size and shape of an unruptured aneurysm and can detect bleeding in the brain.

Cerebrospinal fluid analysis may be ordered if a ruptured aneurysm is suspected. Following application of a local anesthetic, a small amount of this fluid (which protects the brain and spinal cord) is removed from the subarachnoid space—located between the spinal cord and the membranes that surround it—by a spinal needle and tested to detect any bleeding or brain hemorrhage. In individuals with suspected subarachnoid hemorrhage, this procedure is usually done in a hospital.

How are cerebral aneurysms treated?

Not all cerebral aneurysms burst. Some people with very small aneurysms may be monitored to detect any growth or onset of symptoms and to ensure aggressive treatment of coexisting medical problems and risk factors. Each case is unique, and considerations for treating an unruptured aneurysm include the type, size, and location of the aneurysm; risk of rupture; the individual's age, health, and personal and family medical history; and risk of treatment.

Two surgical options are available for treating cerebral aneurysms, both of which carry some risk to the individual (such as possible damage to other blood vessels, the potential for aneurysm recurrence and re-bleeding, and the risk of post-operative stroke).

Microvascular clipping involves cutting off the flow of blood to the aneurysm. Under anesthesia, a section of the skull is removed and the aneurysm is located. The neurosurgeon uses a microscope to isolate the blood vessel that feeds the aneurysm and places a small, metal, clothespin-like clip on the aneurysm's neck, halting its blood supply. The clip remains in the person and prevents the risk of future bleeding. The piece of the skull is then replaced and the scalp is closed. Clipping has been shown to be highly effective, depending on the location, shape, and size of the aneurysm. In general, aneurysms that are completely clipped surgically do not return.

A related procedure is an occlusion, in which the surgeon clamps off (occludes) the entire artery that leads to the aneurysm. This procedure is often performed when the aneurysm has damaged the artery. An occlusion is sometimes accompanied by a bypass, in which a small blood vessel is surgically grafted to the brain artery, rerouting the flow of blood away from the section of the damaged artery.

Endovascular embolization is an alternative to surgery. Once the individual has been anesthetized, the doctor inserts a hollow plastic tube (a catheter) into an artery (usually in the groin) and threads it, using angiography, through the body to the site of the aneurysm. Using a guide wire, detachable coils (spirals of platinum wire) are passed through the catheter and released into the aneurysm. The coils fill the aneurysm, block it from circulation, and cause the blood to clot, which effectively destroys the aneurysm. The procedure may need to be performed more than once during the person's lifetime.

People who receive treatment for an aneurysm must remain in bed until the bleeding stops. Underlying conditions, such as high blood pressure, should be treated. Other treatment for cerebral aneurysm is symptomatic and may include anticonvulsants to prevent seizures and analgesics to treat headache. Vasospasm can be treated with calcium channel-blocking drugs and sedatives may be ordered if the person is restless. A shunt may be surgically inserted into a ventricle several months following rupture if the buildup of cerebrospinal fluid is causing harmful pressure on surrounding tissue. Individuals who have suffered a subarachnoid hemorrhage often need rehabilitative, speech, and occupational therapy to regain lost function and learn to cope with any permanent disability.

Can cerebral aneurysms be prevented?

There are no known ways to prevent a cerebral aneurysm from forming. People with a diagnosed brain aneurysm should carefully control high blood pressure, stop smoking, and avoid cocaine use or other stimulant drugs. They should also consult with a doctor about the benefits and risks of taking aspirin or other drugs that thin the blood. Women should check with their doctors about the use of oral contraceptives.

What is the prognosis?

An unruptured aneurysm may go unnoticed throughout a person's lifetime. A burst aneurysm, however, may be fatal or could lead to hemorrhagic stroke, vasospasm (the leading cause of disability or death following a burst aneurysm), hydrocephalus, coma, or short-term and/or permanent brain damage.

The prognosis for persons whose aneurysm has burst is largely dependent on the age and general health of the individual, other pre-existing neurological conditions, location of the aneurysm, extent of bleeding (and re-bleeding), and time between rupture and medical attention. It is estimated that about 40 percent of individuals whose aneurysm has ruptured do not survive the first 24 hours; up to another 25 percent die from complications within 6 months. People who experience subarachnoid hemorrhage may have permanent neurological damage. Other individuals may recover with little or no neurological deficit. Delayed complications from a burst aneurysm may include hydrocephalus and vasospasm. Early diagnosis and treatment are important.

Individuals who receive treatment for an unruptured aneurysm generally require less rehabilitative therapy and recover more quickly than persons whose aneurysm has burst. Recovery from treatment or rupture may take weeks to months.

Clinical studies suggest that in the first six months after treatment patients treated with endovascular coiling have less disability than those with surgical clipping, but that beyond six months after treatment the amount of disability is about the same. Long-term results of coiling procedures are uncertain and investigators need to conduct more research on this topic, since some aneurysms can recur after coiling. Individuals may want to consult a specialist in both endovascular and surgical repair of aneurysms, to help provide greater understanding of treatment options.

What research is being done?

The National Institute of Neurological Disorders and Stroke (NINDS), a component of the National Institutes of Health (NIH) within the U.S. Department of Health and Human Services, is the nation's primary supporter of research on the brain and nervous system. As part of its mission, the NINDS conducts research on intracranial aneurysms and other vascular lesions of the nervous system and supports studies through grants to medical institutions across the country.

The NINDS sponsored the International Study of Unruptured Intracranial Aneurysms, which included more than 4,000 people at 61 sites in the United States, Canada, and Europe. The findings suggest that the risk of rupture for most very small aneurysms (less than 7 millimeters in size) is small. The results also provide a more comprehensive look at these vascular defects and offer guidance to individuals and physicians facing the difficult decision about whether or not to treat an aneurysm surgically.

The Familial Intracranial Aneurysm Study is a collaborative research effort of scientists in the United States, Canada, Australia, and New Zealand to identify possible genes that may increase the risk of development of aneurysms in blood vessels of the brain. The study will involve 475 families with multiple affected family members. Researchers also hope to determine the effect of environmental factors such as cigarette smoking and high blood pressure on the expression of these genes.

The relationship between intracranial and aortic aneurysm has long been recognized but poorly quantified. Recent genome-wide association studies (GWAS) provide molecular evidence for shared biological function and activities (pathophysiology) of these aneurysms. A specific site on chromosome 9p21 has been identified as increasing the risk for both intracranial and aortic aneurysms. These GWAS data, along with linkage data to other susceptible locations for genes or DNA sequences, indicate that individuals and families harboring one type of aneurysm may be at especially increased risk of the other.

Other scientists are studying additional chromosomes and chromosomal regions to identify aneurysm-related genes.

Aspirin may lessen inflammation in cerebral aneurysms and reduce their incidence of rupture. Scientists using enhanced MRI to monitor the signal generated by macrophages (a type of white blood cell that travels to the injury site during the inflammatory response) hope to determine if daily aspirin intake for three months will reduce the MRI signal changes generated by macrophages in the aneurysm wall.

The incidence of intracranial aneurysms and subarachnoid hemorrhage is significantly higher in women after menopause than in men. Estrogen replacement therapy reduces the risk for subarachnoid hemorrhage in post-menopausal women. Researchers are investigating the role of estrogen in the pathophysiology of intracranial aneurysms.

Other research projects include studies of the effectiveness of microsurgical clipping and endovascular surgery to treat various types of ruptured and unruptured aneurysms, the use of various types of coils to block the flow of blood into the aneurysm, and the aspects of blood flow (hemodynamics), such as blood flow velocity and blood pressure, in initiating cerebral aneurysms.

Chapter 21

Stroke

Introduction

More than 2,400 years ago the father of medicine, Hippocrates, recognized and described stroke—the sudden onset of paralysis. Until recently, modern medicine has had very little power over this disease, but the world of stroke medicine is changing and new and better therapies are being developed every day. Today, some people who have a stroke can walk away from the attack with no or few disabilities *if they are treated promptly*. Doctors can finally offer stroke patients and their families the one thing that until now has been so hard to give: hope.

In ancient times stroke was called *apoplexy*, a general term that physicians applied to anyone suddenly struck down with paralysis. Because many conditions can lead to sudden paralysis, the term apoplexy did not indicate a specific diagnosis or cause. Physicians knew very little about the cause of stroke and the only established therapy was to feed and care for the patient until the attack ran its course.

The first person to investigate the pathological signs of apoplexy was Johann Jacob Wepfer. Born in Schaffhausen, Switzerland, in 1620, Wepfer studied medicine and was the first to identify postmortem signs of bleeding in the brains of patients who died of apoplexy. From autopsy studies he gained knowledge of the *carotid* and *vertebral arteries* that supply the brain with blood. He also was the first person to suggest that apoplexy, in addition to being caused by bleeding in

---

Text in this chapter is excerpted from "Stroke: Hope through Research," National Institute of Neurological Disorders and Stroke (NINDS), March 5, 2015.

the brain, could be caused by a blockage of one of the main arteries supplying blood to the brain; thus stroke became known as a *cerebrovascular disease* ("cerebro" refers to a part of the brain; "vascular" refers to the blood vessels and arteries).

Medical science would eventually confirm Wepfer's hypotheses, but until very recently doctors could offer little in the area of therapy. Over the last two decades basic and clinical investigators, many of them sponsored and funded in part by the National Institute of Neurological Disorders and Stroke (NINDS), have learned a great deal about stroke. They have identified major risk factors for the disease and have developed surgical techniques and drug treatments for the prevention of stroke. But perhaps the most exciting new development in the field of stroke research is the recent approval of a drug treatment that can reverse the course of stroke if given during the first few hours after the onset of symptoms.

Studies with animals have shown that brain injury occurs within minutes of a stroke and can become irreversible within as little as an hour. In humans, brain damage begins from the moment the stroke starts and often continues for days afterward. Scientists now know that there is a very short window of opportunity for treatment of the most common form of stroke. Because of these and other advances in the field of cerebrovascular disease stroke patients now have a chance for survival and recovery.

Cost of Stroke to the United States:

- total cost of stroke to the United States: estimated at about $43 billion/year

- direct costs for medical care and therapy: estimated at about $28 billion/year

- indirect costs from lost productivity and other factors: estimated at about $15 million/year

- average cost of care for a patient up to 90 days after a stroke: $15,000*

- for 10% of patients, cost of care for the first 90 days after a stroke: $35,000*

- percentage of direct cost of care for the first 90 days*:

- initial hospitalization = 43%

- rehabilitation = 16%

- physician costs = 14%
- hospital readmission = 14%
- medications and other expenses = 13%

*From "The Stroke/Brain Attack Reporter's Handbook," National Stroke Association, Englewood, CO, 1997

What is Stroke?

A stroke occurs when the blood supply to part of the brain is suddenly interrupted or when a blood vessel in the brain bursts, spilling blood into the spaces surrounding brain cells. In the same way that a person suffering a loss of blood flow to the heart is said to be having a heart attack, a person with a loss of blood flow to the brain or sudden bleeding in the brain can be said to be having a "brain attack."

Brain cells die when they no longer receive oxygen and nutrients from the blood or when they are damaged by sudden bleeding into or around the brain. *Ischemia* is the term used to describe the loss of oxygen and nutrients for brain cells when there is inadequate blood flow. Ischemia ultimately leads to *infarction*, the death of brain cells which are eventually replaced by a fluid-filled cavity (or *infarct*) in the injured brain.

When blood flow to the brain is interrupted, some brain cells die immediately, while others remain at risk for death. These damaged cells make up the *ischemic penumbra* and can linger in a compromised state for several hours. With timely treatment these cells can be saved.

Even though a stroke occurs in the unseen reaches of the brain, the symptoms of a stroke are easy to spot. They include sudden numbness or weakness, especially on one side of the body; sudden confusion or trouble speaking or understanding speech; sudden trouble seeing in one or both eyes; sudden trouble walking, dizziness, or loss of balance or coordination; or sudden severe headache with no known cause. All of the symptoms of stroke appear suddenly, and often there is more than one symptom at the same time. Therefore stroke can usually be distinguished from other causes of dizziness or headache. These symptoms may indicate that a stroke has occurred and that medical attention is needed immediately.

There are two forms of stroke: *ischemic*—blockage of a blood vessel supplying the brain, and hemorrhagic—bleeding into or around the brain. The following sections describe these forms in detail.

Ischemic Stroke

An ischemic stroke occurs when an artery supplying the brain with blood becomes blocked, suddenly decreasing or stopping blood flow and ultimately causing a brain infarction. This type of stroke accounts for approximately 80 percent of all strokes. Blood clots are the most common cause of artery blockage and brain infarction. The process of clotting is necessary and beneficial throughout the body because it stops bleeding and allows repair of damaged areas of arteries or veins. However, when blood clots develop in the wrong place within an artery they can cause devastating injury by interfering with the normal flow of blood. Problems with clotting become more frequent as people age.

Blood clots can cause ischemia and infarction in two ways. A clot that forms in a part of the body other than the brain can travel through blood vessels and become wedged in a brain artery. This free-roaming clot is called an *embolus* and often forms in the heart. A stroke caused by an embolus is called an *embolic stroke*. The second kind of ischemic stroke, called a *thrombotic stroke*, is caused by *thrombosis*, the formation of a blood clot in one of the cerebral arteries that stays attached to the artery wall until it grows large enough to block blood flow.

Ischemic strokes can also be caused by *stenosis*, or a narrowing of the artery due to the buildup of *plaque* (a mixture of fatty substances, including cholesterol and other lipids) and blood clots along the artery wall. Stenosis can occur in large arteries and small arteries and is therefore called *large vessel disease* or *small vessel disease*, respectively. When a stroke occurs due to small vessel disease, a very small infarction results, sometimes called a *lacunar infarction*, from the French word "lacune" meaning "gap" or "cavity."

The most common blood vessel disease that causes stenosis is *atherosclerosis*. In atherosclerosis, deposits of plaque buildup along the inner walls of large and medium-sized arteries, causing thickening, hardening, and loss of elasticity of artery walls and decreased blood flow.

Hemorrhagic Stroke

In a healthy, functioning brain, neurons do not come into direct contact with blood. The vital oxygen and nutrients the neurons need from the blood come to the neurons across the thin walls of the cerebral capillaries. The glia (nervous system cells that support and protect neurons) form a *blood-brain barrier*, an elaborate meshwork that surrounds blood vessels and capillaries and regulates which elements of the blood can pass through to the neurons.

When an artery in the brain bursts, blood spews out into the surrounding tissue and upsets not only the blood supply but the delicate chemical balance neurons require to function. This is called a hemorrhagic stroke. Such strokes account for approximately 20 percent of all strokes.

Hemorrhage can occur in several ways. One common cause is a bleeding *aneurysm*, a weak or thin spot on an artery wall. Over time, these weak spots stretch or balloon out under high arterial pressure. The thin walls of these ballooning aneurysms can rupture and spill blood into the space surrounding brain cells.

Hemorrhage also occurs when arterial walls break open. Plaque-encrusted artery walls eventually lose their elasticity and become brittle and thin, prone to cracking. *Hypertension*, or *high blood pressure*, increases the risk that a brittle artery wall will give way and release blood into the surrounding brain tissue.

A person with an *arteriovenous malformation (AVM)* also has an increased risk of hemorrhagic stroke. AVMs are a tangle of defective blood vessels and capillaries within the brain that have thin walls and can therefore rupture.

Bleeding from ruptured brain arteries can either go into the substance of the brain or into the various spaces surrounding the brain. *Intracerebral hemorrhage* occurs when a vessel within the brain leaks blood into the brain itself. *Subarachnoid hemorrhage* is bleeding under the meninges, or outer membranes, of the brain into the thin fluid-filled space that surrounds the brain.

The subarachnoid space separates the arachnoid membrane from the underlying pia mater membrane. It contains a clear fluid (*cerebrospinal fluid* or *CSF*) as well as the small blood vessels that supply the outer surface of the brain. In a subarachnoid hemorrhage, one of the small arteries within the subarachnoid space bursts, flooding the area with blood and contaminating the cerebrospinal fluid. Since the CSF flows throughout the cranium, within the spaces of the brain, subarachnoid hemorrhage can lead to extensive damage throughout the brain. In fact, subarachnoid hemorrhage is the most deadly of all strokes.

Transient Ischemic Attacks

A *transient ischemic attack* (TIA), sometimes called a mini-stroke, starts just like a stroke but then resolves leaving no noticeable symptoms or deficits. The occurrence of a TIA is a warning that the person is at risk for a more serious and debilitating stroke. Of the approximately

50,000 Americans who have a TIA each year, about one-third will have an *acute stroke* sometime in the future. The addition of other risk factors compounds a person's risk for a recurrent stroke. The average duration of a TIA is a few minutes. For almost all TIAs, the symptoms go away within an hour. There is no way to tell whether symptoms will be just a TIA or persist and lead to death or disability. The patient should assume that all stroke symptoms signal an emergency and should not wait to see if they go away.

Recurrent Stroke

Recurrent stroke is frequent; about 25 percent of people who recover from their first stroke will have another stroke within 5 years. Recurrent stroke is a major contributor to stroke disability and death, with the risk of severe disability or death from stroke increasing with each stroke recurrence. The risk of a recurrent stroke is greatest right after a stroke, with the risk decreasing with time. About 3 percent of stroke patients will have another stroke within 30 days of their first stroke and one-third of recurrent strokes take place within 2 years of the first stroke.

How Do You Recognize Stroke?

Symptoms of stroke appear suddenly. Watch for these symptoms and be prepared to act quickly for yourself or on behalf of someone you are with:

- Sudden numbness or weakness of the face, arm, or leg, especially on one side of the body.

- Sudden confusion, trouble talking, or understanding speech.

- Sudden trouble seeing in one or both eyes.

- Sudden trouble walking, dizziness, or loss of balance or coordination.

- Sudden severe headache with no known cause.

If you suspect you or someone you know is experiencing any of these symptoms indicative of a stroke, ***do not wait. Call 911 emergency immediately***. There are now effective therapies for stroke that must be administered at a hospital, but they lose their effectiveness if not given within the first 3 hours after stroke symptoms appear. ***Every minute counts!***

How is the Cause of Stroke Determined?

Physicians have several diagnostic techniques and imaging tools to help diagnose the cause of stroke quickly and accurately. The first step in diagnosis is a short neurological examination. When a possible stroke patient arrives at a hospital, a health care professional, usually a doctor or nurse, will ask the patient or a companion what happened and when the symptoms began. Blood tests, an electrocardiogram, and a brain scan, such CT or MRI, will often be done. One test that helps doctors judge the severity of a stroke is the standardized NIH Stroke Scale, developed by the NINDS. Health care professionals use the NIH Stroke Scale to measure a patient's neurological deficits by asking the patient to answer questions and to perform several physical and mental tests. Other scales include the Glasgow Coma Scale, the Hunt and Hess Scale, the Modified Rankin Scale, and the Barthel Index.

Imaging for the Diagnosis of Acute Stroke

Health care professionals also use a variety of imaging devices to evaluate stroke patients. The most widely used imaging procedure is the *computed tomography (CT) scan*. Also known as a CAT scan or computed axial tomography, CT creates a series of cross-sectional images of the head and brain. Because it is readily available at all hours at most major hospitals and produces images quickly, CT is the most commonly used diagnostic technique for acute stroke. CT also has unique diagnostic benefits. It will quickly rule out a hemorrhage, can occasionally show a tumor that might mimic a stroke, and may even show evidence of early infarction. Infarctions generally show up on a CT scan about 6 to 8 hours after the start of stroke symptoms.

If a stroke is caused by hemorrhage, a CT can show evidence of bleeding into the brain almost immediately after stroke symptoms appear. Hemorrhage is the primary reason for avoiding certain drug treatments for stroke, such as thrombolytic therapy, the only proven acute stroke therapy for ischemic stroke. Thrombolytic therapy cannot be used until the doctor can confidently diagnose the patient as suffering from an ischemic stroke because this treatment might increase bleeding and could make a hemorrhagic stroke worse.

Another imaging device used for stroke patients is the *magnetic resonance imaging (MRI) scan*. MRI uses magnetic fields to detect subtle changes in brain tissue content. One effect of stroke is the slowing of water movement, called *diffusion*, through the damaged brain tissue. MRI can show this type of damage within the first hour after the stroke symptoms start. The benefit of MRI over a CT scan is more accurate and earlier diagnosis of infarction, especially for smaller strokes, while showing equivalent accuracy in determining when hemorrhage is present. MRI is more sensitive than CT for other types of brain disease, such as brain tumor, that might mimic a stroke. MRI cannot be performed in patients with certain types of metallic or electronic implants, such as pacemakers for the heart.

Although increasingly used in the emergency diagnosis of stroke, MRI is not immediately available at all hours in most hospitals, where CT is used for acute stroke diagnosis. Also, MRI takes longer to perform than CT, and may not be performed if it would significantly delay treatment.

Other types of MRI scans, often used for the diagnosis of cerebrovascular disease and to predict the risk of stroke, are *magnetic resonance angiography (MRA)* and *functional magnetic resonance imaging (fMRI)*. Neurosurgeons use MRA to detect stenosis (blockage) of the brain arteries inside the skull by mapping flowing blood. Functional MRI uses a magnet to pick up signals from oxygenated blood and can show brain activity through increases in local blood flow. *Duplex Doppler ultrasound and arteriography* are two diagnostic imaging techniques used to decide if an individual would benefit from a surgical procedure called *carotid endarterectomy*. This surgery is used to remove fatty deposits from the carotid arteries and can help prevent stroke.

Doppler ultrasound is a painless, noninvasive test in which sound waves above the range of human hearing are sent into the neck. Echoes bounce off the moving blood and the tissue in the artery and can be formed into an image. Ultrasound is fast, painless, risk-free, and relatively inexpensive compared to MRA and arteriography, but it is not considered to be as accurate as arteriography. Arteriography is an X-ray of the carotid artery taken when a special dye is injected into the artery. The procedure carries its own small risk of causing a stroke and is costly to perform. The benefits of arteriography over MR techniques and ultrasound are that it is extremely reliable and still the best way to measure stenosis of the carotid arteries. Even so, significant advances are being made every day involving noninvasive imaging techniques such as fMRI.

Who is at Risk for Stroke?

Some people are at a higher risk for stroke than others. Unmodifiable risk factors include age, gender, race/ethnicity, and stroke family history. In contrast, other risk factors for stroke, like high blood pressure or cigarette smoking, can be changed or controlled by the person at risk.

Unmodifiable Risk Factors

It is a myth that stroke occurs only in elderly adults. In actuality, stroke strikes all age groups, from fetuses still in the womb to centenarians. It is true, however, that older people have a higher risk for stroke than the general population and that the risk for stroke increases with age. For every decade after the age of 55, the risk of stroke doubles, and two-thirds of all strokes occur in people over 65 years old. People over 65 also have a seven-fold greater risk of dying from stroke than the general population. And the *incidence* of stroke is increasing proportionately with the increase in the elderly population. When the baby boomers move into the over-65 age group, stroke and other diseases will take on even greater significance in the health care field.

Gender also plays a role in risk for stroke. Men have a higher risk for stroke, but more women die from stroke. The stroke risk for men is 1.25 times that for women. But men do not live as long as women, so men are usually younger when they have their strokes and therefore have a higher rate of survival than women. In other words, even though women have fewer strokes than men, women are generally older when they have their strokes and are more likely to die from them.

Stroke seems to run in some families. Several factors might contribute to familial stroke risk. Members of a family might have a genetic tendency for stroke risk factors, such as an inherited predisposition for hypertension or diabetes. The influence of a common lifestyle among family members could also contribute to familial stroke.

The risk for stroke varies among different ethnic and racial groups. The incidence of stroke among African-Americans is almost double that of white Americans, and twice as many African-Americans who have a stroke die from the event compared to white Americans. African-Americans between the ages of 45 and 55 have four to five times the stroke death rate of whites. After age 55 the stroke mortality rate for whites increases and is equal to that of African-Americans.

Compared to white Americans, African-Americans have a higher incidence of stroke risk factors, including high blood pressure and cigarette smoking. African-Americans also have a higher incidence and *prevalence* of some genetic diseases, such as diabetes and sickle cell anemia that predispose them to stroke.

Hispanics and Native Americans have stroke incidence and mortality rates more similar to those of white Americans. In Asian-Americans stroke incidence and mortality rates are also similar to those in white Americans, even though Asians in Japan, China, and other countries of the Far East have significantly higher stroke incidence and mortality rates than white Americans. This suggests that environment and lifestyle factors play a large role in stroke risk.

The "Stroke Belt"

Several decades ago, scientists and statisticians noticed that people in the southeastern United States had the highest stroke mortality rate in the country. They named this region the *stroke belt*. For many years, researchers believed that the increased risk was due to the higher percentage of African-Americans and an overall lower socioeconomic status (SES) in the southern states. A low SES is associated with an overall lower standard of living, leading to a lower standard of health care and therefore an increased risk of stroke. But researchers now know that the higher percentage of African-Americans and the overall lower SES in the southern states does not adequately account for the higher incidence of, and mortality from, stroke in those states. This means that other factors must be contributing to the higher incidence of and mortality from stroke in this region.

Recent studies have also shown that there is a *stroke buckle* in the stroke belt. Three southeastern states, North Carolina, South Carolina, and Georgia, have an extremely high stroke mortality rate, higher than the rate in other stroke belt states and up to two times the stroke mortality rate of the United States overall. The increased risk could be due to geographic or environmental factors or to regional differences in lifestyle, including higher rates of cigarette smoking and a regional preference for salty, high-fat foods.

Other Risk Factors

The most important risk factors for stroke are hypertension, heart disease, diabetes, and cigarette smoking. Others include heavy alcohol consumption, high blood cholesterol levels, illicit drug use, and genetic or congenital conditions, particularly vascular abnormalities. People with more than one risk factor have what is called "amplification of risk." This means that the multiple risk factors compound their destructive effects and create an overall risk greater than the simple cumulative effect of the individual risk factors.

Hypertension

Of all the risk factors that contribute to stroke, the most powerful is hypertension, or high blood pressure. People with hypertension have a risk for stroke that is four to six times higher than the risk for those without hypertension. One-third of the adult U.S. population, about 50 million people (including 40–70 percent of those over age 65) have high blood pressure. Forty to 90 percent of stroke patients have high blood pressure before their stroke event.

A systolic pressure of 120 mm of Hg over a diastolic pressure of 80 mm of Hg* is generally considered normal. Persistently high blood pressure greater than 140 over 90 leads to the diagnosis of the disease called hypertension. The impact of hypertension on the total risk for stroke decreases with increasing age, therefore factors other than hypertension play a greater role in the overall stroke risk in elderly adults. For people without hypertension, the absolute risk of stroke increases over time until around the age of 90, when the absolute risk becomes the same as that for people with hypertension.

* mm of Hg—or millimeters of mercury—is the standard means of expressing blood pressure, which is measured using an instrument called a sphygmomanometer. Using a stethoscope and a cuff that is wrapped around the patient's upper arm, a health professional listens to the sounds of blood rushing through an artery. The first sound registered on the instrument gauge (which measures the pressure of the blood in millimeters on a column of mercury) is called the systolic pressure. This is the maximum pressure produced as the left ventricle of the heart contracts and the blood begins to flow through the artery. The second sound is the diastolic pressure and is the lowest pressure in the artery when the left ventricle is relaxing.

Like stroke, there is a gender difference in the prevalence of hypertension. In younger people, hypertension is more common among men than among women. With increasing age, however, more women than men have hypertension. This hypertension gender-age difference probably has an impact on the incidence and prevalence of stroke in these populations.

Antihypertensive medication can decrease a person's risk for stroke. Recent studies suggest that treatment can decrease the stroke incidence rate by 38 percent and decrease the stroke fatality rate by 40 percent. Common hypertensive agents include adrenergic agents, beta-blockers, angiotensin converting enzyme inhibitors, calcium channel blockers, diuretics, and vasodilators.

Heart Disease

After hypertension, the second most powerful risk factor for stroke is heart disease, especially a condition known as atrial fibrillation. Atrial fibrillation is irregular beating of the left atrium, or left upper chamber, of the heart. In people with atrial fibrillation, the left atrium beats up to four times faster than the rest of the heart. This leads to an irregular flow of blood and the occasional formation of blood clots that can leave the heart and travel to the brain, causing a stroke.

Atrial fibrillation, which affects as many as 2.2 million Americans, increases an individual's risk of stroke by 4 to 6 percent, and about 15 percent of stroke patients have atrial fibrillation before they experience a stroke. The condition is more prevalent in the upper age groups, which means that the prevalence of atrial fibrillation in the United States will increase proportionately with the growth of the elderly population. Unlike hypertension and other risk factors that have a lesser impact on the ever-rising absolute risk of stroke that comes with advancing age, the influence of atrial fibrillation on total risk for stroke increases powerfully with age. In people over 80 years old, atrial fibrillation is the direct cause of one in four strokes.

Other forms of heart disease that increase stroke risk include malformations of the heart valves or the heart muscle. Some valve diseases, like *mitral valve stenosis or mitral annular calcification*, can double the risk for stroke, independent of other risk factors.

Heart muscle malformations can also increase the risk for stroke. Patent foramen ovale (PFO) is a passage or a hole (sometimes called a "shunt") in the heart wall separating the two atria, or upper chambers, of the heart. Clots in the blood are usually filtered out by the lungs, but PFO could allow emboli or blood clots to bypass the lungs and go directly through the arteries to the brain, potentially causing a stroke. Research is currently under way to determine how important PFO is as a cause for stroke. Atrial septal aneurysm (ASA), a congenital (present from birth) malformation of the heart tissue, is a bulging of the septum or heart wall into one of the atria of the heart. Researchers do not know why this malformation increases the risk for stroke. PFO and ASA frequently occur together and therefore amplify the risk for stroke. Two other heart malformations that seem to increase the risk for stroke for unknown reasons are left atrial enlargement and left ventricular hypertrophy. People with left atrial enlargement have a larger than normal left atrium of the heart; those with left ventricular hypertrophy have a thickening of the wall of the left ventricle.

Another risk factor for stroke is cardiac surgery to correct heart malformations or reverse the effects of heart disease. Strokes occurring in this situation are usually the result of surgically dislodged plaques from the aorta that travel through the bloodstream to the arteries in the neck and head, causing stroke. Cardiac surgery increases a person's risk of stroke by about 1 percent. Other types of surgery can also increase the risk of stroke.

Blood Cholesterol Levels

Most people know that high cholesterol levels contribute to heart disease. But many don't realize that a high cholesterol level also contributes to stroke risk. Cholesterol, a waxy substance produced by the liver, is a vital body product. It contributes to the production of hormones and vitamin D and is an integral component of cell membranes. The liver makes enough cholesterol to fuel the body's needs and this natural production of cholesterol alone is not a large contributing factor to atherosclerosis, heart disease, and stroke. Research has shown that the danger from cholesterol comes from a dietary intake of foods that contain high levels of cholesterol. Foods high in saturated fat and cholesterol, like meats, eggs, and dairy products, can increase the amount of total cholesterol in the body to alarming levels, contributing to the risk of atherosclerosis and thickening of the arteries.

Cholesterol is classified as a lipid, meaning that it is fat-soluble rather than water-soluble. Other lipids include fatty acids, glycerides, alcohol, waxes, steroids, and fat-soluble vitamins A, D, and E. Lipids and water, like oil and water, do not mix. Blood is a water-based liquid, therefore cholesterol does not mix with blood. In order to travel through the blood without clumping together, cholesterol needs to be covered by a layer of protein. The cholesterol and protein together are called a *lipoprotein*.

There are two kinds of cholesterol, commonly called the "good" and the "bad." Good cholesterol is *high-density lipoprotein, or HDL*; bad cholesterol is *low-density lipoprotein, or LDL*. Together, these two forms of cholesterol make up a person's *total serum cholesterol* level. Most cholesterol tests measure the level of total cholesterol in the blood and don't distinguish between good and bad cholesterol. For these total serum cholesterol tests, a level of less than 200 mg/dL** is considered safe, while a level of more than 240 is considered dangerous and places a person at risk for heart disease and stroke.

*** mg/dL describes the weight of cholesterol in milligrams in a deciliter of blood. This is the standard way of measuring blood cholesterol levels.*

Most cholesterol in the body is in the form of LDL. LDLs circulate through the bloodstream, picking up excess cholesterol and depositing cholesterol where it is needed (for example, for the production and maintenance of cell membranes). But when too much cholesterol starts circulating in the blood, the body cannot handle the excessive LDLs, which build up along the inside of the arterial walls. The buildup of LDL coating on the inside of the artery walls hardens and turns into arterial plaque, leading to stenosis and atherosclerosis. This plaque blocks blood vessels and contributes to the formation of blood clots. A person's LDL level should be less than 130 mg/dL to be safe. LDL levels between 130 and 159 put a person at a slightly higher risk for atherosclerosis, heart disease, and stroke. A score over 160 puts a person at great risk for a heart attack or stroke.

The other form of cholesterol, HDL, is beneficial and contributes to stroke prevention. HDL carries a small percentage of the cholesterol in the blood, but instead of depositing its cholesterol on the inside of artery walls, HDL returns to the liver to unload its cholesterol. The liver then eliminates the excess cholesterol by passing it along to the kidneys. Currently, any HDL score higher than 35 is considered desirable. Recent studies have shown that high levels of HDL are associated with a reduced risk for heart disease and stroke and that low levels (less than 35 mg/dL), even in people with normal levels of LDL, lead to an increased risk for heart disease and stroke.

A person may lower his risk for atherosclerosis and stroke by improving his cholesterol levels. A healthy diet and regular exercise are the best ways to lower total cholesterol levels. In some cases, physicians may prescribe cholesterol-lowering medication, and recent studies have shown that the newest types of these drugs, called reductase inhibitors or statin drugs, significantly reduce the risk for stroke in most patients with high cholesterol. Scientists believe that statins may work by reducing the amount of bad cholesterol the body produces and by reducing the body's inflammatory immune reaction to cholesterol plaque associated with atherosclerosis and stroke.

Diabetes

Diabetes is another disease that increases a person's risk for stroke. People with diabetes have three times the risk of stroke compared to people without diabetes. The relative risk of stroke from diabetes is highest in the fifth and sixth decades of life and decreases after that. Like hypertension, the relative risk of stroke from diabetes is highest for men at an earlier age and highest for women at an older age. People with diabetes may also have other contributing risk factors that can amplify the overall risk for stroke. For example, the prevalence of hypertension is 40 percent higher in the diabetic population compared to the general population.

Modifiable Lifestyle Risk Factors

Cigarette smoking is the most powerful modifiable stroke risk factor. Smoking almost doubles a person's risk for ischemic stroke, independent of other risk factors, and it increases a person's risk for subarachnoid hemorrhage by up to 3.5 percent. Smoking is directly responsible for a greater percentage of the total number of strokes in young adults than in older adults. Risk factors other than smoking—like hypertension, heart disease, and diabetes—account for more of the total number of strokes in older adults.

Heavy smokers are at greater risk for stroke than light smokers. The relative risk of stroke decreases immediately after quitting smoking, with a major reduction of risk seen after 2 to 4 years. Unfortunately, it may take several decades for a former smoker's risk to drop to the level of someone who never smoked.

Smoking increases the risk of stroke by promoting atherosclerosis and increasing the levels of blood-clotting factors, such as fibrinogen. In addition to promoting conditions linked to stroke, smoking also increases the damage that results from stroke by weakening the *endothelial wall* of the cerebrovascular system. This leads to greater damage to the brain from events that occur in the secondary stage of stroke.

High alcohol consumption is another modifiable risk factor for stroke. Generally, an increase in alcohol consumption leads to an increase in blood pressure. While scientists agree that heavy drinking is a risk for both hemorrhagic and ischemic stroke, in several research studies daily consumption of smaller amounts of alcohol has been found to provide a protective influence against ischemic stroke, perhaps because alcohol decreases the clotting ability of *platelets* in the blood. Moderate alcohol consumption may act in the same way as aspirin to decrease blood clotting and prevent ischemic stroke. Heavy alcohol consumption, though, may seriously deplete platelet numbers and compromise blood clotting and blood viscosity, leading to hemorrhage. In addition, heavy drinking or binge drinking can lead to a rebound effect after the alcohol is purged from the body. The consequences of this rebound effect are that blood viscosity (thickness) and platelet levels skyrocket after heavy drinking, increasing the risk for ischemic stroke.

The use of illicit drugs, such as cocaine and crack cocaine, can cause stroke. Cocaine may act on other risk factors, such as hypertension, heart disease, and vascular disease, to trigger a stroke. It decreases relative cerebrovascular blood flow by up to 30 percent, causes vascular constriction, and inhibits vascular relaxation, leading to narrowing of the arteries. Cocaine also affects the heart, causing arrhythmias and rapid heart rate that can lead to the formation of blood clots.

Marijuana smoking may also be a risk factor for stroke. Marijuana decreases blood pressure and may interact with other risk factors, such as hypertension and cigarette smoking, to cause rapidly fluctuating blood pressure levels, damaging blood vessels.

Other drugs of abuse, such as amphetamines, heroin, and anabolic steroids (and even some common, legal drugs, such as caffeine and L-asparaginase and pseudoephedrine found in over-the-counter decongestants), have been suspected of increasing stroke risk. Many of these drugs are vasoconstrictors, meaning that they cause blood vessels to constrict and blood pressure to rise.

Head and Neck Injuries

Injuries to the head or neck may damage the cerebrovascular system and cause a small number of strokes. Head injury or traumatic brain injury may cause bleeding within the brain leading to damage akin to that caused by a hemorrhagic stroke. Neck injury, when associated with spontaneous tearing of the vertebral or carotid arteries caused by sudden and severe extension of the neck, neck rotation, or pressure on the artery, is a contributing cause of stroke, especially in young adults. This type of stroke is often called "beauty-parlor syndrome," which refers to the practice of extending the neck backwards over a sink for hair-washing in beauty parlors. Neck calisthenics, "bottoms-up" drinking, and improperly performed chiropractic manipulation of the neck can also put strain on the vertebral and carotid arteries, possibly leading to ischemic stroke.

Infections

Recent viral and bacterial infections may act with other risk factors to add a small risk for stroke. The immune system responds to infection by increasing inflammation and increasing the infection-fighting properties of the blood. Unfortunately, this immune response increases the number of clotting factors in the blood, leading to an increased risk of embolic-ischemic stroke.

Genetic Risk Factors

Although there may not be a single genetic factor associated with stroke, genes do play a large role in the expression of stroke risk factors such as hypertension, heart disease, diabetes, and vascular malformations. It is also possible that an increased risk for stroke within a family is due to environmental factors, such as a common sedentary lifestyle or poor eating habits, rather than hereditary factors.

Vascular malformations that cause stroke may have the strongest genetic link of all stroke risk factors. A vascular malformation is an abnormally formed blood vessel or group of blood vessels. One genetic vascular disease called CADASIL, which stands for cerebral autosomal dominant arteriopathy with subcortical infarcts and leukoencephalopathy. CADASIL is a rare, genetically inherited, congenital vascular disease of the brain that causes strokes, subcortical dementia, migraine-like headaches, and psychiatric disturbances. CADASIL is very debilitating and symptoms usually surface around the age of 45. The exact incidence of CADASIL in the United States is unknown.

Medications

Medication or drug therapy is the most common treatment for stroke. The most popular classes of drugs used to prevent or treat stroke are *antithrombotics* (*antiplatelet agents* and *anticoagulants*) and *thrombolytics*.

Antithrombotics prevent the formation of blood clots that can become lodged in a cerebral artery and cause strokes. Antiplatelet drugs prevent clotting by decreasing the activity of platelets, blood cells that contribute to the clotting property of blood. These drugs reduce the risk of blood-clot formation, thus reducing the risk of ischemic stroke. In the context of stroke, physicians prescribe antiplatelet drugs mainly for prevention. The most widely known and used antiplatelet drug is aspirin. Other antiplatelet drugs include clopidogrel, ticlopidine, and dipyridamole. The NINDS sponsors a wide range of clinical trials to determine the effectiveness of antiplatelet drugs for stroke prevention.

Anticoagulants reduce stroke risk by reducing the clotting property of the blood. The most commonly used anticoagulants include *warfarin* (also known as *Coumadin*®), *heparin*, and *enoxaparin* (also known as *Lovenox*). The NINDS has sponsored several trials to test the efficacy of anticoagulants versus antiplatelet drugs. The Stroke Prevention in

Atrial Fibrillation (SPAF) trial found that, although aspirin is an effective therapy for the prevention of a second stroke in most patients with atrial fibrillation, some patients with additional risk factors do better on warfarin therapy. Another study, the Trial of Org 10127 in Acute Stroke Treatment (TOAST), tested the effectiveness of low-molecular weight heparin (Org 10172) in stroke prevention. TOAST showed that heparin anticoagulants are not generally effective in preventing recurrent stroke or improving outcome.

Thrombolytic agents are used to treat an ongoing, acute ischemic stroke caused by an artery blockage. These drugs halt the stroke by dissolving the blood clot that is blocking blood flow to the brain. *Recombinant tissue plasminogen activator (rt-PA)* is a genetically engineered form of t-PA, a thrombolytic substance made naturally by the body. It can be effective if given intravenously within 3 hours of stroke symptom onset, but it should be used only after a physician has confirmed that the patient has suffered an ischemic stroke. Thrombolytic agents can increase bleeding and therefore must be used only after careful patient screening. The NINDS rt-PA Stroke Study showed the efficacy of t-PA and in 1996 led to the first FDA-approved treatment for acute ischemic stroke. Other thrombolytics are currently being tested in clinical trials.

Neuroprotectants are medications that protect the brain from secondary injury caused by stroke. Although no neuroprotectants are FDA-approved for use in stroke at this time, many are in clinical trials. There are several different classes of neuroprotectants that show promise for future therapy, including glutamate antagonists, antioxidants, apoptosis inhibitors, and many others.

Surgery

Surgery can be used to prevent stroke, to treat acute stroke, or to repair vascular damage or malformations in and around the brain. There are two prominent types of surgery for stroke prevention and treatment: carotid endarterectomy and *extracranial/intracranial (EC/IC) bypass*.

Carotid endarterectomy is a surgical procedure in which a doctor removes fatty deposits (plaque) from the inside of one of the carotid arteries, which are located in the neck and are the main suppliers of blood to the brain. As mentioned earlier, the disease atherosclerosis is characterized by the buildup of plaque on the inside of large arteries, and the blockage of an artery by this fatty material is called stenosis.

The NINDS has sponsored two large clinical trials to test the efficacy of carotid endarterectomy: the North American Symptomatic Carotid Endarterectomy Trial (NASCET) and the Asymptomatic Carotid Atherosclerosis Trial (ACAS). These trials showed that carotid endarterectomy is a safe and effective stroke prevention therapy for most people with greater than 50 percent stenosis of the carotid arteries when performed by a qualified and experienced neurosurgeon or vascular surgeon.

Currently, the NINDS is sponsoring the Carotid Revascularization Endarterectomy vs. Stenting Trial (CREST), a large clinical trial designed to test the effectiveness of carotid endarterectomy versus a newer surgical procedure for carotid stenosis called stenting. The procedure involves inserting a long, thin catheter tube into an artery in the leg and threading the catheter through the vascular system into the narrow stenosis of the carotid artery in the neck. Once the catheter is in place in the carotid artery, the radiologist expands the stent with a balloon on the tip of the catheter. The CREST trial will test the effectiveness of the new surgical technique versus the established standard technique of carotid endarterectomy surgery.

EC/IC bypass surgery is a procedure that restores blood flow to a blood-deprived area of brain tissue by rerouting a healthy artery in the scalp to the area of brain tissue affected by a blocked artery. The NINDS-sponsored EC/IC Bypass Study tested the ability of this surgery to prevent recurrent strokes in stroke patients with atherosclerosis. The study showed that, in the long run, EC/IC does not seem to benefit these patients. The surgery is still performed occasionally for patients with aneurysms, some types of small artery disease, and certain vascular abnormalities.

One useful surgical procedure for treatment of brain aneurysms that cause subarachnoid hemorrhage is a technique called *"clipping."* Clipping involves clamping off the aneurysm from the blood vessel, which reduces the chance that it will burst and bleed.

A new therapy that is gaining wide attention is the *detachable coil* technique for the treatment of high-risk intracranial aneurysms. A small platinum coil is inserted through an artery in the thigh and threaded through the arteries to the site of the aneurysm. The coil is then released into the aneurysm, where it evokes an immune response from the body. The body produces a blood clot inside the aneurysm, strengthening the artery walls and reducing the risk of rupture. Once the aneurysm is stabilized, a neurosurgeon can clip the aneurysm with less risk of hemorrhage and death to the patient.

351

Table 21.1. Post-Stroke Rehabilitation

Type	Goal
Physical Therapy (PT)	Relearn walking, sitting, lying down, switching from one type of movement to another
Occupational Therapy (OT)	Relearn eating, drinking, dressing, bathing, cooking, reading, writing, toileting
Speech Therapy	Relearn language and communications skills, including swallowing.
Psychological/Psychiatric Therapy	Alleviate some mental and emotional problems

Rehabilitation Therapy

Stroke is the number one cause of serious adult disability in the United States. Stroke disability is devastating to the stroke patient and family, but therapies are available to help rehabilitate post-stroke patients.

For most stroke patients, physical therapy (PT) is the cornerstone of the rehabilitation process. A physical therapist uses training, exercises, and physical manipulation of the stroke patient's body with the intent of restoring movement, balance, and coordination. The aim of PT is to have the stroke patient relearn simple motor activities such as walking, sitting, standing, lying down, and the process of switching from one type of movement to another.

Another type of therapy involving relearning daily activities is occupational therapy (OT). OT also involves exercise and training to help the stroke patient relearn everyday activities such as eating, drinking, dressing, bathing, cooking, reading and writing, and toileting. The goal of OT is to help the patient become independent or semi-independent.

Speech and language problems arise when brain damage occurs in the language centers of the brain. Due to the brain's great ability to learn and change (called brain *plasticity*), other areas can adapt to take over some of the lost functions. Speech language pathologists help stroke patients relearn language and speaking skills, including swallowing, or learn other forms of communication. Speech therapy is appropriate for any patients with problems understanding speech or written words, or problems forming speech. A speech therapist helps stroke patients help themselves by working to improve language skills, develop alternative ways of communicating, and develop coping skills to deal with the frustration of not being able to communicate fully. With time and patience, a stroke survivor should be able to regain some, and sometimes all, language and speaking abilities.

Many stroke patients require psychological or psychiatric help after a stroke. Psychological problems, such as depression, anxiety, frustration, and anger, are common post-stroke disabilities. Talk therapy, along with appropriate medication, can help alleviate some of the mental and emotional problems that result from stroke. Sometimes it is also beneficial for family members of the stroke patient to seek psychological help as well.

For more information on rehabilitation, contact the National Rehabilitation Information Center, a service of the National Institute on Disability and Rehabilitation Research.

What Disabilities Can Result From a Stroke?

Although stroke is a disease of the brain, it can affect the entire body. Some of the disabilities that can result from a stroke include paralysis, cognitive deficits, speech problems, emotional difficulties, daily living problems, and pain.

Paralysis:

A common disability that results from stroke is complete paralysis on one side of the body, called *hemiplegia*. A related disability that is not as debilitating as paralysis is one-sided weakness or *hemiparesis*. The paralysis or weakness may affect only the face, an arm, or a leg or may affect one entire side of the body and face. A person who suffers a stroke in the left hemisphere of the brain will show right-sided paralysis or paresis. Conversely, a person with a stroke in the right hemisphere of the brain will show deficits on the left side of the body. A stroke patient may have problems with the simplest of daily activities, such as walking, dressing, eating, and using the bathroom. Motor deficits can result from damage to the motor cortex in the frontal lobes of the brain or from damage to the lower parts of the brain, such as the cerebellum, which controls balance and coordination. Some stroke patients also have trouble swallowing, called *dysphagia*.

Cognitive deficits:

Stroke may cause problems with thinking, awareness, attention, learning, judgment, and memory. In some cases of stroke, the patient suffers a "neglect" syndrome. The neglect means that a stroke patient has no knowledge of one side of his or her body, or one side of the visual field, or is unaware of the deficit. A stroke patient may be unaware of his or her surroundings, or may be unaware of the mental deficits that resulted from the stroke.

Language deficits:

Stroke victims often have problems understanding or forming speech. A deficit in understanding or forming speech is called *aphasia*. Aphasia usually occurs along with similar problems in reading or writing. In most people, language problems result from damage to the left hemisphere of the brain. Slurred speech due to weakness or incoordination of the muscles involved in speaking is called *dysarthria*, and is not a problem with language. Because it can result from any weakness or incoordination of the speech muscles, dysarthria can arise from damage to either side of the brain.

Emotional deficits:

A stroke can lead to emotional problems. Stroke patients may have difficulty controlling their emotions or may express inappropriate emotions in certain situations. One common disability that occurs with many stroke patients is depression. Post-stroke depression may be more than a general sadness resulting from the stroke incident. It is a clinical behavioral problem that can hamper recovery and rehabilitation and may even lead to suicide. Post-stroke depression is treated as any depression is treated, with antidepressant medications and therapy.

Pain:

Stroke patients may experience pain, uncomfortable numbness, or strange sensations after a stroke. These sensations may be due to many factors including damage to the sensory regions of the brain, stiff joints, or a disabled limb. An uncommon type of pain resulting from stroke is called *central stroke pain* or *central pain syndrome* (CPS). CPS results from damage to an area in the mid-brain called the thalamus. The pain is a mixture of sensations, including heat and cold, burning, tingling, numbness, and sharp stabbing and underlying aching pain. The pain is often worse in the extremities—the hands and feet—and is made worse by movement and temperature changes, especially cold temperatures. Unfortunately, since most pain medications provide little relief from these sensations, very few treatments or therapies exist to combat CPS.

What Special Risks do Women Face?

Some risk factors for stroke apply only to women. Primary among these are pregnancy, childbirth, and menopause. These risk factors are tied to hormonal fluctuations and changes that affect a woman in different stages of life. Research in the past few decades has shown that high-dose oral contraceptives, the kind used in the 1960s and 1970s, can increase the risk of stroke in women. Fortunately, oral contraceptives with high doses of estrogen are no longer used and have been replaced with safer and more effective oral contraceptives with lower doses of estrogen. Some studies have shown the newer low-dose oral contraceptives may not significantly increase the risk of stroke in women.

Other studies have demonstrated that pregnancy and childbirth can put a woman at an increased risk for stroke. Pregnancy increases the risk of stroke as much as three to 13 times. Of course, the risk of stroke in young women of childbearing years is very small to begin with, so a moderate increase in risk during pregnancy is still a relatively small risk. Pregnancy and childbirth cause strokes in approximately eight in 100,000 women. Unfortunately, 25 percent of strokes during pregnancy end in death, and hemorrhagic strokes, although rare, are still the leading cause of maternal death in the United States. Subarachnoid hemorrhage, in particular, causes one to five maternal deaths per 10,000 pregnancies.

A study sponsored by the NINDS showed that the risk of stroke during pregnancy is greatest in the post-partum period—the 6 weeks following childbirth. The risk of ischemic stroke after pregnancy is about nine times higher and the risk of hemorrhagic stroke is more than 28 times higher for post-partum women than for women who are not pregnant or post-partum. The cause is unknown.

In the same way that the hormonal changes during pregnancy and childbirth are associated with increased risk of stroke, hormonal changes at the end of the childbearing years can increase the risk of stroke. Several studies have shown that menopause, the end of a woman's reproductive ability marked by the termination of her menstrual cycle, can increase a woman's risk of stroke. Fortunately, some studies have suggested that hormone replacement therapy can reduce some of the effects of menopause and decrease stroke risk. Currently, the NINDS is sponsoring the Women's Estrogen for Stroke Trial (WEST), a randomized, placebo-controlled, double-blind trial, to determine whether estrogen therapy can reduce the risk of death or recurrent stroke in postmenopausal women who have a history of a recent TIA or non-disabling stroke. The mechanism by which estrogen can prove beneficial to postmenopausal women could include its role in cholesterol control. Studies have shown that estrogen acts to increase levels of HDL while decreasing LDL levels.

Are Children at Risk For Stroke?

The young have several risk factors unique to them. Young people seem to suffer from hemorrhagic strokes more than ischemic strokes, a significant difference from older age groups where ischemic strokes make up the majority of stroke cases. Hemorrhagic strokes represent 20 percent of all strokes in the United States and young people account for many of these.

Clinicians often separate the "young" into two categories: those younger than 15 years of age, and those 15 to 44 years of age. People 15 to 44 years of age are generally considered young adults and have many of the risk factors mentioned above, such as drug use, alcohol abuse, pregnancy, head and neck injuries, heart disease or heart malformations, and infections. Some other causes of stroke in the young are linked to genetic diseases.

Medical complications that can lead to stroke in children include intracranial infection, brain injury, vascular malformations such as moyamoya syndrome, occlusive vascular disease, and genetic disorders such as sickle cell anemia, tuberous sclerosis, and Marfan's syndrome.

The symptoms of stroke in children are different from those in adults and young adults. A child experiencing a stroke may have seizures, a sudden loss of speech, a loss of expressive language (including body language and gestures), hemiparesis (weakness on one side of the body), hemiplegia (paralysis on one side of the body), dysarthria (impairment of speech), convulsions, headache, or fever. It is a medical emergency when a child shows any of these symptoms.

In children with stroke the underlying conditions that led to the stroke should be determined and managed to prevent future strokes. For example, a recent clinical study sponsored by the National Heart, Lung, and Blood Institute found that giving blood transfusions to young children with sickle cell anemia greatly reduces the risk of stroke. The Institute even suggests attempting to prevent stroke in high-risk children by giving them blood transfusions before they experience a stroke.

Most children who experience a stroke will do better than most adults after treatment and rehabilitation. This is due in part to the immature brain's great plasticity, the ability to adapt to deficits and injury. Children who experience seizures along with stroke do not recover as well as children who do not have seizures. Some children may experience residual hemiplegia, though most will eventually learn how to walk.

What research is being done by the NINDS?

The NINDS is the leading supporter of stroke research in the United States and sponsors a wide range of experimental research studies, from investigations of basic biological mechanisms to studies with animal models and clinical trials.

Currently, NINDS researchers are studying the mechanisms of stroke risk factors and the process of brain damage that results from stroke. Some of this brain damage may be secondary to the initial death of brain cells caused by the lack of blood flow to the brain tissue. This secondary wave of brain injury is a result of a toxic reaction to the primary damage and mainly involves the excitatory neurochemical, glutamate. Glutamate in the normal brain functions as a chemical messenger between brain cells, allowing them to communicate. But an excess amount of glutamate in the brain causes too much activity and brain cells quickly "burn out" from too much excitement, releasing more toxic chemicals, such as caspases, cytokines, monocytes, and oxygen-free radicals. These substances poison the chemical environment of surrounding cells, initiating a cascade of degeneration and programmed cell death, called *apoptosis*. NINDS researchers are studying the mechanisms underlying this secondary insult, which consists mainly of inflammation, toxicity, and a breakdown of the blood vessels that provide blood to the brain. Researchers are also looking for ways to prevent secondary injury to the brain by providing different types of neuroprotection for salvageable cells that prevent inflammation and block some of the toxic chemicals created by dying brain cells. From this research, scientists hope to develop neuroprotective agents to prevent secondary damage. For more information on excitotoxicity, neuroprotection, and the ischemic cascade.

Basic research has also focused on the genetics of stroke and stroke risk factors. One area of research involving genetics is gene therapy. Gene therapy involves putting a gene for a desired protein in certain cells of the body. The inserted gene will then "program" the cell to produce the desired protein. If enough cells in the right areas produce enough protein, then the protein could be therapeutic. Scientists must find ways to deliver the therapeutic DNA to the appropriate cells and must learn how to deliver enough DNA to enough cells so that the tissues produce a therapeutic amount of protein. Gene therapy is in the very early stages of development and there are many problems to overcome, including learning how to penetrate the highly impermeable *blood-brain barrier* and how to halt the host's immune reaction to the virus that carries the gene to the cells. Some of the proteins used for stroke therapy could include neuroprotective proteins, anti-inflammatory proteins, and DNA/cellular repair proteins, among others.

The NINDS supports and conducts a wide variety of studies in animals, from genetics research on zebrafish to rehabilitation research on primates. Much of the Institute's animal research involves rodents, specifically mice and rats. For example, one study of hypertension and stroke uses rats that have been bred to be hypertensive and therefore stroke-prone. By studying stroke in rats, scientists hope to get a better picture of what might be happening in human stroke patients. Scientists can also use animal models to test promising therapeutic interventions for stroke. If a therapy proves to be beneficial to animals, then scientists can consider testing the therapy in human subjects.

One promising area of stroke animal research involves hibernation. The dramatic decrease of blood flow to the brain in hibernating animals is extensive—extensive enough that it would kill a non-hibernating animal. During hibernation, an animal's metabolism slows down, body temperature drops, and energy and oxygen requirements of brain cells decrease. If scientists can discover how animals hibernate without experiencing brain damage, then maybe they can discover ways to stop the brain damage associated with decreased blood flow in stroke patients. Other studies are looking at the role of hypothermia, or decreased body temperature, on metabolism and neuroprotection.

Both hibernation and hypothermia have a relationship to *hypoxia* and *edema*. Hypoxia, or *anoxia*, occurs when there is not enough oxygen available for brain cells to function properly. Since brain cells require large amounts of oxygen for energy requirements, they are especially vulnerable to hypoxia. Edema occurs when the chemical balance of brain tissue is disturbed and water or fluids flow into the brain cells, making them swell and burst, releasing their toxic contents into the surrounding tissues. Edema is one cause of general brain tissue swelling and contributes to the secondary injury associated with stroke.

The basic and animal studies discussed above do not involve people and fall under the category of preclinical research; clinical research involves people. One area of investigation that has made the transition from animal models to clinical research is the study of the mechanisms underlying brain plasticity and the neuronal rewiring that occurs after a stroke.

New advances in imaging and rehabilitation have shown that the brain can compensate for function lost as a result of stroke. When cells in an area of the brain responsible for a particular function die after a stroke, the patient becomes unable to perform that function. For example, a stroke patient with an infarct in the area of the brain responsible for facial recognition becomes unable to recognize faces, a syndrome called facial agnosia. But, in time, the person may come to recognize faces again, even though the area of the brain originally programmed to perform that function remains dead. The plasticity of the brain and the rewiring of the neural connections make it possible for one part of the brain to change functions and take up the more important functions of a disabled part. This rewiring of the brain and restoration of function, which the brain tries to do automatically, can be helped with therapy. Scientists are working to develop new and better ways to help the brain repair itself to restore important functions to the stroke patient.

One example of a therapy resulting from this research is the use of *transcranial magnetic stimulation (TMS)* in stroke rehabilitation. Some evidence suggests that TMS, in which a small magnetic current is delivered to an area of the brain, may possibly increase brain plasticity and speed up recovery of function after a stroke. The TMS device is a small coil which is held outside of the head, over the part of the brain needing stimulation. Currently, several studies at the NINDS are testing whether TMS has any value in increasing motor function and improving functional recovery.

Clinical Trials

Clinical research is usually conducted in a series of trials that become progressively larger. A phase I clinical trial is directly built upon the lessons learned from basic and animal research and is used to test the safety of therapy for a particular disease and to estimate possible efficacy in a few human subjects. A phase II clinical trial usually involves many subjects at several different centers and is used to test safety and possible efficacy on a broader scale, to test different dosing for medications or to perfect techniques for surgery, and to determine the best methodology and outcome measures for the bigger phase III clinical trial to come.

A phase III clinical trial is the largest endeavor in clinical research. This type of trial often involves many centers and many subjects. The trial usually has two patient groups who receive different treatments, but all other standard care is the same and represents the best care available. The trial may compare two treatments, or, if there is only one treatment to test, patients who do not receive the test therapy receive instead a placebo. The patients are told that the additional treatment they are receiving may be either the active treatment or a placebo. Many phase III trials are called double-blind, randomized clinical trials. Double-blind means that neither the subjects nor the doctors and nurses who are treating the subjects and determining the response to the therapy know which treatment a subject receives. Randomization refers to the placing of subjects into one of the treatment groups in a way that can't be predicted by the patients or investigators. These clinical trials usually involve many investigators and take many years to complete. The hypothesis and methods of the trial are very precise and well thought out. Clinical trial designs, as well as the concepts of blinding and randomization, have developed over years of experimentation, trial, and error. At the present time, researchers are developing new designs to maximize the opportunity for all subjects to receive therapy.

Most treatments for general use come out of phase III clinical trials. After one or more phase III trials are finished, and if the results are positive for the treatment, the investigators can petition the FDA for government approval to use the drug or procedure to treat patients. Once the treatment is approved by the FDA, it can be used by qualified doctors throughout the country.

NINDS-Sponsored Stroke Clinical Trials: September 2012

Clinical trials give researchers a way to test new treatments in human subjects. Clinical trials test surgical devices and procedures, medications, rehabilitation therapies, and lifestyle and psychosocial interventions to determine how safe and effective they are and to establish the proper amount or level of treatment. Because of their scope and the need for careful analysis of data and outcomes, clinical trials are usually conducted in three phases and can take several years or more to complete.

- **Phase I** clinical trials are small (involving fewer than 100 people) and are designed to define side effects and tolerance of the medication or therapy.

- **Phase II** trials are conducted with a larger group of subjects and seek to measure the effects of a therapy and establish its proper dosage or level of treatment.

- **Phase III** trials often involve hundreds (sometimes thousands) of volunteer patients who are assigned to treatment and non-treatment groups to test how well the treatment works and how safe it is at the recommended dosage or level of therapy. Many of these trials use a controlled, randomized, double-blind study design. This means that patients are randomly assigned to groups and neither the subject nor the study staff knows to which group a patient belongs. Phase III randomized clinical trials are often called the gold standard of clinical trials.

NINDS conducts clinical trials at the NIH Clinical Center and also provides funding for clinical trials at hospitals and universities across the United States and Canada. Below are findings from some of the largest and most significant recent clinical trials in stroke, as well as summaries of some of the most promising clinical trials in progress.

Findings from Recently Completed Clinical Trials

The Carotid Revascularization Endarterectomy vs. Stenting Trial (CREST)

The use of dilation and stenting techniques similar to those used to unclog and open heart arteries has been proposed as a less invasive alternative to carotid endarterectomy (surgery to remove the buildup of plaque within the carotid artery, which supplies blood to the head and neck). Carotid endarterectomy is considered the gold standard treatment for preventing stroke and other vascular events. Stenting is a newer, less invasive procedure in which an expandable metal stent (tube) is inserted into the carotid artery to keep it open after it has been widened with balloon dilation. The CREST study showed that the overall safety and effectiveness of the two procedures was largely the same—with equal benefits for both men and women, and for people who had previously had a stroke and for those who had not. Physicians will now have more options to tailor treatments for people at risk for stroke.

Carotid Occlusion Surgery Study (COSS)

The goal of this randomized clinical trial was to determine the preventive power of extracranial bypass surgery in a group of stroke survivors who have both a blocked carotid artery and an increased oxygen extraction fraction (or OEF, which indicates how hard the brain has to work to pull oxygen from the blood supply). An increased OEF has been shown to be a powerful and independent risk factor for subsequent stroke. Extracranial bypass surgery uses a healthy blood vessel to detour blood flow around the site of the blocked artery and results in increased blood flow to the brain. The results showed that in spite of the surgical success of improving cerebral blood flow, extra-cranial-intracranial bypass surgery did not demonstrate any benefit in reducing the risk of having a stroke recurrence due to the much better than expected recurrence rate in the non-surgical medical alone group.

Locomotor Experience Applied Post-Stroke (LEAPS)

Only 37 percent of stroke survivors are able to walk after the first week following their stroke. The investigators of the Locomotor Experience Applied Post-Stroke (LEAPS) trial set out to compare the effectiveness of the body-weight supported treadmill training with walking practice started at two different stages—two months post-stroke (early locomotor training) and six months post-stroke (late locomotor training). The locomotor training was also compared against a home exercise program managed by a physical therapist, aimed at enhancing patients' flexibility, range of motion, strength and balance as a way to improve their walking. The primary measure was each group's improvement in walking at one year after the stroke. The study found that stroke patients who had physical therapy at home improved their ability to walk just as well as those who were treated in a training program that requires the use of a body-weight supported treadmill device followed by walking practice. In addition, the study also found that patients continued to improve up to one year after stroke, defying conventional wisdom that recovery occurs early and tops out at six months.

Secondary Prevention of Small Subcortical Strokes (SPS3)

In this trial, investigators are testing new approaches to stroke prevention for people with a history of small subcortical strokes. The trial was designed to compare: 1) aspirin alone vs. combined antiplatelet therapy (aspirin and clopidogrel), and 2) intensive vs. standard blood pressure control. Subcortical strokes, also called lacunar strokes, occur when the thread-like arteries within cerebral tissue become blocked and halt blood flow to the brain. They account for up to one-fifth of all strokes in the U.S. and are especially common among people of Hispanic descent. In the antiplatelet component of SPS3, researchers have found that the combined antiplatelet therapy was about equal to aspirin in reducing stroke risk, but it almost doubled the risk of gastrointestinal bleeding. The blood pressure component of the trial is ongoing.

Stenting vs. Aggressive Medical Management for Preventing Recurrent Stroke in Intracranial Stenosis (SAMMPRIS)

The best treatment for preventing another stroke or TIA in patients with narrowing of a brain artery is uncertain. The purpose of this trial was to compare the safety and effectiveness of aggressive medical treatment (i.e., intensive management of key stroke risk factors including blood pressure, cholesterol, and lifestyle modification) alone to aggressive medical therapy plus a Food and Drug Administration (FDA)-approved intracranial stent to prevent another stroke in individuals who recently had either a transient ischemic attack or non-disabling stroke. The results of this trial, which was stopped early, showed that the group that received the intensive medical management alone had better outcomes than the group who also received the stent. This study provides an answer to a long-standing question by physicians—what to do to prevent a devastating second stroke in a high risk population.

Ongoing Clinical Trials

Albumin in Acute Ischemic Stroke (ALIAS) Trial

Human serum albumin is a protein found in human blood plasma that may have neuroprotective benefit in stroke. The Albumin in Acute Ischemic Stroke trial will compare the use of intravenous albumin administered over a two- hour period to placebo among individuals with acute ischemic stroke, beginning within five hours of stroke onset. Individuals will also receive concurrent treatment with a thrombolytic drug given either intravenously or intra-arterially when appropriate. Patients receiving either albumin or placebo will be followed for one year. The primary outcome will be an assessment of neurological function at three months post-stroke.

Antihypertensive Treatment of Acute Cerebral Hemorrhage (ATACH II)

Intensive blood pressure management following an intracerebral hemorrhage (ICH) may slow the rate and magnitude of the hemorrhage. The primary goal of the Antihypertensive Treatment of Acute Cerebral Hemorrhage trial is to determine the efficacy and safety of intensive systolic blood pressure management in ICH patients treated within three hours of symptom onset. The approach of intensive systolic blood pressure control represents a strategy that can be made widely available without the need of specialized equipment and personnel. Therefore, it has the potential to make a major impact on outcome in patients with ICH.

A Randomized Trial of Unruptured Brain Arteriovenous Malformations (ARUBA)

Arteriovenous malformations (AVMs) are defects of the circulatory system comprised of tangles of arteries and veins that are present from birth. These defects, which can occur in the brain, spinal cord, or other organs, may cause symptoms such as headaches or seizures. AVM that have not ruptured may be left untreated until they become symptomatic or may undergo surgical radiation or endovascular treatment to prevent future rupture. In A Randomized Trial of Unruptured Brain Arteriovenous Malformations (ARUBA), scientists will treat participants with unruptured brain AVMs either conservatively (medical management) or using invasive therapy (surgery, radiation, embolization) and follow their progress for at least five years to compare benefit in terms of reduced risk of subsequent stroke or AVM rupture. The outcome of this trial will indicate the best way to treat individuals with unruptured brain AVMs and offer doctors a more definitive standard of treatment.

Clot Lysis: Evaluating Accelerated Resolution of Intraventricular Hemorrhage, Phase III (CLEAR III)

The objective of the randomized Clot Lysis: Evaluating Accelerated Resolution of Intraventricular Hemorrhage III study is to determine any benefit of the use of the clot-busting drug recombinant tissue plasminogen activator (t-PA) in conjunction with clot removal for intraventricular hemorrhage. The investigators will compare extraventricular draining (surgically inserting tubes that drain fluid from the brain's ventricles) plus t-PA with extraventricular draining plus placebo in managing and treating individuals with small intracerebral hemorrhage and large intraventricular hemorrhage. Participants will receive either t-PA or a placebo every eight hours for up to nine doses. Symptom onset must be within 24 hours prior to a diagnostic CT scan. The neurological function of the two groups will be compared at six months following treatment.

Field Administration of Stroke Therapy Magnesium Trial (FAST-MAG)

Currently, the drug t-PA—the only treatment shown to be effective in treating acute ischemic stroke—must be administered after hospital arrival and within the first three hours of stroke occurrence. There is a need for new treatments that can be administered safely at an earlier time. The purpose of this multicenter, randomized, double-blind trial is to determine if paramedic initiation of the neuroprotective agent magnesium sulfate in the ambulance is an effective and safe treatment for acute stroke. This study will compare magnesium sulfate, an experimental therapy for stroke, vs. placebo among ambulance-transported patients with acute stroke. This trial will also determine if paramedics can safely, effectively and rapidly start neuroprotective therapies for stroke.

Insulin Resistance Intervention after Stroke Trial (IRIS)

The Insulin Resistance Intervention after Stroke (IRIS) trial tests a therapy based on evidence that links insulin resistance to an increased risk for stroke or heart disease. The goal of the trial is to determine if pioglitazone, a drug used to treat Type 2 diabetes, is effective in lowering the risk for stroke and heart attack in a group of nondiabetic men and women who have recently had a stroke and developed insulin resistance. If this intervention is effective, it has the potential to benefit a large number of stroke survivors.

Interdisciplinary Comprehensive Arm Rehabilitation Evaluation (I-CARE)

Building on the positive outcome of the EXCITE clinical trials, investigators in the Interdisciplinary Comprehensive Arm Rehabilitation Evaluation (I-CARE) trial are testing an experimental arm therapy called Accelerated Skills Acquisition Program (ASAP). This therapy combines challenging, intensive, and meaningful practice of tasks of the participant's choice compared to two standard types of therapy (customary arm therapy totaling 30 hours, and customary arm therapy for a duration indicated on the therapy prescription). ASAP is targeted at the acute period of stroke recovery and will enroll participants who are within one to three months after their stroke. Based on compelling scientific data, this combined therapeutic approach is designed to capitalize on the brain's inherent recovery capability to improve upper limb function in people with stroke who have weakness on one side of the body.

Interventional Management of Stroke Trial (IMS III)

The Interventional Management of Stroke Trial (IMS III) is a large study that compares two different strategies for restoring blood flow to the brain in patients who have had a severe ischemic stroke. Patients are randomized to receive either the standard FDA-approved intravenous (IV) treatment of the clot-dissolving drug t-PA alone or a combination approach that provides both standard IV t-PA and an intra-arterial (IA) therapy using either t-PA delivered into the artery directly at the site of the clot or an FDA-approved device to remove the blood clot in the brain. Therapy using both approaches will be initiated within three hours of stroke onset. The trial will measure the ability of participants to live and function independently three months after the stroke. It will also determine and compare the safety and cost effectiveness of the combined IV/IA approach to the standard IV t-PA approach.

Platelet-Oriented Inhibition in New TIA and Minor Ischemic Stroke (POINT) Trial

A transient ischemic attack (TIA) is a brief episode of neurological dysfunction that often is a harbinger of disabling strokes. The primary goal of the Platelet-Oriented Inhibition in New TIA and Minor Ischemic Stroke (POINT) trial is to determine if the drug clopidogrel (used to reduce or prevent blood clots) combined with aspirin is effective in preventing ischemic stroke and myocardial infarction. Individuals over age 18 who can begin treatment within 12 hours of symptom onset will be enrolled. If trial results are positive, treatment with clopidogrel could reduce the burden of stroke in the U.S. and substantially reduce costs of care.

Stroke Hyperglycemia Insulin Network Effort Trial (SHINE)

Nearly 40 percent of patients who experience an ischemic stroke are hyperglycemic upon arriving at the hospital. Current research has indicated that severe or prolonged hyperglycemia is associated with poorer outcome and increased disability. At present there are no clear guidelines for treating this condition. The purpose of this clinical trial is to determine whether tight glucose control of hyperglycemia with three days of intravenous insulin therapy is superior to the standard therapy of glucose control with subcutaneous insulin. The results from this 1,400 participant clinical trial will guide clinical practice all over the nation and the world.

What Stroke Therapies are Available?

Physicians have a wide range of therapies to choose from when determining a stroke patient's best therapeutic plan. The type of stroke therapy a patient should receive depends upon the stage of disease. Generally there are three treatment stages for stroke: prevention, therapy immediately after stroke, and post-stroke rehabilitation. Therapies to prevent a first or recurrent stroke are based on treating an individual's underlying risk factors for stroke, such as hypertension, atrial fibrillation, and diabetes, or preventing the widespread formation of blood clots that can cause ischemic stroke in everyone, whether or not risk factors are present. Acute stroke therapies try to stop a stroke while it is happening by quickly dissolving a blood clot causing the stroke or by stopping the bleeding of a hemorrhagic stroke. The purpose of post-stroke rehabilitation is to overcome disabilities that result from stroke damage.

Therapies for stroke include medications, surgery, or rehabilitation.

Part Five

Congenital Brain Disorders

Chapter 22

Arteriovenous Malformations and Other Vascular Lesions Of The Central Nervous System

What are arteriovenous malformations?

Arteriovenous malformations (AVMs) are defects of the circulatory system that are generally believed to arise during embryonic or fetal development or soon after birth. They are comprised of snarled tangles of arteries and veins. Arteries carry oxygen-rich blood away from the heart to the body's cells; veins return oxygen-depleted blood to the lungs and heart. The absence of capillaries—small blood vessels that connect arteries to veins—creates a short-cut for blood to pass directly from arteries to veins. The presence of an AVM disrupts this vital cyclical process. Although AVMs can develop in many different sites, those located in the brain or spinal cord—the two parts of the central nervous system—can have especially widespread effects on the body.

Text in this chapter is excerpted from "Arteriovenous Malformations and Other Vascular Lesions of the Central Nervous System Fact Sheet," National Institute of Neurological Disorders and Stroke (NINDS), February 23, 2015.

AVMs of the brain or spinal cord (neurological AVMs) are believed to affect approximately 300,000 Americans. They occur in males and females of all racial or ethnic backgrounds at roughly equal rates.

What are the symptoms?

Most people with neurological AVMs experience few, if any, significant symptoms, and the malformations tend to be discovered only incidentally, usually either at autopsy or during treatment for an unrelated disorder. But for about 12 percent of the affected population (about 36,000 of the estimated 300,000 Americans with AVMs), these abnormalities cause symptoms that vary greatly in severity. For a small fraction of the individuals within this group, such symptoms are severe enough to become debilitating or even life-threatening. Each year about 1 percent of those with AVMs will die as a direct result of the AVM.

Seizures and headaches are the most generalized symptoms of AVMs, but no particular type of seizure or headache pattern has been identified. Seizures can be partial or total, involving a loss of control over movement, convulsions, or a change in a person's level of consciousness. Headaches can vary greatly in frequency, duration, and intensity, sometimes becoming as severe as migraines. Sometimes a headache consistently affecting one side of the head may be closely linked to the site of an AVM. More frequently, however, the location of the pain is not specific to the lesion and may encompass most of the head.

AVMs also can cause a wide range of more specific neurological symptoms that vary from person to person, depending primarily upon the location of the AVM. Such symptoms may include muscle weakness or paralysis in one part of the body; a loss of coordination (*ataxia*) that can lead to such problems as gait disturbances; *apraxia*, or difficulties carrying out tasks that require planning; dizziness; visual disturbances such as a loss of part of the visual field; an inability to control eye movement; *papilledema* (swelling of a part of the optic nerve known as the optic disk); various problems using or understanding language (*aphasia*); abnormal sensations such as numbness, tingling, or spontaneous pain (*paresthesia* or *dysesthesia*); memory deficits; and mental confusion, hallucinations, or dementia. Researchers have recently uncovered evidence that AVMs may also cause subtle learning or behavioral disorders in some people during their childhood or adolescence, long before more obvious symptoms become evident.

One of the more distinctive signs indicating the presence of an AVM is an auditory phenomenon called a *bruit*, coined from the French word meaning *noise*. (A *sign* is a physical effect observable by a physician, but not by a patient.) Doctors use this term to describe the rhythmic, whooshing sound caused by excessively rapid blood flow through the arteries and veins of an AVM. The sound is similar to that made by a torrent of water rushing through a narrow pipe. A bruit can sometimes become a symptom when it is especially severe. When audible to individuals, the bruit may compromise hearing, disturb sleep, or cause significant psychological distress.

Symptoms caused by AVMs can appear at any age, but because these abnormalities tend to result from a slow buildup of neurological damage over time they are most often noticed when people are in their twenties, thirties, or forties. If AVMs do not become symptomatic by the time people reach their late forties or early fifties, they tend to remain stable and rarely produce symptoms. In women, pregnancy sometimes causes a sudden onset or worsening of symptoms, due to accompanying cardiovascular changes, especially increases in blood volume and blood pressure.

In contrast to the vast majority of neurological AVMs, one especially severe type causes symptoms to appear at, or very soon after, birth. Called a *vein of Galen defect* after the major blood vessel involved, this lesion is located deep inside the brain. It is frequently associated with *hydrocephalus* (an accumulation of fluid within certain spaces in the brain, often with visible enlargement of the head), swollen veins visible on the scalp, seizures, failure to thrive, and congestive heart failure. Children born with this condition who survive past infancy often remain developmentally impaired.

How do AVMs damage the brain and spinal cord?

AVMs become symptomatic only when the damage they cause to the brain or spinal cord reaches a critical level. This is one of the reasons why a relatively small fraction of people with these lesions experiences significant health problems related to the condition. AVMs damage the brain or spinal cord through three basic mechanisms: by reducing the amount of oxygen reaching neurological tissues; by causing bleeding (hemorrhage) into surrounding tissues; and by compressing or displacing parts of the brain or spinal cord.

AVMs compromise oxygen delivery to the brain or spinal cord by altering normal patterns of blood flow. Arteries and veins are normally interconnected by a series of progressively smaller blood vessels that control and slow the rate of blood flow. Oxygen delivery to surrounding tissues takes place through the thin, porous walls of the smallest of these interconnecting vessels, known as *capillaries*, where the blood flows most slowly. The arteries and veins that make up AVMs, however, lack this intervening capillary network. Instead, arteries dump blood directly into veins through a passageway called a *fistula*. The flow rate is uncontrolled and extremely rapid—too rapid to allow oxygen to be dispersed to surrounding tissues. When starved of normal amounts of oxygen, the cells that make up these tissues begin to deteriorate, sometimes dying off completely.

This abnormally rapid rate of blood flow frequently causes blood pressure inside the vessels located in the central portion of an AVM directly adjacent to the fistula—an area doctors refer to as the *nidus*, from the Latin word for *nest*—to rise to dangerously high levels. The arteries feeding blood into the AVM often become swollen and distorted; the veins that drain blood away from it often become abnormally constricted (a condition called *stenosis*). Moreover, the walls of the involved arteries and veins are often abnormally thin and weak. *Aneurysms*—balloon-like bulges in blood vessel walls that are susceptible to rupture—may develop in association with approximately half of all neurological AVMs due to this structural weakness.

Bleeding can result from this combination of high internal pressure and vessel wall weakness. Such hemorrhages are often microscopic in size, causing limited damage and few significant symptoms. Even many non-symptomatic AVMs show evidence of past bleeding. But massive hemorrhages can occur if the physical stresses caused by extremely high blood pressure, rapid blood flow rates, and vessel wall weakness are great enough. If a large enough volume of blood escapes from a ruptured AVM into the surrounding brain, the result can be a catastrophic stroke. AVMs account for approximately 2 percent of all hemorrhagic strokes that occur each year.

Even in the absence of bleeding or significant oxygen depletion, large AVMs can damage the brain or spinal cord simply by their presence. They can range in size from a fraction of an inch to more than 2.5 inches in diameter, depending on the number and size of the blood vessels making up the lesion. The larger the lesion, the greater the amount of pressure it exerts on surrounding brain or spinal cord structures. The largest lesions may compress several inches of the spinal cord or distort the shape of an entire hemisphere of the brain. Such massive AVMs can constrict the flow of cerebrospinal fluid—a clear liquid that normally nourishes and protects the brain and spinal cord—by distorting or closing the passageways and open chambers (*ventricles*) inside the brain that allow this fluid to circulate freely. As cerebrospinal fluid accumulates, hydrocephalus results. This fluid buildup further increases the amount of pressure on fragile neurological structures, adding to the damage caused by the AVM itself.

Where do neurological AVMs tend to form?

AVMs can form virtually anywhere in the brain or spinal cord—wherever arteries and veins exist. Some are formed from blood vessels located in the *dura mater* or in the *pia mater*, the outermost and innermost, respectively, of the three membranes surrounding the brain and spinal cord. (The third membrane, called the *arachnoid*, lacks blood vessels.) AVMs affecting the spinal cord are of two types, AVMs of the dura mater, which affect the function of the spinal cord by transmitting excess pressure to the venous system of the spinal cord, and AVMs of the spinal cord itself, which affect the function of the spinal cord by hemorrhage, by reducing blood flow to the spinal cord, or by causing excess venous pressure. Spinal AVMs frequently cause attacks of sudden, severe back pain, often concentrated at the roots of nerve fibers where they exit the vertebrae; the pain is similar to that caused by a slipped disk. These lesions also can cause sensory disturbances, muscle weakness, or paralysis in the parts of the body served by the spinal cord or the damaged nerve fibers. Spinal cord injury by the AVM by either of the mechanisms described above can lead to degeneration of the nerve fibers within the spinal cord below the level of the lesion, causing widespread paralysis in parts of the body controlled by those nerve fibers.

Dural and pial AVMs can appear anywhere on the surface of the brain. Those located on the surface of the *cerebral hemispheres*—the uppermost portions of the brain—exert pressure on the *cerebral cortex*, the brain's "gray matter." Depending on their location, these AVMs may damage portions of the cerebral cortex involved with thinking, speaking, understanding language, hearing, taste, touch, or initiating and controlling voluntary movements. AVMs located on the frontal lobe close to the optic nerve or on the occipital lobe, the rear portion of the cerebrum where images are processed, may cause a variety of visual disturbances.

AVMs also can form from blood vessels located deep inside the interior of the cerebrum. These AVMs may compromise the functions of three vital structures: the thalamus, which transmits nerve signals between the spinal cord and upper regions of the brain; the basal ganglia surrounding the thalamus, which coordinate complex movements; and the *hippocampus*, which plays a major role in memory.

AVMs can affect other parts of the brain besides the cerebrum. The hindbrain is formed from two major structures: the *cerebellum*, which is nestled under the rear portion of the cerebrum, and the *brainstem*, which serves as the bridge linking the upper portions of the brain with the spinal cord. These structures control finely coordinated movements, maintain balance, and regulate some functions of internal organs, including those of the heart and lungs. AVM damage to these parts of the hindbrain can result in dizziness, giddiness, vomiting, a loss of the ability to coordinate complex movements such as walking, or uncontrollable muscle tremors.

What are the health consequences of AVMs?

The greatest potential danger posed by AVMs is hemorrhage. Researchers believe that each year between 2 and 4 percent of all AVMs hemorrhage. Most episodes of bleeding remain undetected at the time they occur because they are not severe enough to cause significant neurological damage. But massive, even fatal, bleeding episodes do occur. The present state of knowledge does not permit doctors to predict whether or not any particular person with an AVM will suffer an extensive hemorrhage. The lesions can remain stable or can suddenly begin to grow. In a few cases, they have been observed to regress spontaneously. Whenever an AVM is detected, the individual should be carefully and consistently monitored for any signs of instability that may indicate an increased risk of hemorrhage.

A few physical characteristics appear to indicate a greater-than-usual likelihood of clinically significant hemorrhage. Smaller AVMs have a greater likelihood of bleeding than do larger ones. Impaired drainage by unusually narrow or deeply situated veins also increases the chances of hemorrhage. Pregnancy also appears to increase the likelihood of clinically significant hemorrhage, mainly because of increases in blood pressure and blood volume. Finally, AVMs that have hemorrhaged once are about nine times more likely to bleed again during the first year after the initial hemorrhage than are lesions that have never bled.

The damaging effects of a hemorrhage are related to lesion location. Bleeding from AVMs located deep inside the interior tissues, or *parenchyma*, of the brain typically causes more severe neurological damage than does hemorrhage by lesions that have formed in the dural or pial membranes or on the surface of the brain or spinal cord. (Deeply located bleeding is usually referred to as an *intracerebral* or *parenchymal* hemorrhage; bleeding within the membranes or on the surface of the brain is known as *subdural* or *subarachnoid* hemorrhage.) Thus, location is an important factor to consider when weighing the relative risks of surgical versus non-surgical treatment of AVMs.

What other types of vascular lesions affect the central nervous system?

Besides AVMs, three other main types of vascular lesion can arise in the brain or spinal cord: *cavernous malformations, capillary telangiectasias*, and *venous malformations*. These lesions may form virtually anywhere within the central nervous system, but unlike AVMs, they are not caused by high-velocity blood flow from arteries into veins. In contrast, cavernous malformations, telangiectasias, and venous malformations are all *low-flow* lesions. Instead of a combination of arteries and veins, each one involves only one type of blood vessel. These lesions are less unstable than AVMs and do not pose the same relatively high risk of significant hemorrhage. In general, low-flow lesions tend to cause fewer troubling neurological symptoms and require less aggressive treatment than do AVMs.

- *Cavernous malformations.* These lesions are formed from groups of tightly packed, abnormally thin-walled, small blood vessels that displace normal neurological tissue in the brain or spinal cord. The vessels are filled with slow-moving or stagnant blood that is usually clotted or in a state of decomposition. Like AVMs, cavernous malformations can range in size from a few fractions of an inch to several inches in diameter, depending on the number of blood vessels involved. Some people develop multiple lesions. Although cavernous malformations usually do not hemorrhage as severely as AVMs do, they sometimes leak blood into surrounding neurological tissues because the walls of the involved blood vessels are extremely fragile. Although they are often not as symptomatic as AVMs, cavernous malformations can cause seizures in some people. After AVMs, cavernous malformations are the type of vascular lesion most likely to require treatment.

- *Capillary telangiectasias.* These lesions consist of groups of abnormally swollen capillaries and usually measure less than an inch in diameter. Capillaries are the smallest of all blood vessels, with diameters smaller than that of a human hair; they have the capacity to transport only small quantities of blood, and blood flows through these vessels very slowly. Because of these factors, *telangiectasias* rarely cause extensive damage to surrounding brain or spinal cord tissues. Any isolated hemorrhages that occur are microscopic in size. Thus, the lesions are usually benign. However, in some inherited disorders in which people develop large numbers of these lesions (see below), *telangiectasias* can contribute to the development of nonspecific neurological symptoms such as headaches or seizures.

- *Venous malformations.* These lesions consist of abnormally enlarged veins. The structural defect usually does not interfere with the function of the blood vessels, which is to drain oxygen-depleted blood away from the body's tissues and return it to the lungs and heart. Venous malformations rarely hemorrhage. As with *telangiectasias*, most venous malformations do not produce symptoms, remain undetected, and follow a benign course.

What causes vascular lesions?

Although the cause of these vascular anomalies of the central nervous system is not yet well understood, scientists believe that they most often result from mistakes that occur during embryonic or fetal development. These mistakes may be linked to genetic mutations in some cases. A few types of vascular malformations are known to be hereditary and thus are known to have a genetic basis. Some evidence also suggests that at least some of these lesions are acquired later in life as a result of injury to the central nervous system.

During fetal development, new blood vessels continuously form and then disappear as the human body changes and grows. These changes in the body's vascular map continue after birth and are controlled by *angiogenic factors*, chemicals produced by the body that stimulate new blood vessel formation and growth. Researchers have recently identified changes in the chemical structures of various angiogenic factors in some people who have AVMs or other vascular abnormalities of the central nervous system. However, it is not yet clear how these chemical changes actually cause changes in blood vessel structure.

By studying patterns of familial occurrence, researchers have established that one type of cavernous malformation involving multiple lesion formation is caused by a genetic mutation in chromosome 7. This genetic mutation appears in many ethnic groups, but it is especially frequent in a large population of Hispanic Americans living in the Southwest; these individuals share a common ancestor in whom the genetic change occurred. Some other types of vascular defects of the central nervous system are part of larger medical syndromes known to be hereditary. They include hereditary hemorrhagic telangiectasia (also known as *Osler-Weber-Rendu disease*), *Sturge-Weber syndrome, Klippel-Trenaunay syndrome, Parkes-Weber syndrome*, and *Wyburn-Mason syndrome*.

How are AVMs and other vascular lesions detected?

Physicians now use an array of traditional and new imaging technologies to uncover the presence of AVMs. *Angiography* provides the most accurate pictures of blood vessel structure in AVMs. The technique requires injecting a special water-soluble dye, called a contrast agent, into an artery. The dye highlights the structure of blood vessels so that it can be recorded on conventional X-rays. Although angiography can record fine details of vascular lesions, the procedure is somewhat invasive and carries a slight risk of causing a stroke. Its safety, however, has recently been improved through the development of more precise techniques for delivering dye to the site of an AVM. *Superselective angiography* involves inserting a thin, flexible tube called a catheter into an artery; a physician guides the tip of the catheter to the site of the lesion and then releases a small amount of contrast agent directly into the lesion.

Two of the most frequently employed noninvasive imaging technologies used to detect AVMs are *computed axial tomography (CT)* and *magnetic resonance imaging (MRI)* scans. CT scans use X-rays to create a series of cross-sectional images of the head, brain, or spinal cord and are especially useful in revealing the presence of hemorrhage. MRI imaging, however, offers superior diagnostic information by using magnetic fields to detect subtle changes in neurological tissues. A recently developed application of MRI technology—*magnetic resonance angiography (MRA)*—can record the pattern and velocity of blood flow through vascular lesions as well as the flow of cerebrospinal fluid throughout the brain and spinal cord. CT, MRI, and MRA can provide three-dimensional representations of AVMs by taking images from multiple angles.

How can AVMs and other vascular lesions be treated?

Medication can often alleviate general symptoms such as headache, back pain, and seizures caused by AVMs and other vascular lesions. However, the definitive treatment for AVMs is either surgery or focused irradiation therapy. Venous malformations and capillary *telangiectasias* rarely require surgery; moreover, their structures are diffuse and usually not suitable for surgical correction and they usually do not require treatment anyway. Cavernous malformations are usually well defined enough for surgical removal, but surgery on these lesions is less common than for AVMs because they do not pose the same risk of hemorrhage.

The decision to perform surgery on any individual with an AVM requires a careful consideration of possible benefits versus risks. The natural history of an individual AVM is difficult to predict; however, left untreated, they have the potential of causing significant hemorrhage, which may result in serious neurological deficits or death. On the other hand, surgery on any part of the central nervous system carries its own risks as well; AVM surgery is associated with an estimated 8 percent risk of serious complications or death. There is no easy formula that can allow physicians and their patients to reach a decision on the best course of therapy—all therapeutic decisions must be made on a case-by-case basis.

Today, three surgical options exist for the treatment of AVMs: *conventional surgery, endovascular embolization,* and *radiosurgery.* The choice of treatment depends largely on the size and location of an AVM.

Conventional surgery involves entering the brain or spinal cord and removing the central portion of the AVM, including the fistula, while causing as little damage as possible to surrounding neurological structures. This surgery is most appropriate when an AVM is located in a superficial portion of the brain or spinal cord and is relatively small in size. AVMs located deep inside the brain generally cannot be approached through conventional surgical techniques because there is too great a possibility that functionally important brain tissue will be damaged or destroyed.

Endovascular embolization and radiosurgery are less invasive than conventional surgery and offer safer treatment options for some AVMs located deep inside the brain. In endovascular embolization the surgeon guides a catheter though the arterial network until the tip reaches the site of the AVM. The surgeon then introduces a substance that will plug the fistula, correcting the abnormal pattern of blood flow. This process is known as embolization because it causes an *embolus* (an object or substance) to travel through blood vessels, eventually becoming lodged in a vessel and obstructing blood flow. The embolic materials used to create an artificial blood clot in the center of an AVM include fast-drying biologically inert glues, fibered titanium coils, and tiny balloons. Since embolization usually does not permanently obliterate the AVM, it is usually used as an adjunct to surgery or to radiosurgery to reduce the blood flow through the AVM and make the surgery safer.

Radiosurgery is an even less invasive therapeutic approach. It involves aiming a beam of highly focused radiation directly on the AVM. The high dose of radiation damages the walls of the blood vessels making up the lesion. Over the course of the next several months, the irradiated vessels gradually degenerate and eventually close, leading to the resolution of the AVM.

Embolization frequently proves incomplete or temporary, although in recent years, new embolization materials have led to improved results. Radiosurgery often has incomplete results as well, particularly when an AVM is large, and it poses the additional risk of radiation damage to surrounding normal tissues. Moreover, even when successful, complete closure of an AVM takes place over the course of many months following radiosurgery. During that period, the risk of hemorrhage is still present. However, both techniques now offer the possibility of treating deeply situated AVMs that had previously been inaccessible. And in many individuals, staged embolization followed by conventional surgical removal or by radiosurgery is now performed, resulting in further reductions in mortality and complication rates.

Because so many variables are involved in treating AVMs, doctors must assess the danger posed to individuals largely on a case-by-case basis. The consequences of hemorrhage are potentially disastrous, leading many clinicians to recommend surgical intervention whenever the physical characteristics of an AVM appear to indicate a greater-than-usual likelihood of significant bleeding and resultant neurological damage.

What research is being done?

Within the Federal government, the National Institute of Neurological Disorders and Stroke (NINDS), a division of the National Institutes of Health (NIH), has primary responsibility for sponsoring research on neurological disorders. As part of its mission, the NINDS conducts research on AVMs and other vascular lesions of the central nervous system and supports studies through grants to major medical institutions across the country.

In partnership with the medical school of Columbia University, the NINDS has established a long-term Arteriovenous Study Group to learn more about the natural course of AVMs in patients and to improve the surgical treatment of these lesions.

Another group of NINDS-sponsored researchers is currently studying large populations of patients with AVMs to formulate criteria that will allow doctors to predict more accurately the risk of hemorrhage in individual patients. Of particular importance is the role that high blood pressure within the lesion plays in the onset of hemorrhage. Other scientists are examining the genetic basis of familial cavernous malformations and other hereditary syndromes that cause neurological vascular lesions, including ataxia telangiectasia.

Other scientists are seeking to refine the techniques now available to treat AVMs. Radiosurgery is a special area of interest because this technology is still in its infancy. An ongoing study is closely examining the precise effects that radiation exposure has on vascular tissue in order to improve the predictability and consistency of treatment results.

Finally, several ongoing studies are devoted to developing new non-invasive neuroimaging technologies to increase the effectiveness and safety of AVM surgery. Some scientists are pioneering the use of MRI to measure amounts of oxygen present in the brain tissue of patients with vascular lesions in order to predict the brain's response to surgical therapies. Others are developing a new micro-imager that may be inserted into catheters to increase the accuracy of angiography. In addition, new types of noninvasive imaging devices are being developed that detect functional brain activity through changes in tissue light emission or reflectance. This technology may prove more sensitive than MRI and other imaging devices currently available, giving surgeons a new tool for improving the efficacy and safety of AVM surgery.

Chapter 23

Cephalic Disorders

What are cephalic disorders?

Cephalic disorders are congenital conditions that stem from damage to, or abnormal development of, the budding nervous system. Cephalic is a term that means "head" or "head end of the body." Congenital means the disorder is present at, and usually before, birth. Although there are many congenital developmental disorders, this chapter briefly describes only cephalic conditions.

Cephalic disorders are not necessarily caused by a single factor but may be influenced by hereditary or genetic conditions or by environmental exposures during pregnancy such as medication taken by the mother, maternal infection, or exposure to radiation. Some cephalic disorders occur when the cranial sutures (the fibrous joints that connect the bones of the skull) join prematurely. Most cephalic disorders are caused by a disturbance that occurs very early in the development of the fetal nervous system.

The human nervous system develops from a small, specialized plate of cells on the surface of the embryo. Early in development, this plate of cells forms the neural tube, a narrow sheath that closes between the third and fourth weeks of pregnancy to form the brain and spinal cord of the embryo. Four main processes are responsible for the development of the nervous system: cell proliferation, the process in which

---

Text in this chapter is excerpted from "Cephalic Disorders Fact Sheet," National Institute of Neurological Disorders and Stroke (NINDS), April 16, 2014.

nerve cells divide to form new generations of cells; cell migration, the process in which nerve cells move from their place of origin to the place where they will remain for life; cell differentiation, the process during which cells acquire individual characteristics; and cell death, a natural process in which cells die. Understanding the normal development of the human nervous system, one of the research priorities of the National Institute of Neurological Disorders and Stroke, may lead to a better understanding of cephalic disorders.

Damage to the developing nervous system is a major cause of chronic, disabling disorders and, sometimes, death in infants, children, and even adults. The degree to which damage to the developing nervous system harms the mind and body varies enormously. Many disabilities are mild enough to allow those afflicted to eventually function independently in society. Others are not. Some infants, children, and adults die, others remain totally disabled, and an even larger population is partially disabled, functioning well below normal capacity throughout life.

What are the different kinds of cephalic disorders?

ANENCEPHALY is a neural tube defect that occurs when the cephalic (head) end of the neural tube fails to close, usually between the 23rd and 26th days of pregnancy, resulting in the absence of a major portion of the brain, skull, and scalp. Infants with this disorder are born without a forebrain—the largest part of the brain consisting mainly of the cerebrum, which is responsible for thinking and coordination. The remaining brain tissue is often exposed—not covered by bone or skin.

Infants born with anencephaly are usually blind, deaf, unconscious, and unable to feel pain. Although some individuals with anencephaly may be born with a rudimentary brainstem, the lack of a functioning cerebrum permanently rules out the possibility of ever gaining consciousness. Reflex actions such as breathing and responses to sound or touch may occur. The disorder is one of the most common disorders of the fetal central nervous system. Approximately 1,000 to 2,000 American babies are born with anencephaly each year. The disorder affects females more often than males.

The cause of anencephaly is unknown. Although it is believed that the mother's diet and vitamin intake may play a role, scientists agree that many other factors are also involved.

There is no cure or standard treatment for anencephaly and the prognosis for affected individuals is poor. Most infants do not survive infancy. If the infant is not stillborn, then he or she will usually die within a few hours or days after birth. Anencephaly can often be diagnosed before birth through an ultrasound examination.

Recent studies have shown that the addition of folic acid to the diet of women of child-bearing age may significantly reduce the incidence of neural tube defects. Therefore it is recommended that all women of child-bearing age consume 0.4 mg of folic acid daily.

COLPOCEPHALY is a disorder in which there is an abnormal enlargement of the occipital horns—the posterior or rear portion of the lateral ventricles (cavities or chambers) of the brain. This enlargement occurs when there is an underdevelopment or lack of thickening of the white matter in the posterior cerebrum. Colpocephaly is characterized by microcephaly (abnormally small head) and mental retardation. Other features may include motor abnormalities, muscle spasms, and seizures.

Although the cause is unknown, researchers believe that the disorder results from an intrauterine disturbance that occurs between the second and sixth months of pregnancy. Colpocephaly may be diagnosed late in pregnancy, although it is often misdiagnosed as hydrocephalus (excessive accumulation of cerebrospinal fluid in the brain). It may be more accurately diagnosed after birth when signs of mental retardation, microcephaly, and seizures are present.

There is no definitive treatment for colpocephaly. Anticonvulsant medications can be given to prevent seizures, and doctors try to prevent contractures (shrinkage or shortening of muscles). The prognosis for individuals with colpocephaly depends on the severity of the associated conditions and the degree of abnormal brain development. Some children benefit from special education.

HOLOPROSENCEPHALY is a disorder characterized by the failure of the prosencephalon (the forebrain of the embryo) to develop. During normal development the forebrain is formed and the face begins to develop in the fifth and sixth weeks of pregnancy. Holoprosencephaly is caused by a failure of the embryo's forebrain to divide to form bilateral cerebral hemispheres (the left and right halves of the brain), causing defects in the development of the face and in brain structure and function.

There are three classifications of holoprosencephaly. Alobar holoprosencephaly, the most serious form in which the brain fails to separate, is usually associated with severe facial anomalies. Semilobar holoprosencephaly, in which the brain's hemispheres have a slight tendency to separate, is an intermediate form of the disease. Lobar holoprosencephaly, in which there is considerable evidence of separate brain hemispheres, is the least severe form. In some cases of lobar holoprosencephaly, the patient's brain may be nearly normal.

Holoprosencephaly, once called arhinencephaly, consists of a spectrum of defects or malformations of the brain and face. At the most severe end of this spectrum are cases involving serious malformations of the brain, malformations so severe that they are incompatible with life and often cause spontaneous intrauterine death. At the other end of the spectrum are individuals with facial defects—which may affect the eyes, nose, and upper lip—and normal or near-normal brain development. Seizures and mental retardation may occur.

The most severe of the facial defects (or anomalies) is cyclopia, an abnormality characterized by the development of a single eye, located in the area normally occupied by the root of the nose, and a missing nose or a nose in the form of a proboscis (a tubular appendage) located above the eye.

Ethmocephaly is the least common facial anomaly. It consists of a proboscis separating narrow-set eyes with an absent nose and microphthalmia (abnormal smallness of one or both eyes). Cebocephaly, another facial anomaly, is characterized by a small, flattened nose with a single nostril situated below incomplete or underdeveloped closely set eyes.

The least severe in the spectrum of facial anomalies is the median cleft lip, also called premaxillary agenesis.

Although the causes of most cases of holoprosencephaly remain unknown, researchers know that approximately one-half of all cases have a chromosomal cause. Such chromosomal anomalies as Patau's syndrome (trisomy 13) and Edwards' syndrome (trisomy 18) have been found in association with holoprosencephaly. There is an increased risk for the disorder in infants of diabetic mothers.

There is no treatment for holoprosencephaly and the prognosis for individuals with the disorder is poor. Most of those who survive show no significant developmental gains. For children who survive, treatment is symptomatic. Although it is possible that improved management of diabetic pregnancies may help prevent holoprosencephaly, there is no means of primary prevention.

HYDRANENCEPHALY is a rare condition in which the cerebral hemispheres are absent and replaced by sacs filled with cerebrospinal fluid. Usually the cerebellum and brainstem are formed normally. An infant with hydranencephaly may appear normal at birth. The infant's head size and spontaneous reflexes such as sucking, swallowing, crying, and moving the arms and legs may all seem normal. However, after a few weeks the infant usually becomes irritable and has increased muscle tone (hypertonia). After several months of life, seizures and hydrocephalus may develop. Other symptoms may include visual impairment, lack of growth, deafness, blindness, spastic quadriparesis (paralysis), and intellectual deficits.

Hydranencephaly is an extreme form of porencephaly (a rare disorder, discussed later in this chapter, characterized by a cyst or cavity in the cerebral hemispheres) and may be caused by vascular insult (such as stroke) or injuries, infections, or traumatic disorders after the 12th week of pregnancy.

Diagnosis may be delayed for several months because the infant's early behavior appears to be relatively normal. Transillumination, an examination in which light is passed through body tissues, usually confirms the diagnosis. Some infants may have additional abnormalities at birth, including seizures, myoclonus (involuntary sudden, rapid jerks), and respiratory problems.

There is no standard treatment for hydranencephaly. Treatment is symptomatic and supportive. Hydrocephalus may be treated with a shunt.

The outlook for children with hydranencephaly is generally poor, and many children with this disorder die before age 1. However, in rare cases, children with hydranencephaly may survive for several years or more.

INIENCEPHALY is a rare neural tube defect that combines extreme retroflexion (backward bending) of the head with severe defects of the spine. The affected infant tends to be short, with a disproportionately large head. Diagnosis can be made immediately after birth because the head is so severely retroflexed that the face looks upward. The skin of the face is connected directly to the skin of the chest and the scalp is directly connected to the skin of the back. Generally, the neck is absent.

Most individuals with iniencephaly have other associated anomalies such as anencephaly, cephalocele (a disorder in which part of the cranial contents protrudes from the skull), hydrocephalus, cyclopia, absence of the mandible (lower jaw bone), cleft lip and palate, cardiovascular disorders, diaphragmatic hernia, and gastrointestinal malformation. The disorder is more common among females.

The prognosis for those with iniencephaly is extremely poor. Newborns with iniencephaly seldom live more than a few hours.

The distortion of the fetal body may also pose a danger to the mother's life.

LISSENCEPHALY, which literally means "smooth brain," is a rare brain malformation characterized by microcephaly and the lack of normal convolutions (folds) in the brain. It is caused by defective neuronal migration, the process in which nerve cells move from their place of origin to their permanent location.

The surface of a normal brain is formed by a complex series of folds and grooves. The folds are called gyri or convolutions, and the grooves are called sulci. In children with lissencephaly, the normal convolutions are absent or only partly formed, making the surface of the brain smooth.

Symptoms of the disorder may include unusual facial appearance, difficulty swallowing, failure to thrive, and severe psychomotor retardation. Anomalies of the hands, fingers, or toes, muscle spasms, and seizures may also occur.

Lissencephaly may be diagnosed at or soon after birth. Diagnosis may be confirmed by ultrasound, computed tomography (CT), or magnetic resonance imaging (MRI).

Lissencephaly may be caused by intrauterine viral infections or viral infections in the fetus during the first trimester, insufficient blood supply to the baby's brain early in pregnancy, or a genetic disorder. There are two distinct genetic causes of lissencephaly—X-linked and chromosome 17-linked.

The spectrum of lissencephaly is only now becoming more defined as neuroimaging and genetics has provided more insights into migration disorders. Other causes which have not yet been identified are likely as well.

Lissencephaly may be associated with other diseases including isolated lissencephaly sequence, Miller-Dieker syndrome, and Walker-Warburg syndrome.

Treatment for those with lissencephaly is symptomatic and depends on the severity and locations of the brain malformations. Supportive care may be needed to help with comfort and nursing needs. Seizures may be controlled with medication and hydrocephalus may require shunting. If feeding becomes difficult, a gastrostomy tube may be considered.

The prognosis for children with lissencephaly varies depending on the degree of brain malformation. Many individuals show no significant development beyond a 3- to 5-month-old level. Some may have near-normal development and intelligence. Many will die before the age of 2. Respiratory problems are the most common causes of death.

MEGALENCEPHALY, also called macrencephaly, is a condition in which there is an abnormally large, heavy, and usually malfunctioning brain. By definition, the brain weight is greater than average for the age and gender of the infant or child. Head enlargement may be evident at birth or the head may become abnormally large in the early years of life.

Megalencephaly is thought to be related to a disturbance in the regulation of cell reproduction or proliferation. In normal development, neuron proliferation—the process in which nerve cells divide to form new generations of cells—is regulated so that the correct number of cells is formed in the proper place at the appropriate time.

Symptoms of megalencephaly may include delayed development, convulsive disorders, corticospinal (brain cortex and spinal cord) dysfunction, and seizures. Megalencephaly affects males more often than females.

The prognosis for individuals with megalencephaly largely depends on the underlying cause and the associated neurological disorders. Treatment is symptomatic. Megalencephaly may lead to a condition called macrocephaly (defined later in this chapter). Unilateral megalencephaly or hemimegalencephaly is a rare condition characterized by the enlargement of one-half of the brain. Children with this disorder may have a large, sometimes asymmetrical head. Often they suffer from intractable seizures and mental retardation. The prognosis for those with hemimegalencephaly is poor.

MICROCEPHALY is a neurological disorder in which the circumference of the head is smaller than average for the age and gender of the infant or child. Microcephaly may be congenital or it may develop in the first few years of life. The disorder may stem from a wide variety of conditions that cause abnormal growth of the brain, or from syndromes associated with chromosomal abnormalities.

Infants with microcephaly are born with either a normal or reduced head size. Subsequently the head fails to grow while the face continues to develop at a normal rate, producing a child with a small head, a large face, a receding forehead, and a loose, often wrinkled scalp. As the child grows older, the smallness of the skull becomes more obvious, although the entire body also is often underweight and dwarfed. Development of motor functions and speech may be delayed. Hyperactivity and mental retardation are common occurrences, although the degree of each varies. Convulsions may also occur. Motor ability varies, ranging from clumsiness in some to spastic quadriplegia in others.

Generally there is no specific treatment for microcephaly. Treatment is symptomatic and supportive.

In general, life expectancy for individuals with microcephaly is reduced and the prognosis for normal brain function is poor. The prognosis varies depending on the presence of associated abnormalities.

PORENCEPHALY is an extremely rare disorder of the central nervous system involving a cyst or cavity in a cerebral hemisphere. The cysts or cavities are usually the remnants of destructive lesions, but are sometimes the result of abnormal development. The disorder can occur before or after birth.

Porencephaly most likely has a number of different, often unknown causes, including absence of brain development and destruction of brain tissue. The presence of porencephalic cysts can sometimes be detected by transillumination of the skull in infancy. The diagnosis may be confirmed by CT, MRI, or ultrasonography.

More severely affected infants show symptoms of the disorder shortly after birth, and the diagnosis is usually made before age 1. Signs may include delayed growth and development, spastic paresis (slight or incomplete paralysis), hypotonia (decreased muscle tone), seizures (often infantile spasms), and macrocephaly or microcephaly.

Individuals with porencephaly may have poor or absent speech development, epilepsy, hydrocephalus, spastic contractures (shrinkage or shortening of muscles), and mental retardation. Treatment may include physical therapy, medication for seizure disorders, and a shunt for hydrocephalus. The prognosis for individuals with porencephaly varies according to the location and extent of the lesion. Some patients with this disorder may develop only minor neurological problems and have normal intelligence, while others may be severely disabled. Others may die before the second decade of life.

SCHIZENCEPHALY is a rare developmental disorder characterized by abnormal slits, or clefts, in the cerebral hemispheres. Schizencephaly is a form of porencephaly. Individuals with clefts in both hemispheres, or bilateral clefts, are often developmentally delayed and have delayed speech and language skills and corticospinal dysfunction. Individuals with smaller, unilateral clefts (clefts in one hemisphere) may be weak on one side of the body and may have average or near-average intelligence. Patients with schizencephaly may also have varying degrees of microcephaly, mental retardation, hemiparesis (weakness or paralysis affecting one side of the body), or quadriparesis (weakness or paralysis affecting all four extremities), and may have reduced muscle tone (hypotonia). Most patients have seizures and some may have hydrocephalus.

In schizencephaly, the neurons border the edge of the cleft implying a very early disruption in development. There is now a genetic origin for one type of schizencephaly. Causes of this type may include environmental exposures during pregnancy such as medication taken by the mother, exposure to toxins, or a vascular insult. Often there are associated heterotopias (isolated islands of neurons) which indicate a failure of migration of the neurons to their final position in the brain.

Treatment for individuals with schizencephaly generally consists of physical therapy, treatment for seizures, and, in cases that are complicated by hydrocephalus, a shunt.

The prognosis for individuals with schizencephaly varies depending on the size of the clefts and the degree of neurological deficit.

What are other less common cephalies?

ACEPHALY literally means absence of the head. It is a much rarer condition than anencephaly. The acephalic fetus is a parasitic twin attached to an otherwise intact fetus. The acephalic fetus has a body but lacks a head and a heart; the fetus's neck is attached to the normal twin. The blood circulation of the acephalic fetus is provided by the heart of the twin. The acephalic fetus cannot exist independently of the fetus to which it is attached.

EXENCEPHALY is a condition in which the brain is located outside of the skull. This condition is usually found in embryos as an early stage of anencephaly. As an exencephalic pregnancy progresses, the neural tissue gradually degenerates. It is unusual to find an infant carried to term with this condition because the defect is incompatible with survival.

MACROCEPHALY is a condition in which the head circumference is larger than average for the age and gender of the infant or child. It is a descriptive rather than a diagnostic term and is a characteristic of a variety of disorders. Macrocephaly also may be inherited. Although one form of macrocephaly may be associated with mental retardation, in approximately one-half of cases mental development is normal. Macrocephaly may be caused by an enlarged brain or hydrocephalus. It may be associated with other disorders such as dwarfism, neurofibromatosis, and tuberous sclerosis.

MICRENCEPHALY is a disorder characterized by a small brain and may be caused by a disturbance in the proliferation of nerve cells. Micrencephaly may also be associated with maternal problems such as alcoholism, diabetes, or rubella (German measles). A genetic factor may play a role in causing some cases of micrencephaly. Affected newborns generally have striking neurological defects and seizures. Severely impaired intellectual development is common, but disturbances in motor functions may not appear until later in life.

OTOCEPHALY is a lethal condition in which the primary feature is agnathia—a developmental anomaly characterized by total or virtual absence of the lower jaw. The condition is considered lethal because of a poorly functioning airway. In otocephaly, agnathia may occur alone or together with holoprosencephaly.

Another group of less common cephalic disorders are the craniostenoses. Craniostenoses are deformities of the skull caused by the premature fusion or joining together of the cranial sutures. Cranial sutures are fibrous joints that join the bones of the skull together. The nature of these deformities depends on which sutures are affected.

BRACHYCEPHALY occurs when the coronal suture fuses prematurely, causing a shortened front-to-back diameter of the skull. The coronal suture is the fibrous joint that unites the frontal bone with the two parietal bones of the skull. The parietal bones form the top and sides of the skull.

OXYCEPHALY is a term sometimes used to describe the premature closure of the coronal suture plus any other suture, or it may be used to describe the premature fusing of all sutures. Oxycephaly is the most severe of the craniostenoses.

PLAGIOCEPHALY results from the premature unilateral fusion (joining of one side) of the coronal or lambdoid sutures. The lambdoid suture unites the occipital bone with the parietal bones of the skull. Plagiocephaly is a condition characterized by an asymmetrical distortion (flattening of one side) of the skull. It is a common finding at birth and may be the result of brain malformation, a restrictive intrauterine environment, or torticollis (a spasm or tightening of neck muscles).

SCAPHOCEPHALY applies to premature fusion of the sagittal suture. The sagittal suture joins together the two parietal bones of the skull. Scaphocephaly is the most common of the craniostenoses and is characterized by a long, narrow head.

TRIGONOCEPHALY is the premature fusion of the metopic suture (part of the frontal suture which joins the two halves of the frontal bone of the skull) in which a V-shaped abnormality occurs at the front of the skull. It is characterized by the triangular prominence of the forehead and closely set eyes.

What research is being done?

Within the Federal Government, the National Institute of Neurological Disorders and Stroke (NINDS), one of the National Institutes of Health (NIH), has primary responsibility for conducting and supporting research on normal and abnormal brain and nervous system development, including congenital anomalies. The National Institute of Child Health and Human Development, the National Institute of Mental Health, the National Institute of Environmental Health Sciences, the National Institute of Alcohol Abuse and Alcoholism, and the National Institute on Drug Abuse also support research related to disorders of the developing nervous system. Gaining basic knowledge about how the nervous system develops and understanding the role of genetics in fetal development are major goals of scientists studying congenital neurological disorders.

Scientists are rapidly learning how harmful insults at various stages of pregnancy can lead to developmental disorders. For example, a critical nutritional deficiency or exposure to an environmental insult during the first month of pregnancy (when the neural tube is formed) can produce neural tube defects such as anencephaly.

Scientists are also concentrating their efforts on understanding the complex processes responsible for normal early development of the brain and nervous system and how the disruption of any of these processes results in congenital anomalies such as cephalic disorders. Understanding how genes control brain cell migration, proliferation, differentiation, and death, and how radiation, drugs, toxins, infections, and other factors disrupt these processes will aid in preventing many congenital neurological disorders.

Currently, researchers are examining the mechanisms involved in neurulation—the process of forming the neural tube. These studies will improve our understanding of this process and give insight into how the process can go awry and cause devastating congenital disorders. Investigators are also analyzing genes and gene products necessary for human brain development to achieve a better understanding of normal brain development in humans.

Chapter 24

Spina Bifida

Introduction

The human nervous system develops from a small, specialized plate of cells along the back of an embryo (called the neural plate). Early in development, the edges of this plate begin to curl up toward each other, creating the neural tube—a narrow sheath that closes to form the brain and spinal cord of the embryo. As development progresses, the top of the tube becomes the brain and the remainder becomes the spinal cord. This process is usually complete by the 28th day of pregnancy. But if problems occur during this process, the result can be brain disorders called neural tube defects, including spina bifida.

What is spina bifida?

Spina bifida, which literally means "cleft spine," is characterized by the incomplete development of the brain, spinal cord, and/or meninges (the protective covering around the brain and spinal cord). It is the most common neural tube defect in the United States—affecting 1,500 to 2,000 of the more than 4 million babies born in the country each year. An estimated 166,000 individuals with spina bifida live in the United States.

Text in this chapter is excerpted from "Spina Bifida Fact Sheet," National Institute of Neurological Disorders and Stroke (NINDS), February 23, 2015.

What are the different types of spina bifida?

There are four types of spina bifida: occulta, closed neural tube defects, meningocele, and myelomeningocele.

Occulta is the mildest and most common form in which one or more vertebrae are malformed. The name "occulta," which means "hidden," indicates that a layer of skin covers the malformation, or opening in the vertebrae. This form of spina bifida, present in 10–20 percent of the general population, rarely causes disability or symptoms.

Closed neural tube defects make up the second type of spina bifida. This form consists of a diverse group of defects in which the spinal cord is marked by malformations of fat, bone, or meninges. In most instances there are few or no symptoms; in others the malformation causes incomplete paralysis with urinary and bowel dysfunction.

In the third type, meningocele, spinal fluid and meninges protrude through an abnormal vertebral opening; the malformation contains no neural elements and may or may not be covered by a layer of skin. Some individuals with meningocele may have few or no symptoms while others may experience such symptoms as complete paralysis with bladder and bowel dysfunction.

Myelomeningocele, the fourth form, is the most severe and occurs when the spinal cord/neural elements are exposed through the opening in the spine, resulting in partial or complete paralysis of the parts of the body below the spinal opening. The impairment may be so severe that the affected individual is unable to walk and may have bladder and bowel dysfunction.

What causes spina bifida?

The exact cause of spina bifida remains a mystery. No one knows what disrupts complete closure of the neural tube, causing this malformation to develop. Scientists suspect the factors that cause spina bifida are multiple: genetic, nutritional, and environmental factors all play a role. Research studies indicate that insufficient intake of folic acid—a common B vitamin—in the mother's diet is a key factor in causing spina bifida and other neural tube defects. Prenatal vitamins typically contain folic acid as well as other vitamins. (See heading "Can the disorder be prevented?" on page 400 for more information on folic acid.)

What are the signs and symptoms of spina bifida?

The symptoms of spina bifida vary from person to person, depending on the type and level of involvement. Closed neural tube defects are often recognized early in life due to an abnormal tuft or clump of hair or a small dimple or birthmark on the skin at the site of the spinal malformation.

Meningocele and myelomeningocele generally involve a fluid-filled sac—visible on the back—protruding from the spinal canal. In meningocele, the sac may be covered by a thin layer of skin. In most cases of myelomeningocele, there is no layer of skin covering the sac and an area of abnormally developed spinal cord tissue is usually exposed.

What are the complications of spina bifida?

Complications of spina bifida can range from minor physical problems with little functional impairment to severe physical and mental disabilities. It is important to note, however, that most people with spina bifida are of normal intelligence. Spina bifida's impact is determined by the size and location of the malformation, whether it covered, and which spinal nerves are involved. All nerves located below the malformation are affected to some degree. Therefore, the higher the malformation occurs on the back, the greater the amount of nerve damage and loss of muscle function and sensation.

In addition to abnormal sensation and paralysis, another neurological complication associated with spina bifida is Chiari II malformation—a condition common in children with myelomeningocele—in which the brain stem and the cerebellum (hindbrain) protrude downward into the spinal canal or neck area. This condition can lead to compression of the spinal cord and cause a variety of symptoms including difficulties with feeding, swallowing, and breathing control; choking; and changes in upper arm function (stiffness, weakness).

Chiari II malformation may also result in a blockage of cerebrospinal fluid, causing a condition called hydrocephalus, which is an abnormal buildup of cerebrospinal fluid in and around the brain. Cerebrospinal fluid is a clear liquid that surrounds the brain and spinal cord. The buildup of fluid puts damaging pressure on these structures. Hydrocephalus is commonly treated by surgically implanting a shunt—a hollow tube—in the brain to drain the excess fluid into the abdomen.

Some newborns with myelomeningocele may develop meningitis, an infection in the meninges. Meningitis may cause brain injury and can be life-threatening.

Children with both myelomeningocele and hydrocephalus may have learning disabilities, including difficulty paying attention, problems with language and reading comprehension, and trouble learning math.

Additional problems such as latex allergies, skin problems, gastrointestinal conditions, and depression may occur as children with spina bifida get older.

How is it diagnosed?

In most cases, spina bifida is diagnosed prenatally, or before birth. However, some mild cases may go unnoticed until after birth (postnatal). Very mild forms (spinal bifida occulta), in which there are no symptoms, may never be detected.

Prenatal Diagnosis

The most common screening methods used to look for spina bifida during pregnancy are second trimester (16–18 weeks of gestation) maternal serum alpha fetoprotein (MSAFP) screening and fetal ultrasound. The MSAFP screen measures the level of a protein called alpha-fetoprotein (AFP), which is made naturally by the fetus and placenta. During pregnancy, a small amount of AFP normally crosses the placenta and enters the mother's bloodstream. If abnormally high levels of this protein appear in the mother's bloodstream, it may indicate that the fetus has an "open" (not skin-covered) neural tube defect. The MSAFP test, however, is not specific for spina bifida and requires correct gestational dates to be most accurate; it cannot definitively determine that there is a problem with the fetus. If a high level of AFP is detected, the doctor may request additional testing, such as an ultrasound or amniocentesis to help determine the cause.

The second trimester MSAFP screen described above may be performed alone or as part of a larger, multiple-marker screen. Multiple-marker screens look not only for neural tube defects, but also for other birth defects, including Down syndrome and other chromosomal abnormalities. First trimester screens for chromosomal abnormalities also exist but signs of spina bifida are not evident until the second trimester when the MSAFP screening is performed.

Amniocentesis—an exam in which the doctor removes samples of fluid from the amniotic sac that surrounds the fetus—may also be used to diagnose spina bifida. Although amniocentesis cannot reveal the severity of spina bifida, finding high levels of AFP and other proteins may indicate that the disorder is present.

Postnatal Diagnosis

Mild cases of spina bifida (occulta, closed) not diagnosed during prenatal testing may be detected postnatally by plain film X-ray examination. Individuals with the more severe forms of spina bifida often have muscle weakness in their feet, hips, and legs that result in deformities that may be present at birth. Doctors may use magnetic resonance imaging (MRI) or a computed tomography (CT) scan to get a clearer view of the spinal cord and vertebrae. If hydrocephalus is suspected, the doctor may request a CT scan and/or X-ray of the skull to look for extra cerebrospinal fluid inside the brain.

How is spina bifida treated?

There is no cure for spina bifida. The nerve tissue that is damaged cannot be repaired, nor can function be restored to the damaged nerves. Treatment depends on the type and severity of the disorder. Generally, children with the mildest form need no treatment, although some may require surgery as they grow.

The key early priorities for treating myelomeningocele are to prevent infection from developing in the exposed nerves and tissue through the spinal defect, and to protect the exposed nerves and structures from additional trauma. Typically, a child born with spina bifida will have surgery to close the defect and minimize the risk of infection or further trauma within the first few days of life.

Selected medical centers continue to perform fetal surgery for treatment of myelomeningocele through a National Institutes of Health experimental protocol (Management of Myelomeningocele Study, or MOMS). Fetal surgery is performed in utero (within the uterus) and involves opening the mother's abdomen and uterus and sewing shut the abnormal opening over the developing baby's spinal cord. Some doctors believe the earlier the defect is corrected, the better the baby's outcome. Although the procedure cannot restore lost neurological function, it may prevent additional loss from occurring.

The surgery is considered experimental and there are risks to the fetus as well as to the mother. The major risks to the fetus are those that might occur if the surgery stimulates premature delivery, such as organ immaturity, brain hemorrhage, and death. Risks to the mother include infection, blood loss leading to the need for transfusion, gestational diabetes, and weight gain due to bed rest.

Still, the benefits of fetal surgery are promising, and include less exposure of the vulnerable spinal nerve tissue and bone to the intrauterine environment, in particular the amniotic fluid, which is considered toxic. As an added benefit, doctors have discovered that the procedure may affect the way the fetal hindbrain develops in utero, decreasing the severity of certain complications—such as Chiari II and hydrocephalus—and in some cases, eliminating the need for surgery to implant a shunt.

Twenty to 50 percent of children with myelomeningocele develop a condition called progressive tethering, or tethered cord syndrome; their spinal cord become fastened to an immovable structure—such as overlying membranes and vertebrae—causing the spinal cord to become abnormally stretched with the child's growth. This condition can cause loss of muscle function to the legs, as well as changes in bowel and bladder function. Early surgery on a tethered spinal cord may allow the child to return to their baseline level of functioning and prevent further neurological deterioration.

Some children will need subsequent surgeries to manage problems with the feet, hips, or spine. Individuals with hydrocephalus generally will require additional surgeries to replace the shunt, which can be outgrown or become clogged or infected.

Some individuals with spina bifida require assistive devices such as braces, crutches, or wheelchairs. The location of the malformation on the spine often indicates the type of assistive devices needed. Children with a defect high on the spine will have more extensive paralysis and will often require a wheelchair, while those with a defect lower on the spine may be able to use crutches, leg braces, or walkers. Beginning special exercises for the legs and feet at an early age may help prepare the child for walking with those braces or crutches when he or she is older.

Treatment for bladder and bowel problems typically begins soon after birth, and may include bladder catheterizations and bowel management regimens.

Can the disorder be prevented?

Folic acid, also called folate, is an important vitamin in the development of a healthy fetus. Although taking this vitamin cannot guarantee having a healthy baby, it can help. Recent studies have shown that by adding folic acid to their diets, women of childbearing age significantly reduce the risk of having a child with a neural tube defect, such as spina bifida. Therefore, it is recommended that all women of childbearing age consume 400 micrograms of folic acid daily. Foods high in folic acid include dark green vegetables, egg yolks, and some fruits. Many foods—such as some breakfast cereals, enriched breads, flours, pastas, rice, and other grain products—are now fortified with folic acid. Many multivitamins contain the recommended dosage of folic acid as well.

Women who already have a child with spina bifida, who have spina bifida themselves, or who have already had a pregnancy affected by any neural tube defect are at greater risk of having another child with spina bifida or another neural tube defect; 5–10 times the risk to the general population. These women may benefit from taking a higher daily dose of folic acid before they consider becoming pregnant.

What is the prognosis?

Children with spina bifida can lead active lives. Prognosis, activity, and participation depend on the number and severity of abnormalities and associated personal and environmental factors. Most children with the disorder have normal intelligence and can walk, often with assistive devices. If learning problems develop, appropriate educational interventions are helpful.

What research is being done?

Within the Federal Government, the National Institute of Neurological Disorders and Stroke (NINDS), a part of the National Institutes of Health (NIH), is the Federal Government's leading supporter of research on brain and nervous system disorders. NINDS conducts research in its laboratories at the NIH in Bethesda, Maryland, and supports research through grants to major medical institutions across the country.

In one study supported by NINDS, scientists are looking at the hereditary basis of neural tube defects. The goal of this research is to find the genetic factors that make some children more susceptible to neural tube defects than others. Lessons learned from this research will fill in gaps of knowledge about the causes of neural tube defects and may lead to ways to prevent these disorders. These researchers are also studying gene expression during the process of neural tube closure, which will provide information on the human nervous system during development.

In addition, NINDS-supported scientists are working to identify, characterize, and evaluate genes for neural tube defects. The goal is to understand the genetics of neural tube closure, and to develop information that will translate into improved clinical care, treatment, and genetic counseling.

Other scientists are studying genetic risk factors for spina bifida, especially those that diminish or lessen the function of folic acid in the mother during pregnancy, possibly leading to spina bifida in the fetus. This study will shed light on how folic acid prevents spina bifida and may lead to improved forms of folate supplements.

NINDS also supports and conducts a wide range of basic research studies to understand how the brain and nervous system develop. These studies contribute to a greater understanding of neural tube defects, such as spina bifida, and offer hope for new avenues of treatment for and prevention of these disorders as well as other birth defects.

Another component of the NIH, the Eunice Kennedy Shriver National Institute of Child Health and Human Development (NICHD), is conducting a large 5-year study to determine if fetal surgery to correct spina bifida in the womb is safer and more effective than the traditional surgery—which takes place a few days after birth. Researchers hope this study, called the Management of Myelomeningocele Study or MOMS, will better establish which procedure, prenatal or postnatal, is best for the baby.

Part Six

Brain Tumors

Chapter 25

Idiopathic Intracranial Hypertension (Pseudotumor Cerebri)

What is idiopathic intracranial hypertension?

Intracranial hypertension is a condition due to high pressure within the spaces that surround the brain and spinal cord. These spaces are filled with cerebrospinal fluid (CSF), which cushions the brain from mechanical injury, provides nourishment, and carries away waste.

The most common symptoms of intracranial hypertension are headaches and visual loss, including blind spots, poor peripheral (side) vision, double vision, and short temporary episodes of blindness. Many patients experience permanent vision loss. Other common symptoms include pulsatile tinnitus (ringing in the ears) and neck and shoulder pain.

Intracranial hypertension can be either acute or chronic. In chronic intracranial hypertension, the increased CSF pressure can cause swelling and damage to the optic nerve—a condition called papilledema.

Chronic intracranial hypertension can be caused by many conditions including certain drugs such as tetracycline, a blood clot in the brain, excessive intake of vitamin A, or brain tumor. It can also occur without a detectable cause. This is idiopathic intracranial hypertension (IIH).

Text in this chapter is excerpted from "Idiopathic Intracranial Hypertension," National Eye Institute (NEI), April 2014.

Because the symptoms of IIH can resemble those of a brain tumor, it is sometimes known by the older name pseudotumor cerebri, which means "false brain tumor."

Who is at risk for IIH?

An estimated 100,000 Americans have IIH, and the number is rising as more people become obese or overweight. The disorder is most common in women between the ages of 20 and 50; about 5 percent of those affected are men. Obesity, defined as a body mass index (BMI) greater than 30, is a major risk factor. BMI is a number based on your weight and height. The Centers for Disease Control and Prevention offers an online BMI calculator. A recent gain of 5–15 percent of total body weight is also considered a risk factor for this disorder, even for people with a BMI less than 30.

How is IIH diagnosed?

A thorough medical history and physical exam are needed to identify risk factors for IIH and to evaluate for the many potential causes of increased intracranial pressure. A neurological exam will also be performed. In IIH, the exam is normal except for findings related to increased intracranial pressure, including papilledema, visual loss, and possible weakness in the lateral rectus muscles, which are located near your temples and help turn the eyes outward. Weakness in these muscles can cause the eyes to turn inward, toward the nose, producing double vision.

A number of vision tests may also be performed, including a comprehensive dilated eye exam to look for signs of papilledema. Visual field testing is done to evaluate your peripheral vision. This testing measures the area of space you can see at a given instant without moving your head or eyes.

Brain imaging, including computed tomography (CT) and magnetic resonance imaging (MRI) scans, will be performed to look for a brain tumor, injury, or other potential cause for your symptoms. Normal findings on these exams are essential to a diagnosis of IIH.

A lumbar puncture, also known as a spinal tap, will be performed. In this procedure, a needle is inserted into a CSF-filled sac below the spinal cord in the lower back. The CSF pressure will be measured, and a small amount of CSF will be collected for analysis to look for causes of increased intracranial pressure. The procedure may also cause a temporary reduction in CSF pressure and symptoms.

How is IIH treated?

If a diagnosis of IIH is confirmed, regular visual field tests and comprehensive dilated eye exams are recommended to monitor any changes in vision.

Sustainable weight loss through healthy eating, salt restriction, and exercise is a critical part of treatment for people with IIH who are overweight. Studies show that modest weight loss, around 5–10 percent of total body weight, may be sufficient to reduce signs and symptoms. If lifestyle changes are not successful in reducing weight and relieving IIH, weight loss surgery may be recommended for those with a BMI greater than 40.

For many people, weight loss can be difficult to achieve and maintain. And for those who are able to adjust their weight, relief from IIH tends to be gradual. Acetazolamide (Diamox), a drug that decreases CSF production, is therefore often used as an add-on therapy to weight loss. The drug is taken orally. Common side effects include fatigue, nausea, tingling hands and feet, and a metallic taste, usually triggered by carbonated drinks. These can be reversed by lowering the dose or stopping the drug.

It's important to remember that some medications, such as tetracycline, may help trigger IIH, and that stopping them may lead to improvement.

In rapidly progressive cases that do not respond to other treatments, surgery may be needed to relieve pressure on the optic nerve. Therapeutic shunting, which involves surgically inserting a tube to drain CSF from ventricles or inner brain cavities, can be used to remove excess CSF and lower pressure. In a procedure called optic nerve sheath fenestration, pressure on the optic nerve is relieved by making a small window into the covering that surrounds the nerve just behind the eyeball.

What is the prognosis?

For most people, IIH usually improves with treatment. For others, it progressively worsens with time, or it can resolve and then recur. About 5–10 percent of women with IIH experience disabling vision loss. Most patients do not need surgical treatment.

What research is being done?

For decades, acetazolamide has been the drug of choice for treating IIH, but with little evidence that it helped and no established usage guidelines. The NEI-funded IIH Treatment Trial was designed to investigate the benefits of acetazolamide for IIH in patients with mild visual loss, and balance them against the drug's known side effects. The trial compared acetazolamide plus a weight loss plan, versus the same weight loss plan with a placebo pill, among 161 women and four men who had mild vision loss from IIH. To limit side effects, the dosage was gradually increased to a maximally tolerated dose or up to 4 grams daily. In 2014, the researchers reported that the drug—weight loss combination helped to preserve and even restore vision over a six-month period. The trial will continue for a total of five years.

There is also ongoing research to determine what causes IIH. There have been some reports of IIH in multiple generations within families, suggesting that genes may play a role. Because of its relationship to gender and obesity, there is a strong possibility that hormones contribute to IIH. Some hormones are actually released from fatty tissue, and are being studied as potential factors in the disease. The IIH Treatment Trial includes procedures to address the role of genetics and hormones in IIH.

Chapter 26

Hydrocephalus

What is hydrocephalus?

The term hydrocephalus is derived from the Greek words "hydro" meaning water and "cephalus" meaning head. As the name implies, it is a condition in which the primary characteristic is excessive accumulation of fluid in the brain. Although hydrocephalus was once known as "water on the brain," the "water" is actually cerebrospinal fluid (CSF)—a clear fluid that surrounds the brain and spinal cord. The excessive accumulation of CSF results in an abnormal widening of spaces in the brain called ventricles. This widening creates potentially harmful pressure on the tissues of the brain.

The ventricular system is made up of four ventricles connected by narrow passages. Normally, CSF flows through the ventricles, exits into cisterns (closed spaces that serve as reservoirs) at the base of the brain, bathes the surfaces of the brain and spinal cord, and then reabsorbs into the bloodstream.

CSF has three important life-sustaining functions: 1) to keep the brain tissue buoyant, acting as a cushion or "shock absorber"; 2) to act as the vehicle for delivering nutrients to the brain and removing waste; and 3) to flow between the cranium and spine and compensate for changes in intracranial blood volume (the amount of blood within the brain).

The balance between production and absorption of CSF is critically important. Because CSF is made continuously, medical conditions that

---

Text in this chapter is excerpted from "Hydrocephalus Fact Sheet," National Institute of Neurological Disorders and Stroke (NINDS), February 23, 2015.

block its normal flow or absorption will result in an over-accumulation of CSF. The resulting pressure of the fluid against brain tissue is what causes hydrocephalus.

What are the different types of hydrocephalus?

Hydrocephalus may be congenital or acquired. Congenital hydrocephalus is present at birth and may be caused by either events or influences that occur during fetal development, or genetic abnormalities. Acquired hydrocephalus develops at the time of birth or at some point afterward. This type of hydrocephalus can affect individuals of all ages and may be caused by injury or disease.

Hydrocephalus may also be communicating or non-communicating. Communicating hydrocephalus occurs when the flow of CSF is blocked after it exits the ventricles. This form is called communicating because the CSF can still flow between the ventricles, which remain open. Non-communicating hydrocephalus—also called "obstructive" hydrocephalus—occurs when the flow of CSF is blocked along one or more of the narrow passages connecting the ventricles. One of the most common causes of hydrocephalus is "aqueductal stenosis." In this case, hydrocephalus results from a narrowing of the *aqueduct of Sylvius*, a small passage between the third and fourth ventricles in the middle of the brain.

There are two other forms of hydrocephalus which do not fit exactly into the categories mentioned above and primarily affect adults: hydrocephalus ex-vacuo and Normal Pressure Hydrocephalus (NPH).

Hydrocephalus ex-vacuo occurs when stroke or traumatic injury cause damage to the brain. In these cases, brain tissue may actually shrink. NPH is an abnormal increase of cerebrospinal fluid in the brain's ventricles that may result from a subarachnoid hemorrhage, head trauma, infection, tumor, or complications of surgery. However, many people develop NPH when none of these factors are present. An estimated 375,000 older Americans have NPH.

Who gets this disorder?

The number of people who develop hydrocephalus or who are currently living with it is difficult to establish since the condition occurs in children and adults, and can develop later in life. A 2008 data review by the University of Utah found that, in 2003, hydrocephalus accounted for 0.6 percent of all pediatric hospital admissions in the United States. Some estimates report one to two of every 1,000 babies are born with hydrocephalus.

What causes hydrocephalus?

The causes of hydrocephalus are still not well understood. Hydrocephalus may result from inherited genetic abnormalities (such as the genetic defect that causes aqueductal stenosis) or developmental disorders (such as those associated with neural tube defects including spina bifida and encephalocele). Other possible causes include complications of premature birth such as intraventricular hemorrhage, diseases such as meningitis, tumors, traumatic head injury, or subarachnoid hemorrhage, which block the exit of CSF from the ventricles to the cisterns or eliminate the passageway for CSF within the cisterns.

What are the symptoms?

Symptoms of hydrocephalus vary with age, disease progression, and individual differences in tolerance to the condition. For example, an infant's ability to compensate for increased CSF pressure and enlargement of the ventricles differs from an adult's. The infant skull can expand to accommodate the buildup of CSF because the sutures (the fibrous joints that connect the bones of the skull) have not yet closed.

In infancy, the most obvious indication of hydrocephalus is often a rapid increase in head circumference or an unusually large head size. Other symptoms may include vomiting, sleepiness, irritability, downward deviation of the eyes (also called "sun setting"), and seizures.

Older children and adults may experience different symptoms because their skulls cannot expand to accommodate the buildup of CSF. Symptoms may include headache followed by vomiting, nausea, blurred or double vision, sun setting of the eyes, problems with balance, poor coordination, gait disturbance, urinary incontinence, slowing or loss of developmental progress, lethargy, drowsiness, irritability, or other changes in personality or cognition including memory loss.

Symptoms of normal pressure hydrocephalus include problems with walking, impaired bladder control leading to urinary frequency and/or incontinence, and progressive mental impairment and dementia. An individual with this type of hydrocephalus may have a general slowing of movements or may complain that his or her feet feel "stuck." Because some of these symptoms may also be experienced in other disorders such as Alzheimer's disease, Parkinson's disease, and Creutzfeldt-Jakob disease, normal pressure hydrocephalus is often incorrectly diagnosed and never properly treated. Doctors may use a variety of tests, including brain scans such as computed tomography (CT) and magnetic resonance imaging (MRI), a spinal tap or lumbar catheter, intracranial pressure monitoring, and neuropsychological tests, to help them accurately diagnose normal pressure hydrocephalus and rule out any other conditions.

The symptoms described in this chapter account for the most typical ways in which progressive hydrocephalus is noticeable, but it is important to remember that symptoms vary significantly from person to person.

How is hydrocephalus diagnosed?

Hydrocephalus is diagnosed through clinical neurological evaluation and by using cranial imaging techniques such as ultrasonography, CT, MRI, or pressure-monitoring techniques. A physician selects the appropriate diagnostic tool based on an individual's age, clinical presentation, and the presence of known or suspected abnormalities of the brain or spinal cord.

What is the current treatment?

Hydrocephalus is most often treated by surgically inserting a shunt system. This system diverts the flow of CSF from the CNS to another area of the body where it can be absorbed as part of the normal circulatory process.

A shunt is a flexible but sturdy plastic tube. A shunt system consists of the shunt, a catheter, and a valve. One end of the catheter is placed within a ventricle inside the brain or in the CSF outside the spinal cord. The other end of the catheter is commonly placed within the abdominal cavity, but may also be placed at other sites in the body such as a chamber of the heart or areas around the lung where the CSF can drain and be absorbed. A valve located along the catheter maintains one-way flow and regulates the rate of CSF flow.

A limited number of individuals can be treated with an alternative procedure called third ventriculostomy. In this procedure, a neuroendoscope—a small camera that uses fiber optic technology to visualize small and difficult to reach surgical areas—allows a doctor to view the ventricular surface. Once the scope is guided into position, a small tool makes a tiny hole in the floor of the third ventricle, which allows the CSF to bypass the obstruction and flow toward the site of resorption around the surface of the brain.

What are the possible complications of a shunt system?

Shunt systems are imperfect devices. Complications may include mechanical failure, infections, obstructions, and the need to lengthen or replace the catheter. Generally, shunt systems require monitoring and regular medical follow up. When complications occur, subsequent surgery to replace the failed part or the entire shunt system may be needed.

Some complications can lead to other problems such as over-draining or under-draining. Over-draining occurs when the shunt allows CSF to drain from the ventricles more quickly than it is produced. Over-draining can cause the ventricles to collapse, tearing blood vessels and causing headache, hemorrhage (subdural hematoma), or slit-like ventricles (slit ventricle syndrome). Under-draining occurs when CSF is not removed quickly enough and the symptoms of hydrocephalus recur. Over-drainage and underdrainage of CSF are addressed by adjusting the drainage pressure of the shunt valve; if the shunt has an adjustable pressure valve these changes can be made by placing a special magnet on the scalp over the valve. In addition to the common symptoms of hydrocephalus, infections from a shunt may also produce symptoms such as a low-grade fever, soreness of the neck or shoulder muscles, and redness or tenderness along the shunt tract. When there is reason to suspect that a shunt system is not functioning properly (for example, if the symptoms of hydrocephalus return), medical attention should be sought immediately.

What is the prognosis?

The prognosis for individuals diagnosed with hydrocephalus is difficult to predict, although there is some correlation between the specific cause of the hydrocephalus and the outcome. Prognosis is further clouded by the presence of associated disorders, the timeliness of diagnosis, and the success of treatment. The degree to which relief of CSF pressure following shunt surgery can minimize or reverse damage to the brain is not well understood.

Affected individuals and their families should be aware that hydrocephalus poses risks to both cognitive and physical development. However, many children diagnosed with the disorder benefit from rehabilitation therapies and educational interventions and go on to lead normal lives with few limitations. Treatment by an interdisciplinary team of medical professionals, rehabilitation specialists, and educational experts is critical to a positive outcome. Left untreated, progressive hydrocephalus may be fatal.

The symptoms of normal pressure hydrocephalus usually get worse over time if the condition is not treated, although some people may experience temporary improvements. While the success of treatment with shunts varies from person to person, some people recover almost completely after treatment and have a good quality of life. Early diagnosis and treatment improves the chance of a good recovery.

What research is being done?

The National Institute of Neurological Disorders and Stroke (NINDS) and other institutes of the National Institutes of Health (NIH) conduct research related to hydrocephalus and support additional research through grants to major medical research institutions across the country. Much of this research focuses on finding better ways to prevent, treat, and ultimately cure disorders such as hydrocephalus. The NINDS also conducts and supports a wide range of fundamental studies that explore the complex mechanisms of normal and abnormal brain development.

The Hydrocephalus Clinical Research Network (HCRN, *www.hcrn. org*) is a multi-center collaborative research effort that was borne out of the first NIH workshop on hydrocephalus. NINDS supported the work of HCRN through the Challenge Grant process to advance their studies. HCRN consists of seven pediatric centers that pool their hydrocephalus patient population to more rapidly study the potential for improved treatments. HCRN conducts multiple, simultaneous studies at all of its centers and maintains a substantial registry of patients and procedures.

Chapter 27

Adult Brain Tumors

Chapter Contents

Section 27.1

General Information about Adult Brain Tumors

Text in this section is excerpted from "Adult Brain Tumors
Treatment (PDQ®)," National Cancer Institute at the National
Institutes of Health (NIH), February 25, 2015.

Incidence and Mortality

Estimated new cases and deaths from brain and other nervous
system tumors in the United States in 2015:[1]

- New cases: 22,850.

- Deaths: 15,320.

Brain tumors account for 85% to 90% of all primary central nervous
system (CNS) tumors.[2] Available registry data from the Surveillance,
Epidemiology, and End Results (SEER) database for 2007 indicate that
the combined incidence of primary invasive CNS tumors in the United
States is 6.36 per 100,000 persons per year with an estimated mortality of 4.22 per 100,000 persons per year.[3] Worldwide, approximately
238,000 new cases of brain and other CNS tumors were diagnosed in
the year 2008, with an estimated 175,000 deaths.[4] In general, the
incidence of primary brain tumors is higher in whites than in blacks,
and mortality is higher in males than in females.[2]

Risk Factors

Few definitive observations on environmental or occupational
causes of primary CNS tumors have been made.[2] Exposure to vinyl
chloride may predispose to the development of glioma. Epstein-Barr
virus infection has been implicated in the etiology of primary CNS
lymphoma. Transplant recipients and patients with the acquired
immunodeficiency syndrome have substantially increased risks for
primary CNS lymphoma.[2,5]

Disease Overview

The glial cell tumors, anaplastic astrocytoma and glioblastoma, account for approximately 38% of primary brain tumors. Since anaplastic astrocytomas represent less than 10% of all CNS gliomas, phase III randomized trials restricted to the anaplastic astrocytomas are not practical. Meningiomas and other mesenchymal tumors account for approximately 27% of primary brain tumors.[2]

Other less-common primary brain tumors include the following in decreasing order of frequency:

- Pituitary tumors.
- Schwannomas.
- CNS lymphomas.
- Oligodendrogliomas.
- Ependymomas.
- Low-grade astrocytomas.
- Medulloblastomas.

Schwannomas, meningiomas, and ependymomas account for up to 79% of primary spinal tumors. Other less common primary spinal tumors include sarcomas, astrocytomas, vascular tumors, and chordomas, in decreasing order of frequency. The familial tumor syndromes (and respective chromosomal abnormalities that are associated with CNS neoplasms) include neurofibromatosis type I (17q11), neurofibromatosis type II (22q12), von Hippel-Lindau disease (3p25-26), tuberous sclerosis (9q34, 16p13), Li-Fraumeni syndrome (17p13), Turcot syndrome type 1 (3p21, 7p22), Turcot syndrome type 2 (5q21), and nevoid basal cell carcinoma syndrome (9q22.3).[6,7]

Clinical Presentation

The clinical presentation of various brain tumors is best appreciated by considering the relationship of signs and symptoms to anatomy.[2]

General signs and symptoms include the following:

- Headaches.
- Seizures.

- Visual changes.

- Gastrointestinal symptoms such as nausea, loss of appetite, and vomiting.

- Changes in personality, mood, mental capacity, and concentration.

Whether primary, metastatic, malignant, or benign, brain tumors must be differentiated from other space-occupying lesions such as abscesses, arteriovenous malformations, and infarction, which can have a similar clinical presentation.[8] Other clinical presentations of brain tumors include focal cerebral syndromes such as seizures.[2] Seizures are a presenting symptom in approximately 20% of patients with supratentorial brain tumors and may antedate the clinical diagnosis by months to years in patients with slow-growing tumors. Among all patients with brain tumors, 70% with primary parenchymal tumors and 40% with metastatic brain tumors develop seizures at some time during the clinical course.[9]

Diagnosis

Testing

Computed tomography (CT) and magnetic resonance imaging (MRI) have complementary roles in the diagnosis of CNS neoplasms.[8,10] The speed of CT is desirable for evaluating clinically unstable patients. CT is superior for detecting calcification, skull lesions, and hyperacute hemorrhage (bleeding less than 24-hours old) and helps direct differential diagnosis as well as immediate management. MRI has superior soft-tissue resolution. MRI can better detect isodense lesions, tumor enhancement, and associated findings such as edema, all phases of hemorrhagic states (except hyperacute), and infarction. High-quality MRI is the diagnostic study of choice in the evaluation of intramedullary and extramedullary spinal cord lesions.[2] In post-therapy imaging, single-photon emission computed tomography (SPECT) and positron emission tomography (PET) may be useful in differentiating tumor recurrence from radiation necrosis.[8]

Biopsy confirmation to corroborate the suspected diagnosis of a primary brain tumor is critical, whether before surgery by needle biopsy or at the time of surgical resection, except in cases in which the clinical and radiologic picture clearly point to a benign tumor. Radiologic patterns may be misleading, and a definitive biopsy is needed to rule out other causes of space-occupying lesions, such as metastatic cancer or infection. CT- or MRI-guided stereotactic techniques can be used to place a needle safely and accurately into all but a very few inaccessible locations within the brain.

CNS abnormalities

Specific genetic or chromosomal abnormalities involving deletions of 1p and 19q have been identified for a subset of oligodendroglial tumors, which have a high response rate to chemotherapy.[2,7,11-15] Other CNS tumors are associated with characteristic patterns of altered oncogenes, altered tumor-suppressor genes, and chromosomal abnormalities. Familial tumor syndromes with defined chromosomal abnormalities are associated with gliomas. (Refer to the Section 27.2 of this chapter for more information.)

Metastatic Brain Tumors

Brain metastases outnumber primary neoplasms by at least 10 to 1, and they occur in 20% to 40% of cancer patients.[16] Because no national cancer registry documents brain metastases, the exact incidence is unknown, but it has been estimated that 98,000 to 170,000 new cases are diagnosed in the United States each year.[2,8] This number may be increasing because of the capacity of MRI to detect small metastases and because of prolonged survival resulting from improved systemic therapy.[2,16]

Origins of metastatic brain tumors

The most common primary cancers metastasizing to the brain are lung cancer (50%), breast cancer (15%–20%), unknown primary cancer (10%–15%), melanoma (10%), and colon cancer (5%).[2,16] Eighty percent of brain metastases occur in the cerebral hemispheres, 15% occur in the cerebellum, and 5% occur in the brain stem.[2] Metastases to the brain are multiple in more than 70% of cases, but solitary metastases also occur.[16] Brain involvement can occur with cancers of the nasopharyngeal region by direct extension along the cranial nerves or through the foramina at the base of the skull. Dural metastases may constitute as much as 9% of total CNS metastases.

Primary Brain Tumors

A lesion in the brain should not be assumed to be a metastasis just because a patient has had a previous cancer; such an assumption could result in overlooking appropriate treatment of a curable tumor.

Primary brain tumors rarely spread to other areas of the body, but they can spread to other parts of the brain and to the spinal axis.

Clinical Features

The diagnosis of brain metastases in cancer patients is based on the following:

- Patient history.
- Neurological examination.
- Diagnostic procedures, including a contrast MRI of the brain.

Patients may describe any of the following:

- Headaches.
- Weakness.
- Seizures.
- Sensory defects.
- Gait problems.

Often, family members or friends may notice the following:

- Lethargy.
- Emotional lability.
- Personality change.

A physical examination may show objective neurological findings or only minor cognitive changes. The presence of multiple lesions and a high predilection of primary tumor metastasis may be sufficient to make the diagnosis of brain metastasis. In the case of a solitary lesion or a questionable relationship to the primary tumor, a brain biopsy (via resection or stereotactic biopsy) may be necessary. CT scans with contrast or MRIs with gadolinium are quite sensitive in diagnosing the presence of metastases. PET scanning and spectroscopic evaluation are new strategies to diagnose cerebral metastases and to differentiate the metastases from other intracranial lesions.[17]

References

1. American Cancer Society: Cancer Facts and Figures 2015. Atlanta, Ga: American Cancer Society, 2015. Last accessed January 7, 2015.

2. Mehta M, Vogelbaum MA, Chang S, et al.: Neoplasms of the central nervous system. In: DeVita VT Jr, Lawrence TS, Rosenberg SA: Cancer: Principles and Practice of Oncology. 9th ed. Philadelphia, Pa: Lippincott Williams & Wilkins, 2011, pp 1700-49.

3. Altekruse SF, Kosary CL, Krapcho M, et al.: SEER Cancer Statistics Review, 1975-2007. Bethesda, Md: National Cancer Institute, 2010. Last accessed January 30, 2015.

4. Ferlay J, Shin HR, Bray F, et al.: GLOBOCAN 2008: Cancer Incidence and Mortality Worldwide in 2008. Lyon, France: IARC CancerBase No. 10. Last accessed January 9, 2015.

5. Schabet M: Epidemiology of primary CNS lymphoma. J Neurooncol 43 (3): 199-201, 1999.

6. Behin A, Hoang-Xuan K, Carpentier AF, et al.: Primary brain tumours in adults. Lancet 361 (9354): 323-31, 2003.

7. Kleihues P, Cavenee WK, eds.: Pathology and Genetics of Tumours of the Nervous System. Lyon, France: International Agency for Research on Cancer, 2000.

8. Hutter A, Schwetye KE, Bierhals AJ, et al.: Brain neoplasms: epidemiology, diagnosis, and prospects for cost-effective imaging. Neuroimaging Clin N Am 13 (2): 237-50, x-xi, 2003.

9. Cloughesy T, Selch MT, Liau L: Brain. In: Haskell CM: Cancer Treatment. 5th ed. Philadelphia, Pa: WB Saunders Co, 2001, pp 1106-42.

10. Ricci PE: Imaging of adult brain tumors. Neuroimaging Clin N Am 9 (4): 651-69, 1999.

11. Buckner JC: Factors influencing survival in high-grade gliomas. SeminOncol 30 (6 Suppl 19): 10-4, 2003.

12. DeAngelis LM: Brain tumors. N Engl J Med 344 (2): 114-23, 2001.

13. Ueki K, Nishikawa R, Nakazato Y, et al.: Correlation of histology and molecular genetic analysis of 1p, 19q, 10q, TP53, EGFR, CDK4, and CDKN2A in 91 astrocytic and oligodendroglial tumors. Clin Cancer Res 8 (1): 196-201, 2002.

14. Giordana MT, Ghimenti C, Leonardo E, et al.: Molecular genetic study of a metastatic oligodendroglioma. J Neurooncol 66 (3): 265-71, 2004.

15. Hoang-Xuan K, Capelle L, Kujas M, et al.: Temozolomide as initial treatment for adults with low-grade oligodendrogliomas or oligoastrocytomas and correlation with chromosome 1p deletions. J ClinOncol 22 (15): 3133-8, 2004.

16. Patchell RA: The management of brain metastases. Cancer Treat Rev 29 (6): 533-40, 2003.

17. Schaefer PW, Budzik RF Jr, Gonzalez RG: Imaging of cerebral metastases. NeurosurgClin N Am 7 (3): 393-423, 1996.

Section 27.2

Classification of Adult Brain Tumors

Text in this section is excerpted from "Adult Brain Tumors
Treatment (PDQ®)," National Cancer Institute at the National
Institutes of Health (NIH), February 25, 2015.

This classification is based on the World Health Organization
(WHO) classification of central nervous system (CNS) tumors.[1] The
WHO approach incorporates and interrelates morphology, cytogenet-
ics, molecular genetics, and immunologic markers in an attempt to
construct a cellular classification that is universally applicable and
prognostically valid. Earlier attempts to develop a TNM-based classification were dropped: tumor size (T) is less relevant than tumor
histology and location, nodal status (N) does not apply because the
brain and spinal cord have no lymphatics, and metastatic spread (M)
rarely applies because most patients with CNS neoplasms do not live
long enough to develop metastatic disease.[2]

The WHO grading of CNS tumors establishes a malignancy scale
based on histologic features of the tumor.[3] The histologic grades are
as follows:

WHO grade I includes lesions with low proliferative potential, a
frequently discrete nature, and the possibility of cure following surgical
resection alone.

WHO grade II includes lesions that are generally infiltrating and
low in mitotic activity but recur more frequently than grade I malignant tumors after local therapy. Some tumor types tend to progress
to higher grades of malignancy.

WHO grade III includes lesions with histologic evidence of malignancy, including nuclear atypia and increased mitotic activity. These
lesions have anaplastic histology and infiltrative capacity. They are
usually treated with aggressive adjuvant therapy.

WHO grade IV includes lesions that are mitotically active,
necrosis-prone, and generally associated with a rapid preoperative

and postoperative progression and fatal outcomes. The lesions are usually treated with aggressive adjuvant therapy.

The following table is from the WHO *Classification of Tumours of the Central Nervous System* and lists the tumor types and grades.[4] Tumors limited to the peripheral nervous system are not included.

Table 27.1. WHO Grades of CNS Tumors[a]

	I	II	III	IV
Astrocytic tumors				
Subependymal giant cell astrocytoma	X			
Pilocytic astrocytoma	X			
Pilomyxoid astrocytoma		X		
Diffuse astrocytoma		X		
Pleomorphic xanthoastrocytoma		X		
Anaplastic astrocytoma			X	
Glioblastoma				X
Giant cell glioblastoma				X
Gliosarcoma				X
Oligondendroglial tumors				
Oligodendroglioma		X		
Anaplastic oligodendroglioma			X	
Oligoastrocytic tumors				
Oligoastrocytoma		X		
Anaplastic oligoastrocytoma			X	
Ependymal tumors				
Subependymoma	X			
Myxopapillary ependymoma	X			
Ependymoma		X		
Anaplastic ependymoma			X	
Choroid plexus tumors				
Choroid plexus papilloma	X			
Atypical choroid plexus papilloma		X		
Choroid plexus carcinoma			X	
Other neuroepithelial tumors				
Angiocentric glioma	X			
Chordoid glioma of the third ventricle		X		

	I	II	III	IV
Neuronal and mixed neuronal-glial tumors				
Gangliocytoma	X			
Ganglioglioma	X			
Anaplastic ganglioma			X	
Desmoplastic infantile astrocytoma and ganglioglioma	X			
Dysembryoplastic neuroepithelial tumor	X			
Central neurocytoma		X		
Extraventricular neurocytoma		X		
Cerebellar liponeurocytoma		X		
Paraganglioma of the spinal cord	X			
Papillary glioneuronal tumor	X			
Rosette-forming glioneural tumor of the fourth ventricle	X			
Pineal tumors				
Pineocytoma	X			
Pineal parenchymal tumor of intermediate differentiation		X	X	
Pineoblastoma				X
Papillary tumor of the pineal region		X	X	
Embryonal tumors				
Medulloblastoma				X
CNS primitive neuroectodermal tumor (PNET)				X
Atypical teratoid/rhabdoid tumor				X
Tumors of the cranial and paraspinal nerves				
Schwannoma	X			
Neurofibroma	X			
Perineurioma	X	X	X	
Malignant peripheral nerve sheath tumor (MPNST)		X	X	X
Meningeal tumors				
Meningioma	X			
Atypical meningioma		X		
Anaplastic/malignant meningioma			X	
Hemangiopericytoma		X		
Anaplastic hemangiopericytoma			X	
Hemangioblastoma	X			
Tumors of the sellar region				
Craniopharyngioma	X			

	I	II	III	IV
Granular cell tumor of the neurohypophysis	X			
Pituicytoma	X			
Spindle cell oncocytoma of the adenohypophysis	X			

[a] *Reprinted with permission from Louis, DN, Ohgaki H, Wiestler, OD, Cavenee, WK. World Health Organization Classification of Tumours of the Nervous System. IARC, Lyon, 2007.*

References

1. Kleihues P, Cavenee WK, eds.: Pathology and Genetics of Tumours of the Nervous System. Lyon, France: International Agency for Research on Cancer, 2000.

2. Brain and spinal cord. In: Edge SB, Byrd DR, Compton CC, et al., eds.: AJCC Cancer Staging Manual. 7th ed. New York, NY: Springer, 2010, pp 593-7.

3. Kleihues P, Burger PC, Scheithauer BW: The new WHO classification of brain tumours. Brain Pathol 3 (3): 255-68, 1993.

4. Louis DN, Ohgaki H, Wiestler OD, et al.: The 2007 WHO classification of tumours of the central nervous system. Acta Neuropathol 114 (2): 97-109, 2007.

Section 27.3

Treatment Option Overview

Text in this section is excerpted from "Adult Brain Tumors Treatment (PDQ®)," National Cancer Institute at the National Institutes of Health (NIH), February 25, 2015.

Primary Brain Tumors

Radiation therapy and chemotherapy options vary according to histology and anatomic site of the brain tumor. For glioblastoma, combined modality therapy with resection, radiation, and chemotherapy is standard. Since anaplastic astrocytomas, anaplastic oligodendrogliomas, and anaplastic oligoastrocytomas represent only a small proportion of central nervous system gliomas, phase III randomized trials restricted to them are not generally practical. The natural histories of these tumors are variable, depending on histological and molecular factors; therefore, treatment guidelines are evolving. Therapy involving surgically implanted carmustine-impregnated polymer wafers combined with postoperative external-beam radiation therapy (EBRT) may play a role in the treatment of high-grade gliomas (grade III and IV gliomas) in some patients.[1] Specific treatment options for tumor types are listed below under the tumor types and locations. This section covers general treatment principles.

Dexamethasone, mannitol, and furosemide are used to treat the peritumoral edema associated with brain tumors. Use of anticonvulsants is mandatory for patients with seizures.[2]

Finally, active surveillance is appropriate in some circumstances. With the increasing use of sensitive neuroimaging tools, there has been increased detection of asymptomatic low-grade meningiomas. The majority appear to show minimal growth and can often be safely observed, with therapy deferred until the detection of tumor growth or the development of symptoms.[3,4]

Surgery

For most types of brain tumors in most locations, an attempt at complete or near-complete surgical removal is generally recommended, if possible, within the constraints of preservation of neurologic function and underlying patient health. This recommendation is based on observational evidence that survival is better in patients who undergo tumor resection than in those who have closed biopsy alone.[5,6] However, the benefit of resection has not been tested in randomized trials.

Selection bias can enter into observational studies despite attempts to adjust for patient differences that guide the decision to operate. Therefore, the actual difference in outcome between radical surgery and biopsy alone may not be as large as noted in the retrospective studies.[6] An exception to the general recommendation for attempted resection is the case of deep-seated tumors such as pontine gliomas, which are diagnosed on clinical evidence and treated without initial surgery approximately 50% of the time. In most cases, however, diagnosis by biopsy is preferred. Stereotactic biopsy can be used for lesions that are difficult to reach and resect.

Two primary goals of surgery include:[2]

- Establishing a histologic diagnosis.

- Reducing intracranial pressure by removing as much tumor as is safely possible to preserve neurological function.

However, total elimination of primary malignant intraparenchymal tumors by surgery alone is rarely achievable. Therefore, intraoperative techniques have been developed to reach a balance between removing as much tumor as is practical and the preservation of functional status. For example, craniotomies with stereotactic resections of primary gliomas can be done in cooperative patients while they are awake, with real-time assessment of neurologic function.[7] Resection proceeds until either the magnetic resonance imaging (MRI) signal abnormality being used to monitor the extent of surgery is completely removed or subtle neurologic dysfunction appears (e.g., slight decrease in rapid alternating motor movement or anomia). Likewise, when the tumor is located in or near language centers in the cortex, intraoperative language mapping can be performed by electrode discharge-induced speech arrest while the patient is asked to count or read.[8]

As is the case with several other specialized operations [9,10] in which postoperative mortality has been associated with the number of procedures performed, postoperative mortality after surgery for primary brain tumors may be associated with hospital and/or surgeon volume. [11] Using the Nationwide Inpatient Sample hospital discharge database for the years 1988 to 2000, which represented 20% of inpatient admissions to nonfederal U.S. hospitals, investigators found that large-volume hospitals had lower in-hospital mortality rates after craniotomies for primary brain tumors (odds ratio [OR] = 0.75 for a tenfold higher caseload; 95% confidence interval [CI], 0.62–0.90) and after needle biopsies (OR = 0.54; 95% CI, 0.35–0.83). For example, although there was no specific sharp threshold in mortality outcomes between low-volume hospitals and high-volume hospitals, craniotomy-associated in-hospital mortality was 4.5% for hospitals with five or fewer procedures per year and 1.5% for hospitals with at least 42 procedures per year.

In-hospital mortality rates decreased over the study years (perhaps because the proportion of elective non-emergent operations increased from 45% to 57%), but the decrease was more rapid in high-volume hospitals than in low-volume hospitals. High-volume surgeons also had lower in-hospital patient mortality rates after craniotomy (OR= 0.60; 95% CI, 0.45–0.79).[11] As with any study of volume-outcome associations, these results may not be causal because they may be affected by residual confounding factors, such as referral patterns, private insurance, and patient selection, despite multivariable adjustment.

Radiation Therapy

High-grade tumors

Radiation therapy has a major role in the treatment of patients with high-grade gliomas. A systematic review and meta-analysis of five randomized trials (plus one trial with allocation by birth date) comparing postoperative radiation therapy (PORT) with no radiation therapy showed a statistically significant survival advantage with radiation (risk ratio (RR) = 0.81; 95% CI, 0.74–0.88).[12][Level of evidence: 1iiA] Based on a randomized trial comparing 60 Gray (in 30 fractions over 6 weeks) with 45 Gray (in 25 fractions over 4 weeks) that showed superior survival in the first group (12 months vs. 9 months median survival; hazard ratio [HR] = 0.81; 95% CI, 0.66–0.99), 60 Gray is the accepted standard dose of EBRT for malignant gliomas.[13][Level of evidence: 1iiA]

EBRT using either 3-dimensional conformal radiation therapy or intensity-modulated radiation therapy is considered an acceptable technique in radiation therapy delivery. Typically 2- to 3-cm margins on the MRI-based volumes (T1-weighted and FLAIR [fluid-attenuated inversion recovery]) to create the planning target volume are used. Dose escalation using radiosurgery has not improved outcomes.

A randomized trial tested radiosurgery as a boost added to standard EBRT, but the trial found no improvement in survival, quality of life, or patterns of relapse compared with EBRT without the boost.[14,15]

For the same theoretical reasons, brachytherapy has been used to deliver high doses of radiation locally to the tumor while sparing normal brain tissue. However, this approach is technically demanding and has fallen out of favor with the advent of the above-mentioned techniques.

Low-grade tumors

The role of immediate PORT for low-grade gliomas (i.e., low-grade astrocytoma, oligodendroglioma, mixedoligoastrocytomas) is not as clear as in the case of high-grade tumors. The European Organisation for Research and Treatment of Cancer (EORTC) randomly assigned 311 patients with low-grade gliomas to radiation versus observation in the EORTC-22845 and MRC BR04 trials.[16,17] (On central pathology review, about 25% of the patients on the trial were reported to actually have high-grade tumors.) Most of the control patients received radiation at the time of progression. After a median follow-up of 93 months, median progression-free survival was 5.3 years in the radiation arm versus 3.4 years in the control arm (HR = 0.59; 95% CI, 0.45–0.77).[16,17][Level of evidence: 1iiDiii] However, there was no difference in the overall survival (OS) rate (median survival = 7.4 years vs. 7.2 years; HR = 0.97; 95% CI, 0.71–1.34; P = .87).[16,17][Level of evidence: 1iiA] This was caused by a longer survival after progression in the control arm (3.4 years) than in the radiation arm (1.0 years) (P < .0001). The investigators did not collect reliable quality-of-life measurements, so it is not clear whether the delay in initial relapse in the radiation therapy arm translated into improved function or quality of life.

Repeat radiation therapy (re-irradiation)

Because there are no randomized trials, the role of repeat radiation after disease progression or the development of radiation-induced cancers is also ill defined. The literature is limited to small retrospective case series, which makes interpretation difficult.[18] The decision to use repeat radiation must be made carefully because of the risk of neurocognitive deficits and radiation-induced necrosis. One advantage of radiosurgery is the ability to deliver therapeutic doses to recurrences that may require the re-irradiation of previously irradiated brain tissue beyond tolerable dose limits.

Chemotherapy

Systemic chemotherapy

For many years, the nitrosourea carmustine (BCNU) was the standard chemotherapy added to surgery and radiation for malignant gliomas. This was based upon a randomized trial (RTOG-8302) of 467 patients conducted by the Brain Tumor Study Group that compared four regimens after initial resection, including semustine (methyl-CCNU), radiation therapy, radiation therapy plus carmustine, and radiation therapy plus semustine.[19]

The radiation therapy plus carmustine arm had the best survival rate.[19][Level of evidence: 1iiA] A modest impact on survival using nitrosourea-containing chemotherapy regimens for malignant gliomas was confirmed in a patient-level meta-analysis of 12 randomized trials (combined HR death = 0.85; 95% CI, 0.78–0.91).[20]

However, the oral agent, temozolomide, has since replaced the nitrosoureas as the standard systemic chemotherapy for malignant gliomas based upon a large multicenter trial (NCT00006353) of glioblastoma patients conducted by the EORTC-National Cancer Institute of Canada that showed a survival advantage.[21,22][Level of evidence: 1iiA] (Refer to the Glioblastoma section of the Management of Specific Tumor Types and Locations section of this chapter for more information.)

Localized chemotherapy

Because malignant glioma-related deaths are nearly always the result of an inability to control intracranial disease (rather than the result of distant metastases), the concept of delivering high doses of chemotherapy while avoiding systemic toxicity is attractive. A biodegradable carmustine wafer has been developed for that purpose. The wafers contain 3.85% carmustine, and up to eight wafers are implanted into the tumor bed lining at the time of open resection, with an intended total dose of about 7.7 mg per wafer (61.6 mg maximum per patient) over a period of 2 to 3 weeks. Two randomized, placebo-controlled trials of this focal drug-delivery method have shown an OS advantage associated with the carmustine wafers versus radiation therapy alone. Both trials had an upper age limit of 65 years. The first was a small trial closed because of a lack of continued availability of the carmustine wafers after 32 patients with high-grade gliomas had been entered.[23] Although OS was better in the carmustine-wafer group (median 58.1 vs. 39.9 weeks; P = .012), there was an imbalance in the study arms (only 11 of the16 patients in the carmustine-wafer group vs. 16 of the 16 patients in the placebo-wafer group had Grade IV glioblastoma tumors).

The second study was, therefore, more informative.[24,25] It was a multicenter study of 240 patients with primary malignant gliomas, 207 of whom had glioblastoma. At initial surgery, they received the carmustine versus placebo wafers, followed by radiation therapy (55 Gray–60 Gray). Systemic therapy was not allowed until recurrence, except in the case of anaplastic oligodendrogliomas, of which there were nine patients. Unlike the initial trial, patient characteristics were well balanced between the study arms. Median survival in the two groups was 13.8 months versus 11.6 months; P = .017 (HR = 0.73; 95% CI, 0.56–0.96). A systematic review combining both studies estimated a HR for overall mortality of 0.65; 95% CI, 0.48–0.86; P = .003.[26] [Level of evidence: 1iA]

Treatment Options Under Clinical Evaluation

Patients who have brain tumors that are either infrequently curable or unresectable should be considered candidates for clinical trials.

Heavy-particle radiation, such as proton-beam therapy, carries the theoretical advantage of delivering high doses of ionizing radiation to the tumor bed while sparing surrounding brain tissue. The data are preliminary for this investigational technique, and are not widely available.

Novel biologic therapies under clinical evaluation for patients with brain tumors include the following:[27]

- Dendritic cell vaccination.[28]

- Tyrosine kinase receptor inhibitors.[29]

- Farnesyl transferase inhibitors.

- Viral-based gene therapy.[30,31]

- Oncolytic viruses.

- Epidermal growth factor-receptor inhibitors.

- Vascular endothelial growth factor inhibitors.[27]

- Other antiangiogenesis agents.

Primary Tumors of the Spinal Axis

Surgery and radiation therapy are the primary modalities used to treat tumors of the spinal axis; therapeutic options vary according to the histology of the tumor.[2] The experience with chemotherapy for primary spinal cord tumors is limited; no reports of controlled clinical trials are available for these types of tumors.[2,32] Chemotherapy is indicated for most patients with leptomeningeal involvement (from a primary or metastatic tumor) and positive cerebrospinal fluid (CSF) cytology.[2] Most patients require treatment with corticosteroids, particularly if they are receiving radiation therapy.

Patients who have spinal axis tumors that are either infrequently curable or unresectable should be considered candidates for clinical trials.

Leptomeningeal carcinomatosis (LC)

The management of LC includes the following:

- Intrathecal chemotherapy.

- Intrathecal chemotherapy and systemic chemotherapy.

- Intrathecal chemotherapy and radiation therapy.

- Supportive care.

LC occurs in about 5% of all cancer patients. The most common types include breast tumors (35%), lung tumors (24%), and hematologic malignancies (16%). Diagnosis includes a combination of neurospinal axis imaging and CSF cytology. Median OS is in the range of 10 to 12 weeks.

In a series of 149 patients with metastatic non-small cell lung carcinoma, cytologically proven LC, poor performance status, high protein level in the CSF, and a high initial CSF white blood cell count were significant poor prognostic factors for survival.[33] Patients received active treatment including intrathecal chemotherapy, whole-brain radiation therapy (WBRT), or epidermal growth factor receptor-thymidine kinase-1, or underwent a ventriculoperitoneal shunt procedure.

In a retrospective series of 38 patients with metastatic breast cancer and LC, the proportion of luminal A, B, human epidermal growth factor receptor 2 (HER2)-positive and triple-negative breast cancer subtype was 18.4%, 31.6%, 26.3% and 23.7%, respectively.[34] Patients with triple-negative breast cancer had a shorter interval between metastatic breast cancer diagnosis and the development of LC. Median survival did not differ across breast cancer subtypes. Consideration of intrathecal administration of trastuzumab in patients with HER2-positive LC has also been reported in case reports.[35]

Metastatic Brain Tumors

Approximately 20% to 40% of cancer patients develop brain metastases, with a subsequent median survival generally less than 6 months. Common primary tumors with brain metastases include the following cancers:

- Lung.

- Breast.

- Cancer of unknown primary.

- Melanoma.

- Colon.

- Kidney.

The optimal therapy for patients with brain metastases continues to evolve.[32,36,37] Corticosteroids, anticonvulsants, radiation therapy, radiosurgery, and, possibly, surgical resection have roles in management. Because most cases of brain metastases involve multiple metastases, a mainstay of therapy has historically been WBRT, but stereotactic radiosurgery (SRS) has come into increasingly common use. The role of radiosurgery continues to be defined. Chemotherapy is usually not the primary therapy for most patients; however, it may have a role in the treatment of patients with brain metastases from chemosensitive tumors and can even be curative when combined with radiation for metastatic testicular germ cell tumors.[36,38] Intrathecal chemotherapy is also used for meningeal spread of metastatic tumors.

Treatment for patients with a single metastasis

About 10% to 15% of patients with cancer will have a single brain metastasis. Radiation therapy is the mainstay of palliation for these patients. The extent of extracranial disease can influence treatment of the brain lesions. In the presence of extensive active systemic disease, surgery provides little benefit for OS. In patients with stable minimal extracranial disease, combined modality treatment may be considered, using surgical resection followed by radiation therapy. However, the published literature does not provide clear guidance.

There have been three randomized trials of resection of solitary brain metastases followed by WBRT versus WBRT alone, totaling 195 randomly assigned patients.[39-41] The process that necessarily goes into selecting appropriate patients for surgical resection may account for the small numbers in each trial. In the first trial, performed at a single center, all patients were selected and operated upon by one surgeon. The first two trials showed an improvement in survival in the surgery group, but the third showed a trend in favor of the WBRT-only group. The three trials were combined in a trial-level meta-analysis.[26] The combined analysis did not show a statistically significant difference in OS (HR = 0.72; 95% CI, 0.34–1.53; P = .4); nor was there a statistically significant difference in death from neurologic causes (RRdeath = 0.68; 95% CI, 0.43–1.09; P = .11). None of the trials assessed or reported quality of life. One of the trials reported that combined therapy increased the duration of functionally independent survival.[39][Level of evidence: 1iiD]

The need for WBRT after resection of solitary brain metastases has been tested.[42] Patients in the WBRT group were less likely to have tumor progression in the brain and were significantly less likely to die of neurological causes, but OS was the same, and there was no difference in duration of functional independence.[42] One additional randomized study of observation versus WBRT after either surgery or

SRS for solitary brain metastases was closed because of slow accrual after 19 patients had been entered, so little can be deduced from the trial.[43]

Treatment for patients with oligometastases (1–3 or 4 brain metastases)

A Radiation Therapy Oncology Group (RTOG) study (RTOG-9508) randomly assigned 333 patients with one to three metastases with a maximum diameter of 4 cm to WBRT (37.5 Gy over 3 weeks) with or without a stereotactic boost.[44] Patients with active systemic disease requiring therapy were excluded. The primary endpoint was OS with predefined hypotheses in both the full study population and the 186 patients with a solitary metastasis (and no statistical adjustment of P values for the two separate hypotheses). Mean OS in the combined-therapy and WBRT-alone groups was 5.7 months and 6.5 months, respectively (P = .14). In the subgroup with solitary metastases, OS was better in the combined-therapy group (6.5 months vs. 4.9 months; P =.039 in univariate analysis; P = .053 in a multivariable analysis adjusting for baseline prognostic factors); in patients with multiple metastases, survival was 5.8 months in the combined-therapy group versus 6.7 months in the WBRT-only group (P = .98). (The combined-treatment group had a survival advantage of 2½ months in patients with a single metastasis but not in patients with multiple lesions.) Local control was better in the full population with combined therapy.

At the 6-month follow-up, Karnofsky Performance status (considered a soft endpoint because of its imprecision and subjectivity) was better in the combined-therapy group, but there was no difference in mental status between the treatment groups. Acute and late toxicities were similar in both treatment arms. Quality of life was not assessed.[44] [Levels of evidence: 1iiDii for the full study population and 1iiA for patients with solitary metastases]

The converse question has also been addressed—whether WBRT is necessary after focal treatment (i.e., resection or SRS) of oligometastases. Several randomized trials have been performed that were designed with varying primary endpoints.[45-47] However, the results can be summarized as follows:

1. Studies consistently show that the addition of WBRT to focal therapy decreases the risk of progression and new metastases in the brain.

2. The addition of WBRT does not improve OS.

3. The decrease in risk of intracranial disease progression does not translate into improved functional or neurologic status, nor does it appear to decrease the risk of death from neurologic deterioration.

4. About half or more of the patients who receive focal therapy alone ultimately require salvage therapy, such as WBRT or radiosurgery, compared with about a quarter of the patients who are given up-front WBRT.

5. The impact of better local control associated with WBRT on quality of life has not been reported and remains an open question.

A phase III randomized trial compared adjuvant WBRT with observation after surgery or radiosurgery for a limited number of brain metastases in patients with stable solid tumors.[48] Health-related quality of life was improved in the observation-only arm compared with WBRT. Patients in the observation arm had better mean scores in physical, role, and cognitive functioning at 9 months. In an exploratory analysis, statistically significant worse scores for bladder control, communication deficit, drowsiness, hair loss, motor dysfunction, leg weakness, appetite loss, constipation, nausea/vomiting, pain, and social functioning were observed in patients who underwent WBRT compared with those who underwent observation only.[48][Level of evidence: 1iiC]

The study that had a primary endpoint of learning and neurocognition, using a standardized test for total recall, was stopped by the data and safety monitoring committee because of worse outcomes in the WBRT group.[46]

Given this body of information, focal therapy plus WBRT or focal therapy alone, with close follow-up with serial MRIs and initiation of salvage therapy when clinically indicated, appear to be reasonable treatment options. The pros and cons of each approach should be discussed with the patient.[46][Level of evidence: 1iiD]

Treatment for patients with multiple metastases

Patients with multiple brain metastases may be treated with WBRT. Surgery is indicated to obtain tissue from a metastasis with an unknown primary tumor or to decompress a symptomatic dominant lesion that is causing significant mass effect. SRS in combination with WBRT has been assessed. A meta-analysis of two trials with a total of 358 participants found no statistically significant difference in OS between the

WBRT plus SRS and WBRT alone groups (HR, 0.82; 95% CI, 0.65–1.02). Patients in the WBRT plus SRS group had decreased local failure compared with patients who received WBRT alone (HR, 0.27; 95% CI, 0.14–0.52). Unchanged or improved Karnofsky Performance Scale at 6 months was seen in 43% of patients in the combined therapy group versus only 28% in the WBRT group (P = .03).[49][Level of evidence: 1iiDiii]

References

1. Lallana EC, Abrey LE: Update on the therapeutic approaches to brain tumors. Expert Rev Anticancer Ther 3 (5): 655-70, 2003.

2. Cloughesy T, Selch MT, Liau L: Brain. In: Haskell CM: Cancer Treatment. 5th ed. Philadelphia, Pa: WB Saunders Co, 2001, pp 1106-42.

3. Nakamura M, Roser F, Michel J, et al.: The natural history of incidental meningiomas. Neurosurgery 53 (1): 62-70; discussion 70-1, 2003.

4. Yano S, Kuratsu J; Kumamoto Brain Tumor Research Group: Indications for surgery in patients with asymptomatic meningiomas based on an extensive experience. J Neurosurg 105 (4): 538-43, 2006.

5. Laws ER, Parney IF, Huang W, et al.: Survival following surgery and prognostic factors for recently diagnosed malignant glioma: data from the Glioma Outcomes Project. J Neurosurg 99 (3): 467-73, 2003.

6. Chang SM, Parney IF, Huang W, et al.: Patterns of care for adults with newly diagnosed malignant glioma. JAMA 293 (5): 557-64, 2005.

7. Meyer FB, Bates LM, Goerss SJ, et al.: Awake craniotomy for aggressive resection of primary gliomas located in eloquent brain. Mayo ClinProc 76 (7): 677-87, 2001.

8. Sanai N, Mirzadeh Z, Berger MS: Functional outcome after language mapping for glioma resection. N Engl J Med 358 (1): 18-27, 2008.

9. Begg CB, Cramer LD, Hoskins WJ, et al.: Impact of hospital volume on operative mortality for major cancer surgery. JAMA 280 (20): 1747-51, 1998.

10. Birkmeyer JD, Finlayson EV, Birkmeyer CM: Volume standards for high-risk surgical procedures: potential benefits of the Leapfrog initiative. Surgery 130 (3): 415-22, 2001.

11. Barker FG 2nd, Curry WT Jr, Carter BS: Surgery for primary supratentorial brain tumors in the United States, 1988 to 2000: the effect of provider caseload and centralization of care. Neuro Oncol 7 (1): 49-63, 2005.

12. Laperriere N, Zuraw L, Cairncross G, et al.: Radiotherapy for newly diagnosed malignant glioma in adults: a systematic review. RadiotherOncol 64 (3): 259-73, 2002.

13. Bleehen NM, Stenning SP: A Medical Research Council trial of two radiotherapy doses in the treatment of grades 3 and 4 astrocytoma. The Medical Research Council Brain Tumour Working Party. Br J Cancer 64 (4): 769-74, 1991.

14. Tsao MN, Mehta MP, Whelan TJ, et al.: The American Society for Therapeutic Radiology and Oncology (ASTRO) evidence-based review of the role of radiosurgery for malignant glioma. Int J RadiatOncolBiolPhys 63 (1): 47-55, 2005.

15. Souhami L, Seiferheld W, Brachman D, et al.: Randomized comparison of stereotactic radiosurgery followed by conventional radiotherapy with carmustine to conventional radiotherapy with carmustine for patients with glioblastoma multiforme: report of Radiation Therapy Oncology Group 93-05 protocol. Int J RadiatOncolBiolPhys 60 (3): 853-60, 2004.

16. Karim AB, Afra D, Cornu P, et al.: Randomized trial on the efficacy of radiotherapy for cerebral low-grade glioma in the adult: European Organization for Research and Treatment of Cancer Study 22845 with the Medical Research Council study BRO4: an interim analysis. Int J RadiatOncolBiolPhys 52 (2): 316-24, 2002.

17. van den Bent MJ, Afra D, de Witte O, et al.: Long-term efficacy of early versus delayed radiotherapy for low-grade astrocytoma and oligodendroglioma in adults: the EORTC 22845 randomised trial. Lancet 366 (9490): 985-90, 2005.

18. Paulino AC, Mai WY, Chintagumpala M, et al.: Radiation-induced malignant gliomas: is there a role for reirradiation? Int J RadiatOncolBiolPhys 71 (5): 1381-7, 2008.

19. Walker MD, Green SB, Byar DP, et al.: Randomized comparisons of radiotherapy and nitrosoureas for the treatment of malignant glioma after surgery. N Engl J Med 303 (23): 1323-9, 1980.

20. Stewart LA: Chemotherapy in adult high-grade glioma: a systematic review and meta-analysis of individual patient data from 12 randomised trials. Lancet 359 (9311): 1011-8, 2002.

21. Stupp R, Mason WP, van den Bent MJ, et al.: Radiotherapy plus concomitant and adjuvant temozolomide for glioblastoma. N Engl J Med 352 (10): 987-96, 2005.

22. Stupp R, Hegi ME, Mason WP, et al.: Effects of radiotherapy with concomitant and adjuvant temozolomide versus radiotherapy alone on survival in glioblastoma in a randomised phase III study: 5-year analysis of the EORTC-NCIC trial. Lancet Oncol 10 (5): 459-66, 2009.

23. Valtonen S, Timonen U, Toivanen P, et al.: Interstitial chemotherapy with carmustine-loaded polymers for high-grade gliomas: a randomized double-blind study. Neurosurgery 41 (1): 44-8; discussion 48-9, 1997.

24. Westphal M, Hilt DC, Bortey E, et al.: A phase 3 trial of local chemotherapy with biodegradable carmustine (BCNU) wafers (Gliadel wafers) in patients with primary malignant glioma. Neuro-oncol 5 (2): 79-88, 2003.

25. Westphal M, Ram Z, Riddle V, et al.: Gliadel wafer in initial surgery for malignant glioma: long-term follow-up of a multicenter controlled trial. ActaNeurochir (Wien) 148 (3): 269-75; discussion 275, 2006.

26. Hart MG, Grant R, Garside R, et al.: Chemotherapeutic wafers for high grade glioma. Cochrane Database Syst Rev (3): CD007294, 2008.

27. Fine HA: Promising new therapies for malignant gliomas. Cancer J 13 (6): 349-54, 2007 Nov-Dec.

28. Fecci PE, Mitchell DA, Archer GE, et al.: The history, evolution, and clinical use of dendritic cell-based immunization strategies in the therapy of brain tumors. J Neurooncol 64 (1-2): 161-76, 2003 Aug-Sep.

29. Newton HB: Molecular neuro-oncology and development of targeted therapeutic strategies for brain tumors. Part 1: Growth factor and Ras signaling pathways. Expert Rev Anticancer Ther 3 (5): 595-614, 2003.

30. Kew Y, Levin VA: Advances in gene therapy and immunotherapy for brain tumors. CurrOpinNeurol 16 (6): 665-70, 2003.

31. Chiocca EA, Aghi M, Fulci G: Viral therapy for glioblastoma. Cancer J 9 (3): 167-79, 2003 May-Jun.

32. Mehta M, Vogelbaum MA, Chang S, et al.: Neoplasms of the central nervous system. In: DeVita VT Jr, Lawrence TS, Rosenberg SA: Cancer: Principles and Practice of Oncology. 9th ed. Philadelphia, Pa: Lippincott Williams & Wilkins, 2011, pp 1700-49. Lee SJ, Lee JI, Nam DH, et al.: Leptomeningeal carcinomatosis in non-small-cell lung cancer patients: impact on survival and correlated prognostic factors. J Thorac Oncol 8 (2): 185-91, 2013.

33. Torrejón D, Oliveira M, Cortes J, et al.: Implication of breast cancer phenotype for patients with leptomeningeal carcinomatosis. Breast 22 (1): 19-23, 2013.

34. Bartsch R, Berghoff AS, Preusser M: Optimal management of brain metastases from breast cancer. Issues and considerations. CNS Drugs 27 (2): 121-34, 2013.

35. Patchell RA: The management of brain metastases. Cancer Treat Rev 29 (6): 533-40, 2003.

36. Soffietti R, Cornu P, Delattre JY, et al.: EFNS Guidelines on diagnosis and treatment of brain metastases: report of an EFNS Task Force. Eur J Neurol 13 (7): 674-81, 2006.

37. Ogawa K, Yoshii Y, Nishimaki T, et al.: Treatment and prognosis of brain metastases from breast cancer. J Neurooncol 86 (2): 231-8, 2008.

38. Patchell RA, Tibbs PA, Walsh JW, et al.: A randomized trial of surgery in the treatment of single metastases to the brain. N Engl J Med 322 (8): 494-500, 1990.

39. Vecht CJ, Haaxma-Reiche H, Noordijk EM, et al.: Treatment of single brain metastasis: radiotherapy alone or combined with neurosurgery? Ann Neurol 33 (6): 583-90, 1993.

40. Mintz AH, Kestle J, Rathbone MP, et al.: A randomized trial to assess the efficacy of surgery in addition to radiotherapy in patients with a single cerebral metastasis. Cancer 78 (7): 1470-6, 1996.

41. Patchell RA, Tibbs PA, Regine WF, et al.: Postoperative radiotherapy in the treatment of single metastases to the brain: a randomized trial. JAMA 280 (17): 1485-9, 1998.

42. Roos DE, Wirth A, Burmeister BH, et al.: Whole brain irradiation following surgery or radiosurgery for solitary brain metastases: mature results of a prematurely closed randomized Trans-Tasman Radiation Oncology Group trial (TROG 98.05). RadiotherOncol 80 (3): 318-22, 2006.

43. Andrews DW, Scott CB, Sperduto PW, et al.: Whole brain radiation therapy with or without stereotactic radiosurgery boost for patients with one to three brain metastases: phase III results of the RTOG 9508 randomised trial. Lancet 363 (9422): 1665-72, 2004.

44. Aoyama H, Shirato H, Tago M, et al.: Stereotactic radiosurgery plus whole-brain radiation therapy vs stereotactic radiosurgery alone for treatment of brain metastases: a randomized controlled trial. JAMA 295 (21): 2483-91, 2006.

45. Chang EL, Wefel JS, Hess KR, et al.: Neurocognition in patients with brain metastases treated with radiosurgery or radiosurgery plus whole-brain irradiation: a randomised controlled trial. Lancet Oncol 10 (11): 1037-44, 2009.

46. Kocher M, Soffietti R, Abacioglu U, et al.: Adjuvant whole-brain radiotherapy versus observation after radiosurgery or surgical resection of one to three cerebral metastases: results of the EORTC 22952-26001 study. J ClinOncol 29 (2): 134-41, 2011.

47. Soffietti R, Kocher M, Abacioglu UM, et al.: A European Organisation for Research and Treatment of Cancer phase III trial of adjuvant whole-brain radiotherapy versus observation in patients with one to three brain metastases from solid tumors after surgical resection or radiosurgery: quality-of-life results. J ClinOncol 31 (1): 65-72, 2013.

48. Patil CG, Pricola K, Sarmiento JM, et al.: Whole brain radiation therapy (WBRT) alone versus WBRT and radiosurgery for the treatment of brain metastases. Cochrane Database Syst Rev 9: CD006121, 2012.

Section 27.4

Management of Specific Tumor Types and Locations

Text in this section is excerpted from "Adult Brain Tumors
Treatment (PDQ®)," National Cancer Institute at the National
Institutes of Health (NIH), February 25, 2015.

Brain Stem Gliomas

Standard treatment options:

- Radiation therapy.

Patients with brain stem gliomas have relatively poor prognoses
that correlate with histology (when biopsies are performed), location,
and extent of tumor. The overall median survival time of patients in
studies has been 44 to 74 weeks.

Current Clinical Trials

Check for U.S. clinical trials from NCI's list of cancer clinical trials
that are now accepting patients with adult brain stem glioma. The list
of clinical trials can be further narrowed by location, drug, intervention, and other criteria.

Pineal Astrocytic Tumors

Standard treatment options:

1. Surgery plus radiation therapy for patients with pilocytic or
   diffuse astrocytoma.

2. Surgery plus radiation therapy and chemotherapy for patients
   with higher grade tumors.

Depending on the degree of anaplasia, patients with pineal astrocytomas vary in prognoses. Higher grades have worse prognoses.

Pilocytic Astrocytomas

Standard treatment options:

1. Surgery alone if the tumor is totally resectable.

2. Surgery followed by radiation therapy to known or suspected residual tumor.

This astrocytic tumor is classified as a World Health Organization (WHO) grade I tumor and is often curable.

Diffuse Astrocytomas (WHO grade II)

Standard treatment options:

- Surgery plus radiation therapy; however, some controversy exists. Some physicians treat these patients with surgery alone if the patient is younger than 35 years and if the tumor does not contrast-enhance on a computed tomographic scan.[1]

This WHO grade II astrocytic tumor is less often curable than is a pilocytic astrocytoma.

Anaplastic Astrocytomas (WHO grade III)

Standard treatment options:

1. Surgery plus radiation therapy.

2. Surgery plus radiation therapy and chemotherapy.

Patients with anaplastic astrocytomas (WHO grade III) have a low cure rate with standard local treatment. Because anaplastic astrocytomas represent less than 10% of all central nervous system gliomas, phase III randomized trials restricted to patients with them are not practical. However, because these tumors are often aggressive, they are frequently managed the same way as glioblastomas, with surgery and radiation, and often with chemotherapy, even though it is not known whether the improved survival with chemotherapy in glioblastoma can be extrapolated to anaplastic astrocytomas.

Postoperative radiation alone has been compared with postoperative chemotherapy alone in patients with anaplastic gliomas (i.e., 144 astrocytomas, 91 oligoastrocytomas, and 39 oligodendrogliomas) with crossover to the other modality at the time of tumor progression. Of the 139 patients randomly assigned to radiation therapy, 135 were randomly assigned to chemotherapy with a 32-week course of either procarbazine + lomustine + vincristine (PCV) or single-agent temozolomide (2:1:1 randomization). The order of the modalities did not affect time to treatment failure (TTF) or overall survival (OS).[2] [Levels of evidence: 1iiA and 1iiD] Neither TTF nor OS differed across the treatment arms.

Patients with anaplastic astrocytomas are appropriate candidates for clinical trials designed to improve local control by adding newer forms of treatment to standard treatment. Information about ongoing clinical trials is available from the NCI Web site.

Glioblastomas

Standard treatment options for patients with newly diagnosed disease:

1. Surgery plus radiation therapy.

2. Surgery plus radiation therapy and chemotherapy.

3. Carmustine-impregnated polymer implanted during initial surgery.

4. Radiation therapy and concurrent chemotherapy.

The standard-of-care treatment for patients with newly diagnosed glioblastoma is surgery followed by concurrent radiation therapy and daily temozolomide, and then followed by six cycles of temozolomide. This standard therapy is based on a large, multicenter, randomized trial (NCT00006353) conducted by the European Organization for Research and Treatment of Cancer (EORTC) and National Cancer Institute of Canada (NCIC), which reported a survival benefit with concurrent radiation therapy and temozolomide compared with radiation therapy alone.[3,4][Level of evidence: 1iiA] In that study, 573 patients with glioblastoma were randomly assigned to receive standard radiation to the tumor volume with a 2- to 3-cm margin (60 Gray, 2 Gray per fraction, over 6 weeks) alone or with temozolomide (75 mg/m2 orally per day during radiation therapy for up to 49 days, followed by a 4-week break and then up to six cycles of five daily doses every 28 days at a dose of 150 mg/m2, increasing to 200 mg/m2 after the first cycle). Patients in the combined therapy group were given prophylactic therapy for pneumocystis carinii during the period of concomitant radiation therapy and temozolomide. OS was statistically significantly better in the combined radiation therapy–temozolomide group (hazard ratio [HR]death, 0.6; 95% confidence interval [CI], 0.5–0.7; OS at 3 years was 16.0% vs. 4.4%).

O6-methylguanine–DNA methyltransferase (MGMT) promoter DNA methylation

A companion molecular, correlation subset study to the EORTC-NCIC trial provided strong evidence that epigenetic silencing of the MGMT DNA-repair gene by promoter DNA methylation was associated with increased OS in patients with newly diagnosed glioblastoma.[5] MGMT promoter methylation was an independent favorable prognostic factor (P < .001 by the log-rank test; HR, 0.45; 95% CI, 0.32–0.61). The median OS for MGMT-methylated patients was 18.2 months (95% CI, 15.5–22.0), compared with 12.2 months (95% CI, 11.4–13.5) for MGMT-unmethylated patients.

Dose-dense temozolomide

MGMT DNA-repair activity has been proposed as a major mechanism of resistance to alkylating agents. Intracellular depletion of MGMT has been hypothesized to enhance treatment response, and protracted temozolomide schedules have been shown to deplete intracellular MGMT in peripheral blood mononuclear cells. To test whether protracted temozolomide enhances treatment response in patients with newly diagnosed glioblastoma, a multicenter, randomized, phase III trial conducted by the Radiation Therapy Oncology Group (RTOG), EORTC, and the North Central Cancer Therapy Group, RTOG 0525 (NCT00304031), compared standard adjuvant temozolomide treatment (days 1–5 of a 28-day cycle) with a dose-dense schedule (days 1–21 of a 28-day cycle). All patients were treated with surgery followed by radiation therapy and concurrent daily temozolomide. Patients were then randomly assigned to receive either standard adjuvant temozolomide or dose-dense temozolomide.[6][Level of evidence: 1iiA]

Among 833 randomly assigned patients, no statistically significant difference between standard and dose-dense temozolomide was observed for median OS (16.6 months for standard temozolomide vs. 14.9 months for dose-dense temozolomide; HR, 1.03; P = .63) or median progression-free survival (PFS) (5.5 vs. 6.7 months; HR, 0.87; P = .06). MGMT status was determined in 86% of randomly assigned patients, and no difference in efficacy was observed in either the MGMT-methylated or MGMT-unmethylated subsets. However, this study confirmed the strong prognostic effect of MGMT methylation because the median OS was 21.2 months (95% CI, 17.9–24.8) for methylated patients versus 14 months (95% CI, 12.9–14.7) (HR, 1.74; P < .001) for unmethylated patients.

In summary, there was no survival advantage for the use of dose-dense temozolomide versus standard-dose temozolomide in newly diagnosed glioblastoma patients, regardless of MGMT status. The efficacy of dose-dense temozolomide for patients who have recurrent glioblastoma, however, is yet to be determined.

Bevacizumab in newly diagnosed glioblastoma

In 2013, final data from two multicenter, phase III, randomized, double-blind, placebo-controlled trials of bevacizumab in patients who have newly diagnosed glioblastoma were reported: RTOG 0825 (NCT00884741) and the Roche-sponsored AVAglio (NCT00943826). [7,8][Level of evidence: 1iA] Patients in both studies were randomly assigned to receive standard therapy (chemoradiation with temozolomide) or standard therapy plus bevacizumab. OS and PFS were coprimary endpoints in both trials, and these outcomes were similar. Bevacizumab did not improve OS in either study (median OS was 16–17 months for each arm in both studies); however, it increased median PFS to a similar degree (AVAglio study: 10.6 vs. 6.2 months; HR, 0.64; P < .0001; RTOG 0825 study: 10.7 vs. 7.3 months; HR, 0.79; P = .007). The PFS result in the AVAglio study was statistically significant and associated with clinical benefit because bevacizumab-treated patients remained functionally independent for longer (9.0 months vs. 6.0 months) and went longer before their Karnofsky Performance scale deteriorated (HR, 0.65; P < .0001). Furthermore, bevacizumab-treated patients went longer before corticosteroids were initiated (12.3 vs. 3.7 months; HR, 0.71; P = .002), and a larger proportion of patients was able to discontinue corticosteroids if they were already taking them (66% vs. 47%). However, the PFS result in the RTOG 0825 trial did not meet the prespecified significance level (P = .004). Of note, there was significant crossover in both trials (approximately 40% of RTOG 0825 patients and approximately 30% of AVAglio patients received bevacizumab at the first sign of disease progression).

The two trials had contradictory results in health-related quality of life (HRQoL) and neurocognitive outcomes studies. In the mandatory HRQoL studies in the AVAglio trial, bevacizumab-treated patients experienced improved HRQoL, but bevacizumab-treated patients in the elective RTOG 0825 studies showed more decline in patient-reported HRQoL and neurocognitive function. The reasons for these discrepancies are unclear.

On the basis of these results, there is no definite evidence that the addition of bevacizumab to standard therapy is beneficial for all newly diagnosed glioblastoma patients. It is yet to be determined whether certain subgroups may benefit from the addition of bevacizumab.

For patients with glioblastoma (WHO grade IV), the cure rate is very low with standard local treatment. These patients are appropriate candidates for clinical trials designed to improve local control by adding newer forms of treatment to standard treatment. Information about ongoing clinical trials is available from the NCI Web site.

Oligodendroglial Tumors

Oligodendrogliomas

Standard treatment options:

Surgery plus radiation therapy; however, some controversy exists concerning the timing of radiation therapy. A study (EORTC-22845) of 300 patients who had surgery and were randomly assigned to either radiation therapy or watch and wait did not show a difference in OS in the two groups.[9][Level of evidence: 1iiA]

Patients who have oligodendrogliomas (WHO grade II) generally have better prognoses than do patients who have diffuse astrocytomas; however, most of the oligodendrogliomas eventually progress.

Anaplastic oligodendrogliomas

Standard treatment options:

1. Surgery plus radiation therapy.

2. Surgery plus radiation therapy plus chemotherapy.[10]

3. Patients with an allelic loss at 1p and 19q have a higher than average response rate to PCV chemotherapy.

Mature results from the European Organisation for Research and Treatment of Cancer (EORTC) Brain Tumor Group Study 26951 (NCT00002840), a phase III, randomized study with 11.7 years of follow up demonstrated increased OS and progression-free survival in patients with anaplastic oligodendroglial tumors with six cycles of adjuvant PCV chemotherapy after radiation therapy compared with radiation therapy alone.[11] The OS was significantly longer in the radiation therapy and PCV arm (42.3 months vs. 30.6 months; HR, 0.75; 95% CI, 0.60–0.95). 1p/19q-codeleted tumors derived more benefit from adjuvant PCV chemotherapy compared with non-1p/19q-deleted tumors.[11][Level of evidence: 1iiA]

In contrast, the Radiation Therapy Oncology Group (RTOG) trial (RTOG-9402 [NCT00002569]) demonstrated no differences in median survival by treatment arm between an 8-week, intensive PCV chemotherapy regimen followed by immediate involved-field-plus-radiation therapy and radiation therapy alone.[12] However, in an unplanned subgroup analysis, patients with 1p/19q codeleted anaplastic oligodendroglioma and mixed anaplastic astrocytoma demonstrated a median survival of 14.7 years versus 7.3 years (HR, 0.59; 95% CI, 0.37–0.95; P = .03). For patients with noncodeleted tumors, there was no difference in median survival by treatment arm (2.6 vs. 2.7 years; HR, 0.85; 95% CI, 0.58–1.23; P = .39).[12][Level of evidence: 1iiA]

On the basis of these data, CODEL, a study that randomly assigned patients to radiation therapy alone (control arm), radiation therapy with temozolomide, and temozolomide alone (exploratory arm), was halted because radiation therapy alone was no longer considered adequate treatment in patients with anaplastic oligodendroglioma with 1p/19q codeletion.[13] A comparison between temozolomide and PCV chemotherapy in anaplastic oligodendroglioma has not been done, although in the setting of grade 3 anaplastic gliomas, no survival difference was seen between PCV chemotherapy and temozolomide.[2,14]

Patients with anaplastic oligodendrogliomas (WHO grade III) have a low cure rate with standard local treatment, but their prognoses are generally better than are the prognoses of patients with anaplastic astrocytomas. Since anaplastic oligodendrogliomas are uncommon, phase III randomized trials restricted to patients with them are not practical. Patients with these tumors are generally managed with the following:

- Postoperative radiation therapy (PORT) alone, with chemotherapy at progression.

- Postoperative chemotherapy with radiation at progression.

- PORT plus chemotherapy, even though the combination of radiation plus chemotherapy is not known to be superior in outcome to sequential modality therapy.

PORT alone has been compared with postoperative chemotherapy alone in patients with anaplastic gliomas (i.e., 144 astrocytomas, 91 oligoastrocytomas, and 39 oligodendrogliomas) with crossover to the other modality at the time of tumor progression. Of the 139 patients randomly assigned to radiation therapy, 135 were randomly assigned to chemotherapy with a 32-week course of either PCV or single-agent temozolomide (2:1:1 randomization). The order of the modalities did not affect TTF or OS.[2][Levels of evidence: 1iiA and 1iiD]. Neither TTF nor OS differed across the treatment arms.

These patients are appropriate candidates for clinical trials designed to improve local control by adding newer forms of treatment. Information about ongoing clinical trials is available from the NCI Web site.

Mixed Gliomas

Standard treatment options:

1. Surgery plus radiation therapy.

2. Surgery plus radiation therapy plus chemotherapy.

Patients with mixed glial tumors, which include oligoastrocytoma (WHO grade II) and anaplastic oligoastrocytoma (WHO grade III), have prognoses similar to that for astrocytic tumors of corresponding grades and are often treated as such.

Ependymal Tumors

Grade I and II ependymal tumors

Standard treatment options:

1. Surgery alone if the tumor is totally resectable.

2. Surgery followed by radiation therapy to known or suspected residual tumor.

Ependymomas (WHO grade II) and ependymal tumors (WHO grade I), i.e., subependymoma and myxopapillaryependymomas, are often curable.

Anaplastic ependymomas

Standard treatment options:

- Surgery plus radiation therapy.[15]

Patients with anaplastic ependymomas (WHO grade III) have variable prognoses that depend on the location and extent of disease. Frequently, but not invariably, patients with anaplastic ependymomas have worse prognoses than do those patients with lower-grade ependymal tumors.

Embryonal Cell Tumors: Medulloblastomas

Standard treatment options:

- Surgery plus craniospinal radiation therapy for good-risk patients.[16]

Treatment options under clinical evaluation:

- Surgery plus craniospinal radiation therapy and various chemotherapy regimens are being evaluated for poor-risk patients.[16]

Medulloblastoma occurs primarily in children, but it also occurs with some frequency in adults.[17] Other embryonal tumors are pediatric conditions. (Refer to the PDQ summary on Childhood Central Nervous System Embryonal Tumors Treatment at cdc.gov for more information.)

Pineal Parenchymal Tumors

Standard treatment options:

1. Surgery plus radiation therapy for pineocytoma.

2. Surgery plus radiation therapy and chemotherapy for pineoblastoma.

Pineocytoma (WHO grade II), pineoblastoma (WHO grade IV), and pineal parenchymal tumors of intermediate differentiation are diverse tumors that require special consideration. Pineocytomas are slow-growing tumors, and patients with them carry variable prognoses for cure. Pineoblastomas are more rapidly growing tumors, and patients with them have worse prognoses. Pineal parenchymal tumors of intermediate differentiation have unpredictable growth and clinical behavior.

Meningeal Tumors

Grade I meningiomas

Standard treatment options:

1. Active surveillance with deferred treatment, especially for incidentally discovered asymptomatic tumors.[18,19]

2. Surgery.

3. Stereotactic radiosurgery for tumors less than 3 cm.

4. Surgery plus radiation therapy is used in selected cases, such as for patients with known or suspected residual disease or with recurrence after previous surgery.

5. Fractionated radiation therapy for patients with unresectable tumors.[20]

WHO grade I meningiomas are usually curable when the mengiomas are resectable. With the increasing use of sensitive neuroimaging tools, there has been greater detection of asymptomatic low-grade meningiomas. The majority appear to show minimal growth and can often be safely observed while therapy is deferred until growth or the development of symptoms.[18,19]

Grade II and III meningiomas and hemangiopericytomas

Standard treatment options:

- Surgery plus radiation therapy.

The prognoses for patients with meningiomas (WHO grade II) (i.e., atypical, clear cell, and chordoid), meningiomas (WHO grade III) (i.e., anaplastic/malignant, rhabdoid, and papillary), and hemangiopericytomas are worse than are those for patients with low-grade meningiomas because complete resections are less commonly feasible, and the proliferative capacity is greater.

Germ Cell Tumors

The prognoses and treatment of patients with germ cell tumors—which include germinoma, embryonal carcinoma, choriocarcinoma, and teratoma—depend on tumor histology, tumor location, presence and amount of biological markers, and surgical resectability.

Tumors of the Sellar Region: Craniopharyngiomas

Standard treatment options:

1. Surgery alone if the tumor is totally resectable.

2. Debulking surgery plus radiation therapy if the tumor is unresectable.

Craniopharyngiomas (WHO grade I) are often curable.

Current Clinical Trials

Check for U.S. clinical trials from NCI's list of cancer clinical trials that are now accepting patients with adult brain tumor. The list of clinical trials can be further narrowed by location, drug, intervention, and other criteria.

References

1. Kaye AH, Walker DG: Low grade astrocytomas: controversies in management. J ClinNeurosci 7 (6): 475-83, 2000.

2. Wick W, Hartmann C, Engel C, et al.: NOA-04 randomized phase III trial of sequential radiochemotherapy of anaplastic glioma with procarbazine, lomustine, and vincristine or temozolomide. J ClinOncol 27 (35): 5874-80, 2009.

3. Stupp R, Mason WP, van den Bent MJ, et al.: Radiotherapy plus concomitant and adjuvant temozolomide for glioblastoma. N Engl J Med 352 (10): 987-96, 2005.

4. Stupp R, Hegi ME, Mason WP, et al.: Effects of radiotherapy with concomitant and adjuvant temozolomide versus radiotherapy alone on survival in glioblastoma in a randomised phase III study: 5-year analysis of the EORTC-NCIC trial. Lancet Oncol 10 (5): 459-66, 2009.

5. Hegi ME, Diserens AC, Gorlia T, et al.: MGMT gene silencing and benefit from temozolomide in glioblastoma. N Engl J Med 352 (10): 997-1003, 2005.

6. Gilbert MR, Wang M, Aldape KD, et al.: Dose-dense temozolomide for newly diagnosed glioblastoma: a randomized phase III clinical trial. J ClinOncol 31 (32): 4085-91, 2013.

7. Gilbert MR, Dignam JJ, Armstrong TS, et al.: A randomized trial of bevacizumab for newly diagnosed glioblastoma. N Engl J Med 370 (8): 699-708, 2014.

8. Chinot OL, Wick W, Mason W, et al.: Bevacizumab plus radiotherapy-temozolomide for newly diagnosed glioblastoma. N Engl J Med 370 (8): 709-22, 2014.

9. van den Bent MJ, Afra D, de Witte O, et al.: Long-term efficacy of early versus delayed radiotherapy for low-grade astrocytoma and oligodendroglioma in adults: the EORTC 22845 randomised trial. Lancet 366 (9490): 985-90, 2005.

10. van den Bent MJ, Chinot O, Boogerd W, et al.: Second-line chemotherapy with temozolomide in recurrent oligodendroglioma after PCV (procarbazine, lomustine and vincristine) chemotherapy: EORTC Brain Tumor Group phase II study 26972. Ann Oncol 14 (4): 599-602, 2003.

11. van den Bent MJ, Brandes AA, Taphoorn MJ, et al.: Adjuvant procarbazine, lomustine, and vincristine chemotherapy in newly diagnosed anaplastic oligodendroglioma: long-term follow-up of EORTC brain tumor group study 26951. J ClinOncol 31 (3): 344-50, 2013.

12. Cairncross G, Wang M, Shaw E, et al.: Phase III trial of chemoradiotherapy for anaplastic oligodendroglioma: long-term results of RTOG 9402. J ClinOncol 31 (3): 337-43, 2013.

13. Gilbert MR: Minding the Ps and Qs: perseverance and quality studies lead to major advances in patients with anaplastic oligodendroglioma. J ClinOncol 31 (3): 299-300, 2013.

14. Brada M, Stenning S, Gabe R, et al.: Temozolomide versus procarbazine, lomustine, and vincristine in recurrent high-grade glioma. J ClinOncol 28 (30): 4601-8, 2010.

15. Oya N, Shibamoto Y, Nagata Y, et al.: Postoperative radiotherapy for intracranial ependymoma: analysis of prognostic factors and patterns of failure. J Neurooncol 56 (1): 87-94, 2002.

16. Brandes AA, Franceschi E, Tosoni A, et al.: Long-term results of a prospective study on the treatment of medulloblastoma in adults. Cancer 110 (9): 2035-41, 2007.

17. Brandes AA, Ermani M, Amista P, et al.: The treatment of adults with medulloblastoma: a prospective study. Int J RadiatOncolBiolPhys 57 (3): 755-61, 2003.

18. Nakamura M, Roser F, Michel J, et al.: The natural history of incidental meningiomas. Neurosurgery 53 (1): 62-70; discussion 70-1, 2003.

19. Yano S, Kuratsu J; Kumamoto Brain Tumor Research Group: Indications for surgery in patients with asymptomatic meningiomas based on an extensive experience. J Neurosurg 105 (4): 538-43, 2006.

20. Debus J, Wuendrich M, Pirzkall A, et al.: High efficacy of fractionated stereotactic radiotherapy of large base-of-skull meningiomas: long-term results. J ClinOncol 19 (15): 3547-53, 2001.

Section 27.5

Recurrent Adult Brain Tumors

Text in this section is excerpted from "Adult Brain Tumors
Treatment (PDQ®)," National Cancer Institute at the National
Institutes of Health (NIH), February 25, 2015.

Surgery

Re-resection of recurrent brain tumors is used in some patients.
However, the majority of patients do not qualify because of a deteriorating condition or technically inoperable tumors. The evidence is
limited to non-controlled studies and case series on patients who are
healthy enough and have small enough tumors to technically debulk.
The impact of reoperation versus patient selection on survival is not
known.

Localized Chemotherapy

Carmustine wafers have been investigated in the setting of recurrent malignant gliomas, but the impact on survival is less clear than
at the time of initial diagnosis and resection. In a multicenter randomized, placebo-controlled trial, 222 patients with recurrent malignant
primary brain tumors requiring reoperation were randomly assigned to
receive implanted carmustine wafers or placebo biodegradable wafers.[1]
Approximately half of the patients had received prior systemic chemotherapy. The two treatment groups were well balanced at baseline. Median survival was 31 versus 23 weeks in the two groups. The
statistical significance between the two overall survival (OS) curves
depended upon the method of analysis. The hazard ratio (HR) for risk
of dying in the direct intention-to-treat comparison between the two
groups was 0.83 (95% confidence interval [CI], 0.63–1.10; P = .19).
The baseline characteristics were similar in the two groups, but the
investigators did an additional analysis, adjusting for prognostic factors, because they felt that even small differences in baseline characteristics could have a powerful influence on outcomes. In the adjusted
proportional hazards model, the HR for risk of death was 0.67 (95%

CI, 0.51–0.90, P = .006). The investigators put their emphasis on this latter analysis and reported this as a positive trial.[1][Level of evidence: 1iA] However, a Cochrane Collaboration systematic review of chemotherapeutic wafers for high-grade glioma focused on the unadjusted analysis and reported the same trial as negative.[2]

Systemic Chemotherapy

Bevacizumab

In 2009, the U.S. Food and Drug Administration (FDA) granted accelerated approval of bevacizumab monotherapy for patients with progressive glioblastoma. The indication was granted under the FDA's accelerated approval program that permits the use of certain surrogate endpoints or an effect on a clinical endpoint other than survival or irreversible morbidity as bases for approvals of products intended for serious or life-threatening illnesses or conditions. The approval was based on the demonstration of improved objective response rates observed in two historically controlled, single-arm, or non-comparative phase II trials.[3,4][Level of evidence: 3iiiDiv]

The FDA independently reviewed an open-label, multicenter, non-comparative phase II study that randomly assigned 167 recurrent glioblastoma multiforme (GBM) patients to receive bevacizumab alone or bevacizumab in combination with irinotecan,[3] although only efficacy data from the bevacizumab monotherapy arm (n = 85) were used to support drug approval. According to the FDA analysis of this study, tumor responses were observed in 26% of patients treated with bevacizumab alone, and the median duration of response in these patients was 4.2 months. On the basis of this externally controlled trial, the incidence of adverse events associated with bevacizumab did not appear to be significantly increased in GBM patients. The FDA independently assessed another single-arm, single-institution trial in which 56 recurrent glioblastoma patients were treated with bevacizumab alone.[4] Responses were observed in 20% of patients, and the median duration of response was 3.9 months.

Currently, however, no data are available from prospective, randomized controlled trials demonstrating improvement in health outcomes, such as disease-related symptoms or increased survival with the use of bevacizumab to treat glioblastoma. On the basis of these data and FDA approval, bevacizumab monotherapy has become standard therapy for recurrent glioblastoma.

Systemic chemotherapy

Systemic therapy (e.g., temozolomide, lomustine, or the combination of procarbazine, a nitrosourea, and vincristine in patients who have not previously received the drugs) has been used at the time of recurrence of primary malignant brain tumors. However, it has not been tested in controlled studies. Patient-selection factors likely play a strong role in determining outcomes, so the impact of therapy on survival is not clear.

Radiation Therapy

Because there are no randomized trials, the role of repeat radiation after disease progression or the development of radiation-induced cancers is also ill defined. Interpretation is difficult because the literature is limited to small retrospective case series.[5] The decision must be made carefully because of the risk of neurocognitive deficits and radiation necrosis.

Patients who have recurrent brain tumors are rarely curable and should be considered candidates for clinical trials when they have exhausted standard therapy. Information about ongoing clinical trials is available from the NCI Web site.

Current Clinical Trials

Check for U.S. clinical trials from NCI's list of cancer clinical trials that are now accepting patients with recurrent adult brain tumor. The list of clinical trials can be further narrowed by location, drug, intervention, and other criteria.

References

1. Brem H, Piantadosi S, Burger PC, et al.: Placebo-controlled trial of safety and efficacy of intraoperative controlled delivery by biodegradable polymers of chemotherapy for recurrent gliomas. The Polymer-brain Tumor Treatment Group. Lancet 345 (8956): 1008-12, 1995.

2. Hart MG, Grant R, Garside R, et al.: Chemotherapeutic wafers for high grade glioma. Cochrane Database Syst Rev (3): CD007294, 2008.

3. Friedman HS, Prados MD, Wen PY, et al.: Bevacizumab alone and in combination with irinotecan in recurrent glioblastoma. J ClinOncol 27 (28): 4733-40, 2009.

4. Kreisl TN, Kim L, Moore K, et al.: Phase II trial of single-agent bevacizumab followed by bevacizumab plus irinotecan at tumor progression in recurrent glioblastoma. J ClinOncol 27 (5): 740-5, 2009.

5. Paulino AC, Mai WY, Chintagumpala M, et al.: Radiation-induced malignant gliomas: is there a role for reirradiation? Int J RadiatOncolBiolPhys 71 (5): 1381-7, 2008.

Part Seven

Seizures

Chapter 28

Seizures and Epilepsy

Introduction

Few experiences match the drama of a convulsive seizure. A person having a severe seizure may cry out, fall to the floor unconscious, twitch or move uncontrollably, drool, or even lose bladder control. Within minutes, the attack is over, and the person regains consciousness but is exhausted and dazed. This is the image most people have when they hear the word epilepsy. However, this type of seizure—a generalized tonic-clonic seizure—is only one kind of epilepsy. There are many other kinds, each with a different set of symptoms.

Epilepsy was one of the first brain disorders to be described. It was mentioned in ancient Babylon more than 3,000 years ago. The strange behavior caused by some seizures has contributed through the ages to many superstitions and prejudices. The word epilepsy is derived from the Greek word for "attack." People once thought that those with epilepsy were being visited by demons or gods. However, in 400 B.C., the early physician Hippocrates suggested that epilepsy was a disorder of the brain—and we now know that he was right.

Text in this chapter is excerpted from "Seizures and Epilepsy: Hope through Research," National Institute of Neurological Disorders and Stroke (NINDS), February 13, 2015.

What is epilepsy?

Epilepsy is a brain disorder in which clusters of nerve cells, or neurons, in the brain sometimes signal abnormally. Neurons normally generate electrochemical impulses that act on other neurons, glands, and muscles to produce human thoughts, feelings, and actions. In epilepsy, the normal pattern of neuronal activity becomes disturbed, causing strange sensations, emotions, and behavior, or sometimes convulsions, muscle spasms, and loss of consciousness. During a seizure, neurons may fire as many as 500 times a second, much faster than normal. In some people, this happens only occasionally; for others, it may happen up to hundreds of times a day.

More than 2 million people in the United States—about 1 in 100—have experienced an unprovoked seizure or been diagnosed with epilepsy. For about 80 percent of those diagnosed with epilepsy, seizures can be controlled with modern medicines and surgical techniques. However, about 25 to 30 percent of people with epilepsy will continue to experience seizures even with the best available treatment. Doctors call this situation intractable epilepsy. Having a seizure does not necessarily mean that a person has epilepsy. Only when a person has had two or more seizures is he or she considered to have epilepsy.

Epilepsy is not contagious and is not caused by mental illness or mental retardation. Some people with mental retardation may experience seizures, but seizures do not necessarily mean the person has or will develop mental impairment. Many people with epilepsy have normal or above-average intelligence. Famous people who are known or rumored to have had epilepsy include the Russian writer Dostoyevsky, the philosopher Socrates, the military general Napoleon, and the inventor of dynamite, Alfred Nobel, who established the Nobel Prize. Several Olympic medalists and other athletes also have had epilepsy. Seizures sometimes do cause brain damage, particularly if they are severe. However, most seizures do not seem to have a detrimental effect on the brain. Any changes that do occur are usually subtle, and it is often unclear whether these changes are caused by the seizures themselves or by the underlying problem that caused the seizures.

While epilepsy cannot currently be cured, for some people it does eventually go away. One study found that children with idiopathic epilepsy, or epilepsy with an unknown cause, had a 68 to 92 percent chance of becoming seizure-free by 20 years after their diagnosis. The odds of becoming seizure-free are not as good for adults or for children with severe epilepsy syndromes, but it is nonetheless possible that seizures may decrease or even stop over time. This is more likely if the epilepsy has been well-controlled by medication or if the person has had epilepsy surgery.

What causes epilepsy?

Epilepsy is a disorder with many possible causes. Anything that disturbs the normal pattern of neuron activity—from illness to brain damage to abnormal brain development—can lead to seizures.

Epilepsy may develop because of an abnormality in brain wiring, an imbalance of nerve signaling chemicals called neurotransmitters, or some combination of these factors. Researchers believe that some people with epilepsy have an abnormally high level of excitatory neurotransmitters that increase neuronal activity, while others have an abnormally low level of inhibitory neurotransmitters that decrease neuronal activity in the brain. Either situation can result in too much neuronal activity and cause epilepsy. One of the most-studied neurotransmitters that plays a role in epilepsy is GABA, or gamma-aminobutyric acid, which is an inhibitory neurotransmitter. Research on GABA has led to drugs that alter the amount of this neurotransmitter in the brain or change how the brain responds to it. Researchers also are studying excitatory neurotransmitters such as glutamate.

In some cases, the brain's attempts to repair itself after a head injury, stroke, or other problem may inadvertently generate abnormal nerve connections that lead to epilepsy. Abnormalities in brain wiring that occur during brain development also may disturb neuronal activity and lead to epilepsy.

Research has shown that the cell membrane that surrounds each neuron plays an important role in epilepsy. Cell membranes are crucial for a neuron to generate electrical impulses. For this reason, researchers are studying details of the membrane structure, how molecules move in and out of membranes, and how the cell nourishes and repairs the membrane. A disruption in any of these processes may lead to epilepsy. Studies in animals have shown that, because the brain continually adapts to changes in stimuli, a small change in neuronal activity, if repeated, may eventually lead to full-blown epilepsy. Researchers are investigating whether this phenomenon, called kindling, may also occur in humans.

In some cases, epilepsy may result from changes in non-neuronal brain cells called glia. These cells regulate concentrations of chemicals in the brain that can affect neuronal signaling.

About half of all seizures have no known cause. However, in other cases, the seizures are clearly linked to infection, trauma, or other identifiable problems.

Genetic Factors

Research suggests that genetic abnormalities may be some of the most important factors contributing to epilepsy. Some types of epilepsy have been traced to an abnormality in a specific gene. Many other types of epilepsy tend to run in families, which suggests that genes influence epilepsy. Some researchers estimate that more than 500 genes could play a role in this disorder. However, it is increasingly clear that, for many forms of epilepsy, genetic abnormalities play only a partial role, perhaps by increasing a person's susceptibility to seizures that are triggered by an environmental factor.

Several types of epilepsy have now been linked to defective genes for ion channels, the "gates" that control the flow of ions in and out of cells and regulate neuron signaling. Another gene, which is missing in people with progressive myoclonus epilepsy, codes for a protein called cystatin B. This protein regulates enzymes that break down other proteins. Another gene, which is altered in a severe form of epilepsy called Lafora disease, has been linked to a gene that helps to break down carbohydrates.

While abnormal genes sometimes cause epilepsy, they also may influence the disorder in subtler ways. For example, one study showed that many people with epilepsy have an abnormally active version of a gene that increases resistance to drugs. This may help explain why anticonvulsant drugs do not work for some people. Genes also may control other aspects of the body's response to medications and each person's susceptibility to seizures, or seizure threshold. Abnormalities in the genes that control neuronal migration—a critical step in brain development—can lead to areas of misplaced or abnormally formed neurons, or dysplasia, in the brain that can cause epilepsy. In some cases, genes may contribute to development of epilepsy even in people with no family history of the disorder. These people may have a newly developed abnormality, or mutation, in an epilepsy-related gene.

Other Disorders

In many cases, epilepsy develops as a result of brain damage from other disorders. For example, brain tumors, alcoholism, and Alzheimer's disease frequently lead to epilepsy because they alter the normal workings of the brain. Strokes, heart attacks, and other conditions that deprive the brain of oxygen also can cause epilepsy in some cases. About 32 percent of all cases of newly developed epilepsy in elderly people appears to be due to cerebrovascular disease, which reduces the supply of oxygen to brain cells. Meningitis, AIDS, viral encephalitis, and other infectious diseases can lead to epilepsy, as can hydrocephalus—a condition in which excess fluid builds up in the brain. Epilepsy also can result from intolerance to wheat gluten (also known as celiac disease), or from a parasitic infection of the brain called neurocysticercosis. Seizures may stop once these disorders are treated successfully. However, the odds of becoming seizure-free after the primary disorder is treated are uncertain and vary depending on the type of disorder, the brain region that is affected, and how much brain damage occurred prior to treatment.

Epilepsy is associated with a variety of developmental and metabolic disorders, including cerebral palsy, neurofibromatosis, pyruvate dependency, tuberous sclerosis, Landau-Kleffner syndrome, and autism. Epilepsy is just one of a set of symptoms commonly found in people with these disorders.

Head Injury

In some cases, head injury can lead to seizures or epilepsy. Safety measures such as wearing seat belts in cars and using helmets when riding a motorcycle or playing competitive sports can protect people from epilepsy and other problems that result from head injury.

Prenatal injury and developmental problems

The developing brain is susceptible to many kinds of injury. Maternal infections, poor nutrition, and oxygen deficiencies are just some of the conditions that may take a toll on the brain of a developing baby. These conditions may lead to cerebral palsy, which often is associated with epilepsy, or they may cause epilepsy that is unrelated to any other disorders. About 20 percent of seizures in children are due to cerebral palsy or other neurological abnormalities. Abnormalities in genes that control development also may contribute to epilepsy. Advanced brain imaging has revealed that some cases of epilepsy that occur with no obvious cause may be associated with areas of dysplasia in the brain that probably develop before birth.

Poisoning

Seizures can result from exposure to lead, carbon monoxide, and many other poisons. They also can result from exposure to street drugs and from overdoses of antidepressants and other medications.

Seizures are often triggered by factors such as lack of sleep, alcohol consumption, stress, or hormonal changes associated with the menstrual cycle. These seizure triggers do not cause epilepsy but can provoke first seizures or cause breakthrough seizures in people who otherwise experience good seizure control with their medication. Sleep deprivation in particular is a universal and powerful trigger of seizures. For this reason, people with epilepsy should make sure to get enough sleep and should try to stay on a regular sleep schedule as much as possible. For some people, light flashing at a certain speed or the flicker of a computer monitor can trigger a seizure; this problem is called photosensitive epilepsy. Smoking cigarettes also can trigger seizures. The nicotine in cigarettes acts on receptors for the excitatory neurotransmitter acetylcholine in the brain, which increases neuronal firing. Seizures are not triggered by sexual activity except in very rare instances.

What are the different kinds of seizures?

Doctors have described more than 30 different types of seizures. Seizures are divided into two major categories—focal seizures and generalized seizures. However, there are many different types of seizures in each of these categories.

Focal Seizures

Focal seizures, also called partial seizures, occur in just one part of the brain. About 60 percent of people with epilepsy have focal seizures. These seizures are frequently described by the area of the brain in which they originate. For example, someone might be diagnosed with focal frontal lobe seizures.

In a simple focal seizure, the person will remain conscious but experience unusual feelings or sensations that can take many forms. The person may experience sudden and unexplainable feelings of joy, anger, sadness, or nausea. He or she also may hear, smell, taste, see, or feel things that are not real.

In a complex focal seizure, the person has a change in or loss of consciousness. His or her consciousness may be altered, producing a dreamlike experience. People having a complex focal seizure may display strange, repetitious behaviors such as blinks, twitches, mouth movements, or even walking in a circle. These repetitious movements are called automatisms. More complicated actions, which may seem purposeful, can also occur involuntarily. Patients may also continue activities they started before the seizure began, such as washing dishes in a repetitive, unproductive fashion. These seizures usually last just a few seconds.

Some people with focal seizures, especially complex focal seizures, may experience auras—unusual sensations that warn of an impending seizure. These auras are actually simple focal seizures in which the person maintains consciousness. The symptoms an individual person has, and the progression of those symptoms, tend to be stereotyped, or similar every time.

The symptoms of focal seizures can easily be confused with other disorders. For instance, the dreamlike perceptions associated with a complex focal seizure may be misdiagnosed as migraine headaches, which also may cause a dreamlike state. The strange behavior and sensations caused by focal seizures also can be mistaken for symptoms of narcolepsy, fainting, or even mental illness. It may take many tests and careful monitoring by an experienced physician to tell the difference between epilepsy and other disorders.

Generalized Seizures

Generalized seizures are a result of abnormal neuronal activity on both sides of the brain. These seizures may cause loss of consciousness, falls, or massive muscle spasms.

There are many kinds of generalized seizures. In absence seizures, the person may appear to be staring into space and/or have jerking or twitching muscles. These seizures are sometimes referred to as petit mal seizures, which is an older term. Tonic seizures cause stiffening of muscles of the body, generally those in the back, legs, and arms. Clonic seizures cause repeated jerking movements of muscles on both sides of the body. Myoclonic seizures cause jerks or twitches of the upper body, arms, or legs. Atonic seizures cause a loss of normal muscle tone. The affected person will fall down or may drop his or her head involuntarily. Tonic-clonic seizures cause a mixture of symptoms, including stiffening of the body and repeated jerks of the arms and/or legs as well as loss of consciousness. Tonic-clonic seizures are sometimes referred to by an older term: grand mal seizures.

Not all seizures can be easily defined as either focal or generalized. Some people have seizures that begin as focal seizures but then spread to the entire brain. Other people may have both types of seizures but with no clear pattern.

Society's lack of understanding about the many different types of seizures is one of the biggest problems for people with epilepsy. People who witness a non-convulsive seizure often find it difficult to understand that behavior which looks deliberate is not under the person's control. In some cases, this has led to the affected person being arrested or admitted to a psychiatric hospital. To combat these problems, people everywhere need to understand the many different types of seizures and how they may appear.

What are the different kinds of epilepsy?

Just as there are many different kinds of seizures, there are many different kinds of epilepsy. Doctors have identified hundreds of different epilepsy syndromes—disorders characterized by a specific set of symptoms that include epilepsy. Some of these syndromes appear to be hereditary. For other syndromes, the cause is unknown. Epilepsy syndromes are frequently described by their symptoms or by where in the brain they originate. People should discuss the implications of their type of epilepsy with their doctors to understand the full range of symptoms, the possible treatments, and the prognosis.

People with absence epilepsy have repeated absence seizures that cause momentary lapses of consciousness. These seizures almost always begin in childhood or adolescence, and they tend to run in families, suggesting that they may be at least partially due to a defective gene or genes. Some people with absence seizures have purposeless movements during their seizures, such as a jerking arm or rapidly blinking eyes. Others have no noticeable symptoms except for brief times when they are "out of it." Immediately after a seizure, the person can resume whatever he or she was doing. However, these seizures may occur so frequently that the person cannot concentrate in school or other situations. Childhood absence epilepsy usually stops when the child reaches puberty. Absence seizures usually have no lasting effect on intelligence or other brain functions.

Temporal lobe epilepsy, or TLE, is the most common epilepsy syndrome with focal seizures. These seizures are often associated with auras. TLE often begins in childhood. Research has shown that repeated temporal lobe seizures can cause a brain structure called the hippocampus to shrink over time. The hippocampus is important for memory and learning. While it may take years of temporal lobe seizures for measurable hippocampal damage to occur, this finding underlines the need to treat TLE early and as effectively as possible.

Neocortical epilepsy is characterized by seizures that originate from the brain's cortex, or outer layer. The seizures can be either focal or generalized. They may include strange sensations, visual hallucinations, emotional changes, muscle spasms, convulsions, and a variety of other symptoms, depending on where in the brain the seizures originate.

There are many other types of epilepsy, each with its own characteristic set of symptoms. Many of these, including Lennox-Gastaut syndrome and Rasmussen's encephalitis, begin in childhood. Children with Lennox-Gastaut syndrome have severe epilepsy with several different types of seizures, including atonic seizures, which cause sudden falls and are also called drop attacks. This severe form of epilepsy can be very difficult to treat effectively. Rasmussen's encephalitis is a progressive type of epilepsy in which half of the brain shows continual inflammation. It sometimes is treated with a radical surgical procedure called hemispherectomy (see the section on Surgery). Some childhood epilepsy syndromes, such as childhood absence epilepsy, tend to go into remission or stop entirely during adolescence, whereas other syndromes such as juvenile myoclonic epilepsy and Lennox-Gastaut syndrome are usually present for life once they develop. Seizure syndromes do not always appear in childhood, however.

Epilepsy syndromes that are easily treated, do not seem to impair cognitive functions or development, and usually stop spontaneously are often described as benign. Benign epilepsy syndromes include benign infantile encephalopathy and benign neonatal convulsions. Other syndromes, such as early myoclonic encephalopathy, include neurological and developmental problems. However, these problems may be caused by underlying neurodegenerative processes rather than by the seizures. Epilepsy syndromes in which the seizures and/or the person's cognitive abilities get worse over time are called progressive epilepsy.

Several types of epilepsy begin in infancy. The most common type of infantile epilepsy is infantile spasms, clusters of seizures that usually begin before the age of 6 months. During these seizures the infant may bend and cry out. Anticonvulsant drugs often do not work for infantile spasms, but the seizures can be treated with ACTH (adrenocorticotropic hormone) or prednisone.

When are seizures not epilepsy?

While any seizure is cause for concern, having a seizure does not by itself mean a person has epilepsy. First seizures, febrile seizures, nonepileptic events, and eclampsia are examples of seizures that may not be associated with epilepsy.

First Seizures

Many people have a single seizure at some point in their lives. Often these seizures occur in reaction to anesthesia or a strong drug, but they also may be unprovoked, meaning that they occur without any obvious triggering factor. Unless the person has suffered brain damage or there is a family history of epilepsy or other neurological abnormalities, these single seizures usually are not followed by additional seizures. One recent study that followed patients for an average of 8 years found that only 33 percent of people have a second seizure within 4 years after an initial seizure. People who did not have a second seizure within that time remained seizure-free for the rest of the study. For people who did have a second seizure, the risk of a third seizure was about 73 percent on average by the end of 4 years.

When someone has experienced a first seizure, the doctor will usually order an electroencephalogram, or EEG, to determine what type of seizure the person may have had and if there are any detectable abnormalities in the person's brain waves. The doctor also may order brain scans to identify abnormalities that may be visible in the brain. These tests may help the doctor decide whether or not to treat the person with antiepileptic drugs. In some cases, drug treatment after the first seizure may help prevent future seizures and epilepsy. However, the drugs also can cause detrimental side effects, so doctors prescribe them only when they feel the benefits outweigh the risks. Evidence suggests that it may be beneficial to begin anticonvulsant medication once a person has had a second seizure, as the chance of future seizures increases significantly after this occurs.

Febrile Seizures

Sometimes a child will have a seizure during the course of an illness with a high fever. These seizures are called febrile seizures (febrile is derived from the Latin word for "fever") and can be very alarming to the parents and other caregivers. In the past, doctors usually prescribed a course of anticonvulsant drugs following a febrile seizure in the hope of preventing epilepsy. However, most children who have a febrile seizure do not develop epilepsy, and long-term use of anticonvulsant drugs in children may damage the developing brain or cause other detrimental side effects. Experts at a 1980 consensus conference coordinated by the National Institutes of Health concluded that preventive treatment after a febrile seizure is generally not warranted unless certain other conditions are present: a family history of epilepsy, signs of nervous system impairment prior to the seizure, or a relatively prolonged or complicated seizure. The risk of subsequent non-febrile seizures is only 2 to 3 percent unless one of these factors is present.

Researchers have now identified several different genes that influence the risk of febrile seizures in certain families. Studying these genes may lead to new understanding of how febrile seizures occur and perhaps point to ways of preventing them.

Nonepileptic Events

Sometimes people appear to have seizures, even though their brains show no seizure activity. This type of phenomenon has various names, including nonepileptic events and pseudoseizures. Both of these terms essentially mean something that looks like a seizure but isn't one. Nonepileptic events that are psychological in origin may be referred to as psychogenic seizures. Psychogenic seizures may indicate dependence, a need for attention, avoidance of stressful situations, or specific psychiatric conditions. Some people with epilepsy have psychogenic seizures in addition to their epileptic seizures. Other people who have psychogenic seizures do not have epilepsy at all. Psychogenic seizures cannot be treated in the same way as epileptic seizures. Instead, they are often treated by mental health specialists.

Other nonepileptic events may be caused by narcolepsy, Tourette syndrome, cardiac arrhythmia, and other medical conditions with symptoms that resemble seizures. Because symptoms of these disorders can look very much like epileptic seizures, they are often mistaken for epilepsy. Distinguishing between true epileptic seizures and nonepileptic events can be very difficult and requires a thorough medical assessment, careful monitoring, and knowledgeable health professionals. Improvements in brain scanning and monitoring technology may improve diagnosis of nonepileptic events in the future.

Eclampsia

Eclampsia is a life-threatening condition that can develop in pregnant women. Its symptoms include sudden elevations of blood pressure and seizures. Pregnant women who develop unexpected seizures should be rushed to a hospital immediately. Eclampsia can be treated in a hospital setting and usually does not result in additional seizures or epilepsy once the pregnancy is over.

How is epilepsy diagnosed?

Doctors have developed a number of different tests to determine whether a person has epilepsy and, if so, what kind of seizures the person has. In some cases, people may have symptoms that look very much like a seizure but in fact are nonepileptic events caused by other disorders. Even doctors may not be able to tell the difference between these disorders and epilepsy without close observation and intensive testing.

EEG Monitoring

An EEG records brain waves detected by electrodes placed on the scalp. This is the most common diagnostic test for epilepsy and can detect abnormalities in the brain's electrical activity. People with epilepsy frequently have changes in their normal pattern of brain waves, even when they are not experiencing a seizure. While this type of test can be very useful in diagnosing epilepsy, it is not foolproof. Some people continue to show normal brain wave patterns even after they have experienced a seizure. In other cases, the unusual brain waves are generated deep in the brain where the EEG is unable to detect them. Many people who do not have epilepsy also show some unusual brain activity on an EEG. Whenever possible, an EEG should be performed within 24 hours of a patient's first seizure. Ideally, EEGs should be performed while the patient is sleeping as well as when he or she is awake, because brain activity during sleep is often quite different than at other times.

Video monitoring is often used in conjunction with EEG to determine the nature of a person's seizures. It also can be used in some cases to rule out other disorders such as cardiac arrhythmia or narcolepsy that may look like epilepsy.

Brain Scans

One of the most important ways of diagnosing epilepsy is through the use of brain scans. The most commonly used brain scans include CT (computed tomography), PET (positron emission tomography) and MRI (magnetic resonance imaging). CT and MRI scans reveal the structure of the brain, which can be useful for identifying brain tumors, cysts, and other structural abnormalities. PET and an adapted kind of MRI called functional MRI (fMRI) can be used to monitor the brain's activity and detect abnormalities in how it works. SPECT (single photon emission computed tomography) is a relatively new kind of brain scan that is sometimes used to locate seizure foci in the brain.

In some cases, doctors may use an experimental type of brain scan called a magnetoencephalogram, or MEG. MEG detects the magnetic signals generated by neurons to allow doctors to monitor brain activity at different points in the brain over time, revealing different brain functions. While MEG is similar in concept to EEG, it does not require electrodes and it can detect signals from deeper in the brain than an EEG. Doctors also are experimenting with brain scans called magnetic resonance spectroscopy (MRS) that can detect abnormalities in the brain's biochemical processes, and with near-infrared spectroscopy, a technique that can detect oxygen levels in brain tissue.

Medical History

Taking a detailed medical history, including symptoms and duration of the seizures, is still one of the best methods available to determine if a person has epilepsy and what kind of seizures he or she has. The doctor will ask questions about the seizures and any past illnesses or other symptoms a person may have had. Since people who have suffered a seizure often do not remember what happened, caregivers' accounts of the seizure are vital to this evaluation.

Blood Tests

Doctors often take blood samples for testing, particularly when they are examining a child. These blood samples are often screened for metabolic or genetic disorders that may be associated with the seizures. They also may be used to check for underlying problems such as infections, lead poisoning, anemia, and diabetes that may be causing or triggering the seizures.

Developmental, Neurological, and Behavioral Tests

Doctors often use tests devised to measure motor abilities, behavior, and intellectual capacity as a way to determine how the epilepsy is affecting that person. These tests also can provide clues about what kind of epilepsy the person has.

Can epilepsy be prevented?

Many cases of epilepsy can be prevented by wearing seatbelts and bicycle helmets, putting children in car seats, and other measures that prevent head injury and other trauma. Prescribing medication after first or second seizures or febrile seizures also may help prevent epilepsy in some cases. Good prenatal care, including treatment of high blood pressure and infections during pregnancy, can prevent brain damage in the developing baby that may lead to epilepsy and other neurological problems later. Treating cardiovascular disease, high blood pressure, infections, and other disorders that can affect the brain during adulthood and aging also may prevent many cases of epilepsy. Finally, identifying the genes for many neurological disorders can provide opportunities for genetic screening and prenatal diagnosis that may ultimately prevent many cases of epilepsy.

How can epilepsy be treated?

Accurate diagnosis of the type of epilepsy a person has is crucial for finding an effective treatment. There are many different ways to treat epilepsy. Currently available treatments can control seizures at least some of the time in about 80 percent of people with epilepsy. However, another 20 percent—about 600,000 people with epilepsy in the United States—have intractable seizures, and another 400,000 feel they get inadequate relief from available treatments. These statistics make it clear that improved treatments are desperately needed.

Doctors who treat epilepsy come from many different fields of medicine. They include neurologists, pediatricians, pediatric neurologists, internists, and family physicians, as well as neurosurgeons and doctors called epileptologists who specialize in treating epilepsy. People who need specialized or intensive care for epilepsy may be treated at large medical centers and neurology clinics at hospitals or by neurologists in private practice. Many epilepsy treatment centers are associated with university hospitals that perform research in addition to providing medical care.

Once epilepsy is diagnosed, it is important to begin treatment as soon as possible. Research suggests that medication and other treatments may be less successful in treating epilepsy once seizures and their consequences become established.

Medications

By far the most common approach to treating epilepsy is to prescribe antiepileptic drugs. The first effective antiepileptic drugs were bromides, introduced by an English physician named Sir Charles Locock in 1857. He noticed that bromides had a sedative effect and seemed to reduce seizures in some patients. More than 20 different antiepileptic drugs are now on the market, all with different benefits and side effects. The choice of which drug to prescribe, and at what dosage, depends on many different factors, including the type of seizures a person has, the person's lifestyle and age, how frequently the seizures occur, and, for a woman, the likelihood that she will become pregnant. People with epilepsy should follow their doctor's advice and share any concerns they may have regarding their medication.

Doctors seeing a patient with newly developed epilepsy often prescribe carbamazepine, valproate, lamotrigine, oxcarbazepine, or phenytoin first, unless the epilepsy is a type that is known to require a different kind of treatment. For absence seizures, ethosuximide is often the primary treatment. Other commonly prescribed drugs include clonazepam, phenobarbital, and primidone. Some relatively new epilepsy drugs include tiagabine, gabapentin, topiramate, levetiracetam, and felbamate. Other drugs are used in combination with one of the standard drugs or for intractable seizures that do not respond to other medications. A few drugs, such as fosphenytoin, are approved for use only in hospital settings to treat specific problems such as status epilepticus (see heading, "Are There Special Risks Associated With Epilepsy?"). For people with stereotyped recurrent severe seizures that can be easily recognized by the person's family, the drug diazepam is now available as a gel that can be administered rectally by a family member. This method of drug delivery may be able to stop prolonged or repeated seizures before they develop into status epilepticus.

For most people with epilepsy, seizures can be controlled with just one drug at the optimal dosage. Combining medications usually amplifies side effects such as fatigue and decreased appetite, so doctors usually prescribe monotherapy, or the use of just one drug, whenever possible. Combinations of drugs are sometimes prescribed if monotherapy fails to effectively control a patient's seizures.

The number of times a person needs to take medication each day is usually determined by the drug's half-life, or the time it takes for half the drug dose to be metabolized or broken down into other substances in the body. Some drugs, such as phenytoin and phenobarbital, only need to be taken once a day, while others such as valproate must be taken two or three times a day.

Most side effects of antiepileptic drugs are relatively minor, such as fatigue, dizziness, or weight gain. However, severe and life-threatening side effects such as allergic reactions can occur. Epilepsy medication also may predispose people to developing depression or psychoses. People with epilepsy should consult a doctor immediately if they develop any kind of rash while on medication, or if they find themselves depressed or otherwise unable to think in a rational manner. Other danger signs that should be discussed with a doctor immediately are extreme fatigue, staggering or other movement problems, and slurring of words. People with epilepsy should be aware that their epilepsy medication can interact with many other drugs in potentially harmful ways. For this reason, people with epilepsy should always tell doctors who treat them which medications they are taking. Women also should know that some antiepileptic drugs can interfere with the effectiveness of oral contraceptives, and they should discuss this possibility with their doctors.

Since people can become more sensitive to medications as they age, they may need to have their blood levels of medication checked occasionally to see if the dose needs to be adjusted. The effects of a particular medication also sometimes wear off over time, leading to an increase in seizures if the dose is not adjusted. People should know that some citrus fruit, in particular grapefruit juice, may interfere with breakdown of many drugs. This can cause too much of the drug to build up in their bodies, often worsening the side effects.

People taking epilepsy medication should be sure to check with their doctor and/or seek a second medical opinion if their medication does not appear to be working or if it causes unexpected side effects.

Tailoring the dosage of antiepileptic drugs

When a person starts a new epilepsy drug, it is important to tailor the dosage to achieve the best results. People's bodies react to medications in very different and sometimes unpredictable ways, so it may take some time to find the right drug at the right dose to provide optimal control of seizures while minimizing side effects. A drug that has no effect or very bad side effects at one dose may work very well at another dose. Doctors will usually prescribe a low dose of the new drug initially and monitor blood levels of the drug to determine when the best possible dose has been reached.

Generic versions are available for many antiepileptic drugs. The chemicals in generic drugs are exactly the same as in the brand-name drugs, but they may be absorbed or processed differently in the body because of the way they are prepared. Therefore, patients should always check with their doctors before switching to a generic version of their medication.

Discontinuing medication

Some doctors will advise people with epilepsy to discontinue their antiepileptic drugs after 2 years have passed without a seizure. Others feel it is better to wait for 4 to 5 years. Discontinuing medication should

always be done with a doctor's advice and supervision. It is very important to continue taking epilepsy medication for as long as the doctor prescribes it. People also should ask the doctor or pharmacist ahead of time what they should do if they miss a dose. Discontinuing medication without a doctor's advice is one of the major reasons people who have been seizure-free begin having new seizures. Seizures that result from suddenly stopping medication can be very serious and can lead to status epilepticus. Furthermore, there is some evidence that uncontrolled seizures trigger changes in neurons that can make it more difficult to treat the seizures in the future.

The chance that a person will eventually be able to discontinue medication varies depending on the person's age and his or her type of epilepsy. More than half of children who go into remission with medication can eventually stop their medication without having new seizures. One study showed that 68 percent of adults who had been seizure-free for 2 years before stopping medication were able to do so without having more seizures and 75 percent could successfully discontinue medication if they had been seizure-free for 3 years. However, the odds of successfully stopping medication are not as good for people with a family history of epilepsy, those who need multiple medications, those with focal seizures, and those who continue to have abnormal EEG results while on medication.

Surgery

When seizures cannot be adequately controlled by medications, doctors may recommend that the person be evaluated for surgery. Surgery for epilepsy is performed by teams of doctors at medical centers. To decide if a person may benefit from surgery, doctors consider the type or types of seizures he or she has. They also take into account the brain region involved and how important that region is for everyday behavior. Surgeons usually avoid operating in areas of the brain that are necessary for speech, language, hearing, or other important abilities. Doctors may perform tests such as a Wada test (administration of the drug amobarbital into the carotid artery) to find areas of the brain that control speech and memory. They often monitor the patient intensively prior to surgery in order to pinpoint the exact location in the brain where seizures begin. They also may use implanted electrodes to record brain activity from the surface of the brain. This yields better information than an external EEG.

A 1990 National Institutes of Health consensus conference on surgery for epilepsy concluded that there are three broad categories of epilepsy that can be treated successfully with surgery. These include focal seizures, seizures that begin as focal seizures before spreading to the rest of the brain, and unilateral multifocal epilepsy with infantile hemiplegia (such as Rasmussen's encephalitis). Doctors generally recommend surgery only after patients have tried two or three different medications without success, or if there is an identifiable brain lesion—a damaged or dysfunctional area—believed to cause the seizures.

A study published in 2000 compared surgery to an additional year of treatment with antiepileptic drugs in people with longstanding temporal lobe epilepsy. The results showed that 64 percent of patients receiving surgery became seizure-free, compared to 8 percent of those who continued with medication only. Because of this study and other evidence, the American Academy of Neurology (AAN) now recommends surgery for TLE when antiepileptic drugs are not effective. However, the study and the AAN guidelines do not provide guidance on how long seizures should occur, how severe they should be, or how many drugs should be tried before surgery is considered. A nationwide study is now underway to determine how soon surgery for TLE should be performed.

If a person is considered a good candidate for surgery and has seizures that cannot be controlled with available medication, experts generally agree that surgery should be performed as early as possible. It can be difficult for a person who has had years of seizures to fully re-adapt to a seizure-free life if the surgery is successful. The person may never have had an opportunity to develop independence, and he or she may have had difficulties with school and work that could have been avoided with earlier treatment. Surgery should always be performed with support from rehabilitation specialists and counselors who can help the person deal with the many psychological, social, and employment issues he or she may face.

While surgery can significantly reduce or even halt seizures for some people, it is important to remember that any kind of surgery carries some amount of risk (usually small). Surgery for epilepsy does not always successfully reduce seizures and it can result in cognitive or personality changes, even in people who are excellent candidates for surgery. Patients should ask their surgeon about his or her experience, success rates, and complication rates with the procedure they are considering.

Even when surgery completely ends a person's seizures, it is important to continue taking seizure medication for some time to give the brain time to re-adapt. Doctors generally recommend medication for 2 years after a successful operation to avoid new seizures.

Surgery to treat underlying conditions

In cases where seizures are caused by a brain tumor, hydrocephalus, or other conditions that can be treated with surgery, doctors may operate to treat these underlying conditions. In many cases, once the underlying condition is successfully treated, a person's seizures will disappear as well.

Surgery to remove a seizure focus

The most common type of surgery for epilepsy is removal of a seizure focus, or small area of the brain where seizures originate. This type of surgery, which doctors may refer to as a lobectomy or lesionectomy, is appropriate only for focal seizures that originate in just one area of the brain. In general, people have a better chance of becoming seizure-free after surgery if they have a small, well-defined seizure focus. Lobectomies have a 55–70 percent success rate when the type of epilepsy and the seizure focus is well-defined. The most common type of lobectomy is a temporal lobe resection, which is performed for people with temporal lobe epilepsy. Temporal lobe resection leads to a significant reduction or complete cessation of seizures about 70–90 percent of the time.

Multiple subpial transection

When seizures originate in part of the brain that cannot be removed, surgeons may perform a procedure called a multiple subpial transection. In this type of operation, which has been commonly performed since 1989, surgeons make a series of cuts that are designed to prevent seizures from spreading into other parts of the brain while leaving the person's normal abilities intact. About 70 percent of patients who undergo a multiple subpial transection have satisfactory improvement in seizure control.

Corpus callosotomy

Corpus callosotomy, or severing the network of neural connections between the right and left halves, or hemispheres, of the brain, is done primarily in children with severe seizures that start in one half of the brain and spread to the other side. Corpus callosotomy can end drop attacks and other generalized seizures. However, the procedure does not stop seizures in the side of the brain where they originate, and these focal seizures may even increase after surgery.

Hemispherectomy and hemispherotomy

These procedures remove half of the brain's cortex, or outer layer. They are used predominantly in children who have seizures that do not respond to medication because of damage that involves only half the brain, as occurs with conditions such as Rasmussen's encephalitis, Sturge-Weber syndrome, and hemimegalencephaly. While this type of surgery is very radical and is performed only as a last resort, children often recover very well from the procedure, and their seizures usually cease altogether. With intense rehabilitation, they often recover nearly normal abilities. Since the chance of a full recovery is best in young children, hemispherectomy should be performed as early in a child's life as possible. It is rarely performed in children older than 13.

Devices

The vagus nerve stimulator was approved by the U.S. Food and Drug Administration (FDA) in 1997 for use in people with seizures that are not well-controlled by medication. The vagus nerve stimulator is a battery-powered device that is surgically implanted under the skin of the chest, much like a pacemaker, and is attached to the vagus nerve in the lower neck. This device delivers short bursts of electrical energy to the brain via the vagus nerve. On average, this stimulation reduces seizures by about 20–40 percent. Patients usually cannot stop taking epilepsy medication because of the stimulator, but they often experience fewer seizures and they may be able to reduce the dose of their medication. Side effects of the vagus nerve stimulator are generally mild but may include hoarseness, ear pain, a sore throat, or nausea. Adjusting the amount of stimulation can usually eliminate most side effects, although the hoarseness typically persists. The batteries in the vagus nerve stimulator need to be replaced about once every 5 years; this requires a minor operation that can usually be performed as an outpatient procedure.

Several new devices may become available for epilepsy in the future. Researchers are studying whether transcranial magnetic stimulation (TMS), a procedure which uses a strong magnet held outside the head to influence brain activity, may reduce seizures. They also hope to develop implantable devices that can deliver drugs to specific parts of the brain.

Diet

Studies have shown that, in some cases, children may experience fewer seizures if they maintain a strict diet rich in fats and low in carbohydrates. This unusual diet, called the ketogenic diet, causes the body to break down fats instead of carbohydrates to survive. This condition is called ketosis. One study of 150 children whose seizures were poorly controlled by medication found that about one-fourth of the children had a 90 percent or better decrease in seizures with the ketogenic diet, and another half of the group had a 50 percent or better decrease in their seizures. Moreover, some children can discontinue the ketogenic diet after several years and remain seizure-free. The ketogenic diet is not easy to maintain, as it requires strict adherence to an unusual and limited range of foods. Possible side effects include retarded growth due to nutritional deficiency and a buildup of uric acid in the blood, which can lead to kidney stones. People who try the ketogenic diet should seek the guidance of a dietician to ensure that it does not lead to serious nutritional deficiency.

Researchers are not sure how ketosis inhibits seizures. One study showed that a byproduct of ketosis called beta-hydroxybutyrate (BHB) inhibits seizures in animals. If BHB also works in humans, researchers may eventually be able to develop drugs that mimic the seizure-inhibiting effects of the ketogenic diet.

Other Treatment Strategies

Researchers are studying whether biofeedback—a strategy in which individuals learn to control their own brain waves—may be useful in controlling seizures. However, this type of therapy is controversial and most studies have shown discouraging results. Taking large doses of vitamins generally does not help a person's seizures and may even be harmful in some cases. But a good diet and some vitamin supplements, particularly folic acid, may help reduce some birth defects and medication-related nutritional deficiencies. Use of non-vitamin supplements such as melatonin is controversial and can be risky. One study showed that melatonin may reduce seizures in some children, while another found that the risk of seizures increased measurably with melatonin. Most non-vitamin supplements such as those found in health food stores are not regulated by the FDA, so their true effects and their interactions with other drugs are largely unknown.

How does epilepsy affect daily life?

Most people with epilepsy lead outwardly normal lives. Approximately 80 percent can be significantly helped by modern therapies, and some may go months or years between seizures. However, the condition can and does affect daily life for people with epilepsy, their family, and their friends. People with severe seizures that resist treatment have, on average, a shorter life expectancy and an increased risk of cognitive impairment, particularly if the seizures developed in early childhood. These impairments may be related to the underlying conditions that cause epilepsy or to epilepsy treatment rather than the epilepsy itself.

Behavior and Emotions

It is not uncommon for people with epilepsy, especially children, to develop behavioral and emotional problems. Sometimes these problems are caused by embarrassment or frustration associated with epilepsy. Other problems may result from bullying, teasing, or avoidance in school and other social settings. In children, these problems can be minimized if parents encourage a positive outlook and independence, do not reward negative behavior with unusual amounts of attention, and try to stay attuned to their child's needs and feelings. Families must learn to accept and live with the seizures without blaming or resenting the affected person. Counseling services can help families cope with epilepsy in a positive manner. Epilepsy support groups also can help by providing a way for people with epilepsy and their family members to share their experiences, frustrations, and tips for coping with the disorder.

People with epilepsy have an increased risk of poor self-esteem, depression, and suicide. These problems may be a reaction to a lack of understanding or discomfort about epilepsy that may result in cruelty or avoidance by other people. Many people with epilepsy also live with an ever-present fear that they will have another seizure.

Driving and Recreation

For many people with epilepsy, the risk of seizures restricts their independence, in particular the ability to drive. Most states and the District of Columbia will not issue a driver's license to someone with epilepsy unless the person can document that they have gone a specific amount of time without a seizure (the waiting period varies from a few months to several years). Some states make exceptions for this policy when seizures don't impair consciousness, occur only during sleep, or have long auras or other warning signs that allow the person to avoid driving when a seizure is likely to occur. Studies show that the risk of having a seizure-related accident decreases as the length of time since the last seizure increases. One study found that the risk of having a seizure-related motor vehicle accident is 93 percent less in people who wait at least 1 year after their last seizure before driving, compared to people who wait for shorter intervals.

The risk of seizures also restricts people's recreational choices. For instance, people with epilepsy should not participate in sports such as skydiving or motor racing where a moment's inattention could lead to injury. Other activities, such as swimming and sailing, should be done only with precautions and/or supervision. However, jogging, football, and many other sports are reasonably safe for a person with epilepsy. Studies to date have not shown any increase in seizures due to sports, although these studies have not focused on any activity in particular. There is some evidence that regular exercise may even improve seizure control in some people. Sports are often such a positive factor in life that it is best for the person to participate, although the person with epilepsy and the coach or other leader should take appropriate safety precautions. It is important to take steps to avoid potential sports-related problems such as dehydration, overexertion, and hypoglycemia, as these problems can increase the risk of seizures.

Education and Employment

By law, people with epilepsy or other handicaps in the United States cannot be denied employment or access to any educational, recreational, or other activity because of their seizures. However, one survey showed that only about 56 percent of people with epilepsy finish high school and about 15 percent finish college—rates much lower than those for the general population. The same survey found that about 25 percent of working-age people with epilepsy are unemployed. These numbers indicate that significant barriers still exist for people with epilepsy in school and work. Restrictions on driving limit the employment opportunities for many people with epilepsy, and many find it difficult to face the misunderstandings and social pressures they encounter in public situations. Antiepileptic drugs also may cause side effects that interfere with concentration and memory. Children with epilepsy may need extra time to complete schoolwork, and they sometimes may need to have instructions or other information repeated for them. Teachers should be told what to do if a child in their classroom has a seizure, and parents should work with the school system to find reasonable ways to accommodate any special needs their child may have.

Pregnancy and Motherhood

Women with epilepsy are often concerned about whether they can become pregnant and have a healthy child. This is usually possible. While some seizure medications and some types of epilepsy may reduce a person's interest in sexual activity, most people with epilepsy can become pregnant. Moreover, women with epilepsy have a 90 percent or better chance of having a normal, healthy baby, and the risk of birth defects is only about 4 to 6 percent. The risk that children of parents with epilepsy will develop epilepsy themselves is only about 5 percent unless the parent has a clearly hereditary form of the disorder. Parents who are worried that their epilepsy may be hereditary may wish to consult a genetic counselor to determine what the risk might be. Amniocentesis and high-level ultrasound can be performed during pregnancy to ensure that the baby is developing normally, and a procedure called a maternal serum alpha-fetoprotein test can be used for prenatal diagnosis of many conditions if a problem is suspected.

There are several precautions women can take before and during pregnancy to reduce the risks associated with pregnancy and delivery. Women who are thinking about becoming pregnant should talk with their doctors to learn any special risks associated with their epilepsy and the medications they may be taking. Some seizure medications, particularly valproate, trimethadione, and phenytoin, are known to increase the risk of having a child with birth defects such as cleft palate, heart problems, or finger and toe defects. For this reason, a woman's doctor may advise switching to other medications during pregnancy. Whenever possible, a woman should allow her doctor enough time to properly change medications, including phasing in the new medications and checking to determine when blood levels are stabilized, before she tries to become pregnant. Women should also begin prenatal vitamin supplements—especially with folic acid, which may reduce the risk of some birth defects—well before pregnancy. Women who discover that they are pregnant but have not already spoken with their doctor about ways to reduce the risks should do so as soon as possible. However, they should continue taking seizure medication as prescribed until that time to avoid preventable seizures. Seizures during pregnancy can harm the developing baby or lead to miscarriage, particularly if the seizures are severe. Nevertheless, many women who have seizures during pregnancy have normal, healthy babies.

Women with epilepsy sometimes experience a change in their seizure frequency during pregnancy, even if they do not change medications. About 25 to 40 percent of women have an increase in their seizure frequency while they are pregnant, while other women may have fewer seizures during pregnancy. The frequency of seizures during pregnancy may be influenced by a variety of factors, including the woman's increased blood volume during pregnancy, which can dilute the effect of medication. Women should have their blood levels of seizure medications monitored closely during and after pregnancy, and the medication dosage should be adjusted accordingly.

Pregnant women with epilepsy should take prenatal vitamins and get plenty of sleep to avoid seizures caused by sleep deprivation. They also should take vitamin K supplements after 34 weeks of pregnancy to reduce the risk of a blood-clotting disorder in infants called neonatal coagulopathy that can result from fetal exposure to epilepsy medications. Finally, they should get good prenatal care, avoid tobacco, caffeine, alcohol, and illegal drugs, and try to avoid stress.

Labor and delivery usually proceed normally for women with epilepsy, although there is a slightly increased risk of hemorrhage, eclampsia, premature labor, and cesarean section. Doctors can administer antiepileptic drugs intravenously and monitor blood levels of anticonvulsant medication during labor to reduce the risk that the labor will trigger a seizure. Babies sometimes have symptoms of withdrawal from the mother's seizure medication after they are born, but these problems wear off in a few weeks or months and usually do not cause serious or long-term effects. A mother's blood levels of anticonvulsant medication should be checked frequently after delivery as medication often needs to be decreased.

Epilepsy medications need not influence a woman's decision about breast-feeding her baby. Only minor amounts of epilepsy medications are secreted in breast milk, usually not enough to harm the baby and much less than the baby was exposed to in the womb. On rare occasions, the baby may become excessively drowsy or feed poorly, and these problems should be closely monitored. However, experts believe the benefits of breast-feeding outweigh the risks except in rare circumstances.

To increase doctors' understanding of how different epilepsy medications affect pregnancy and the chances of having a healthy baby, Massachusetts General Hospital has begun a nationwide registry for women who take antiepileptic drugs while pregnant. Women who enroll in this program are given educational materials on pre-conception planning and perinatal care and are asked to provide information about the health of their children (this information is kept confidential). Women and physicians can contact this registry by calling 1-888-233-2334 or 617-726-1742 (fax: 617-724-8307).

Women with epilepsy should be aware that some epilepsy medications can interfere with the effectiveness of oral contraceptives. Women who wish to use oral contraceptives to prevent pregnancy should discuss this with their doctors, who may be able to prescribe a different kind of antiepileptic medication or suggest other ways of avoiding an unplanned pregnancy.

Are there special risks associated with epilepsy?

Although most people with epilepsy lead full, active lives, they are at special risk for two life-threatening conditions: status epilepticus and sudden unexplained death in epilepsy (SUDEP).

Status Epilepticus

Status epilepticus is a potentially life-threatening condition in which a person either has an abnormally prolonged seizure or does not fully regain consciousness between recurring seizures. Although there is no strict definition for the time at which a seizure turns into status epilepticus, most people agree that any seizure lasting longer than 5 minutes should, for practical purposes, be treated as though it was status epilepticus. There is some evidence that 5 minutes is sufficient to damage neurons and that seizures are unlikely to end on their own by that time.

Status epilepticus affects about 195,000 people each year in the United States and results in about 42,000 deaths. While people with epilepsy are at an increased risk for status epilepticus, about 75 percent of people who develop this condition have no previous seizure history. These cases often result from tumors, trauma, or other problems that affect the brain and may be life-threatening.

While most seizures do not require emergency medical treatment, someone with a prolonged seizure lasting more than 5 minutes may be in status epilepticus and should be taken to an emergency room immediately. It is important to treat a person with status epilepticus as soon as possible. (See also http://www.ninds.nih.gov/news_and_events/news_articles/RAMPART_results.htm)

The mortality rate of status epilepticus can be fairly high (about 20 percent), especially if treatment is not initiated quickly. One study showed that 80 percent of people in status epilepticus who received medication within 30 minutes of seizure onset eventually stopped having seizures, whereas only 40 percent recovered if 2 hours had passed before they received medication. Doctors in a hospital setting can treat status epilepticus with several different drugs and can undertake emergency life-saving measures, such as administering oxygen, if necessary. With optimal neurological care, adherence to a medication regimen, and a good prognosis (no known underlying uncontrolled brain or other organic disease) an individual in good health—even someone who has been diagnosed with epilepsy—can survive with minimal or no brain damage, and can decrease their risk of death, and even avoid these seizures in the future.

Status epilepticus can be divided into two categories: convulsive (in which outward signs of a seizure are observed) and nonconvulsive (which has no outward signs and is diagnosed by an abnormal EEG). Nonconvulsive status epilepticus may appear as a sustained episode of confusion or agitation in someone who does not ordinarily have that kind of mental impairment. While this type of episode may not seem as severe as convulsive status epilepticus, it should still be treated as an emergency.

Sudden Unexplained Death

For reasons that are poorly understood, people with epilepsy have an increased risk of dying suddenly for no discernible reason. This condition, called sudden unexplained death in epilepsy, can occur in people without epilepsy, but epilepsy increases the risk about two-fold. SUDEP can occur at any age. Researchers are still unsure why sudden unexplained death occurs; it may not be a direct result of a seizure. Recent research points to abnormal heart and respiratory function due to gene abnormalities. Not taking the prescribed dose of medication on a regular basis may increase the risk of SUDEP in individuals with epilepsy, especially those who are taking more than one medication for their epilepsy. One study suggested that use of more than two anticonvulsant drugs may be a risk factor. However, it is not clear whether the use of multiple drugs causes the sudden death, or whether people who use multiple anticonvulsants have a greater risk of death because they have more severe types of epilepsy.

What research is being done on epilepsy?

Scientists are studying the underlying causes of the epilepsies in children, adults and the elderly, as well as following brain trauma, stroke, and brain tumors.

Ongoing research is focused on developing new model systems that can be used to more quickly screen potential new treatments for the epilepsies. Scientists continue to study how neurotransmitters interact

487

with brain cells to control nerve firing and how non-neuronal cells in the brain contribute to seizures. New genetic information may allow doctors to prevent the epilepsies or to predict which treatments will be most beneficial to an individual with specific type(s) of the epilepsies. Researchers are continually improving MRI and other brain scans to assist in the diagnosis of the epilepsies and the ability to identify the source (focus) of the seizures in the brain.

Researchers funded by the National Institutes of Health have developed a flexible brain implant that could one day be used to treat seizures. In animal studies, the researchers used the device—a type of electrode array that conforms to the brain's surface—to take an unprecedented look at the brain activity underlying seizures. This research will help determine which individuals are candidates to undergo brain surgery as a treatment for epilepsy.

One new research initiative is focused on the identification of genes that may influence or cause the epilepsies.

Researchers are studying the cause(s) and risk factors that lead to sudden and unexpected death in individuals with epilepsy. Other scientists are investigating novel, innovative approaches to studying the epilepsies. Two new areas of research in the epilepsies include prevention of seizures (anti-epileptogenesis) and the role of inflammation in epilepsy. Researchers are exploring the causes of epilepsy in individuals with specific genetic disorders (Dravet Syndrome, Tuberous Sclerosis Complex, Rett Syndrome), as well as after traumatic brain injury, stroke, or a brain tumor in order to understand the underlying mechanisms that lead to seizures. This research will provide the opportunity to develop new therapies designed to prevent epilepsy from developing in those individuals who are at high risk.

Although little is known about the role of inflammation in the epilepsies, researchers are examining whether activation of the innate immune system and associated inflammatory reactions in the brain may mediate some of the molecular and structural changes occurring during and after seizure activity. Whether the immune response that takes place in the brain is beneficial or toxic is still an open and intriguing question that is being addressed.

Chapter 29

Febrile Seizures

What are febrile seizures?

Febrile seizures are convulsions brought on by a fever in infants or small children. During a febrile seizure, a child often loses consciousness and shakes, moving limbs on both sides of the body. Less commonly, the child becomes rigid or has twitches in only a portion of the body, such as an arm or a leg, or on the right or the left side only. Most febrile seizures last a minute or two, although some can be as brief as a few seconds while others last for more than 15 minutes.

The majority of children with febrile seizures have rectal temperatures greater than 102 degrees Fahrenheit. Most febrile seizures occur during the first day of a child's fever. Children prone to febrile seizures are not considered to have epilepsy, since epilepsy is characterized by recurrent seizures that are not triggered by fever.

How common are febrile seizures?

Approximately one in every 25 children will have at least one febrile seizure, and more than one-third of these children will have additional febrile seizures before they outgrow the tendency to have them. Febrile seizures usually occur in children between the ages of 6 months

---

Text in this chapter is excerpted from "Febrile Seizures Fact Sheet," National Institute of Neurological Disorders and Stroke (NINDS), February 23, 2015.

and 5 years and are particularly common in toddlers. Children rarely develop their first febrile seizure before the age of 6 months or after 3 years of age. The older a child is when the first febrile seizure occurs, the less likely that child is to have more.

What makes a child prone to recurrent febrile seizures?

A few factors appear to boost a child's risk of having recurrent febrile seizures, including young age (less than 15 months) during the first seizure, frequent fevers, and having immediate family members with a history of febrile seizures. If the seizure occurs soon after a fever has begun or when the temperature is relatively low, the risk of recurrence is higher. A long initial febrile seizure does not substantially boost the risk of recurrent febrile seizures, either brief or long.

Are febrile seizures harmful?

Although they can be frightening to parents, the vast majority of febrile seizures are short and harmless. During a seizure, there is a small chance that the child may be injured by falling or may choke from food or saliva in the mouth. Using proper first aid for seizures can help avoid these hazards (see heading "What should be done for a child having a febrile seizure?").

There is no evidence that short febrile seizures cause brain damage. Large studies have found that children with febrile seizures have normal school achievement and perform as well on intellectual tests as their siblings who don't have seizures. Even when seizures are very long (more than 1 hour), most children recover completely, but a few might be at risk of subsequent seizures without fever (epilepsy).

In other words, between 95 and 98 percent of children who experience febrile seizures do not go on to develop epilepsy. However, although the absolute risk remains small, some groups of children—including those with cerebral palsy, delayed development, or other neurological abnormalities—have an increased risk of developing epilepsy. The type of febrile seizure also matters; children who have prolonged febrile seizures (particularly lasting more than an hour) or seizures that affect only part of the body, or that recur within 24 hours, are at a somewhat higher risk. Among children who don't have any of these risk factors, only one in 100 develops epilepsy after a febrile seizure.

What should be done for a child having a febrile seizure?

Seizures are frightening, but it is important that parents and care-givers stay calm and carefully observe the child. To prevent accidental injury, the child should be placed on a protected surface such as the floor or ground. The child should not be held or restrained during a convulsion. To prevent choking, the child should be placed on his or her side or stomach. When possible, gently remove any objects from the child's mouth. Never place anything in the child's mouth during a convulsion. Objects placed in the mouth can be broken and obstruct the child's airway. Look at your watch when the seizure starts. If the seizure lasts 10 minutes, the child should be taken immediately to the nearest medical facility. Once the seizure has ended, the child should be taken to his or her doctor to check for the source of the fever. This is especially urgent if the child shows symptoms of stiff neck, extreme lethargy, or abundant vomiting.

How are febrile seizures diagnosed and treated?

Before diagnosing febrile seizures in infants and children, doctors sometimes perform tests to be sure that seizures are not caused by something other than simply the fever itself. For example, if a doctor suspects the child has meningitis (an infection of the membranes surrounding the brain), a spinal tap may be needed to check for signs of the infection in the cerebrospinal fluid (fluid that bathes the brain and spinal cord). If there has been severe diarrhea or vomiting, dehydration could be responsible for seizures. Also, doctors often perform other tests such as examining the blood and urine to pinpoint the cause of the child's fever.

A child who has a febrile seizure usually doesn't need to be hospitalized. If the seizure is prolonged or is accompanied by a serious infection, or if the source of the infection cannot be determined, a doctor may recommend that the child be hospitalized for observation.

How are febrile seizures prevented?

If a child has a fever most parents will use fever-lowering drugs such as acetaminophen or ibuprofen to make the child more comfort-able, although there are no studies that prove that this will reduce the risk of a seizure.

Prolonged daily use of oral anticonvulsants, such as phenobarbital or valproate, to prevent febrile seizures is usually not recommended because of their potential for side effects and questionable effectiveness for preventing such seizures.

Children especially prone to febrile seizures may be treated with the drug diazepam orally or rectally, whenever they have a fever. The majority of children with febrile seizures do not need to be treated with medication, but in some cases a doctor may decide that medicine given only while the child has a fever may be the best alternative. This medication may lower the risk of having another febrile seizure. It is usually well tolerated, although it occasionally can cause drowsiness, a lack of coordination, or hyperactivity. Children vary widely in their susceptibility to such side effects.

In addition, some children are prone to having very long (lasting an hour or more) febrile seizures. When a child has had a long febrile seizure, subsequent ones might also be long. Because very long febrile convulsions are associated with increased risk of developing epilepsy, some doctors will suggest the child be treated with a rectal form of the drug diazepam to stop the seizure and prevent it from becoming long. The parents of a child who had a very long febrile seizure may wish to consult their doctor about this possibility.

What research is being done on febrile seizures?

The National Institute of Neurological Disorders and Stroke (NINDS), a part of the National Institutes of Health (NIH), sponsors research on all forms of febrile seizures in medical centers throughout the country. NINDS-supported scientists are exploring environmental and genetic risk factors that may make children susceptible to febrile seizures. Scientists are also working to pinpoint factors that can help predict which children are likely to have recurrent or long-lasting febrile seizures.

Investigators continue to monitor the long-term impact that febrile seizures might have on intelligence, behavior, school achievement, and the development of epilepsy. For example, scientists conducting studies in animals are assessing the effects of febrile seizures, and especially very long seizures, on measures of intelligence and on the development of epilepsy. In particular they are trying to see if they can predict which children experiencing a very long febrile seizure might be at a higher risk for these problems, and how this risk can be lessened or prevented.

Investigators also continue to explore which drugs can effectively treat or prevent febrile seizures and to check for side effects of these medicines.

Chapter 30

Infantile Spasms

What is X-linked infantile spasm syndrome?

X-linked infantile spasm syndrome is a seizure disorder character-ized by a type of seizure known as infantile spasms. The spasms usually appear before the age of 1. Several types of spasms have been described, but the most commonly reported involves bending at the waist and neck with extension of the arms and legs (sometimes called a jackknife spasm). Each spasm lasts only seconds, but they occur in clusters sev-eral minutes long. Although individuals are not usually affected while they are sleeping, the spasms commonly occur just after awakening. Infantile spasms usually disappear by age 5, but many children then develop other types of seizures that recur throughout their lives.

Most babies with X-linked infantile spasm syndrome have charac-teristic results on an electroencephalogram (EEG), a test used to mea-sure the electrical activity of the brain. The EEG of these individuals typically shows an irregular pattern known as hypsarrhythmia, and this finding can help differentiate infantile spasms from other types of seizures.

Because of the recurrent seizures, babies with X-linked infantile spasm syndrome stop developing normally and begin to lose skills

---

This chapter includes excerpts from "X-linked Infantile Spasm Syndrome," Genetics Home Reference, March 10, 2015; and text from "Infantile Spasms Infor-mation Page," National Institutes of Neurological Disorders and Stroke (NINDS), February 13, 2015.

they have acquired (developmental regression), such as sitting, rolling over, and babbling. Subsequently, development in affected children is delayed. Most affected individuals also have intellectual disability throughout their lives.

How common is X-linked infantile spasm syndrome?

Infantile spasms are estimated to affect 1 to 1.6 in 100,000 individuals. This estimate includes X-linked infantile spasm syndrome as well as infantile spasms that have other causes.

What genes are related to X-linked infantile spasm syndrome?

X-linked infantile spasm syndrome is caused by mutations in either the ARX gene or the CDKL5 gene. The proteins produced from these genes play a role in the normal functioning of the brain. The ARX protein is involved in the regulation of other genes that contribute to brain development. The CDKL5 protein is thought to regulate the activity of at least one protein that is critical for normal brain function. Researchers are working to determine how mutations in either of these genes lead to seizures and intellectual disability.

Infantile spasms can have non-genetic causes, such as brain malformations, other disorders that affect brain function, or brain damage. In addition, changes in genes that are not located on the X chromosome cause infantile spasms in rare cases.

How do people inherit X-linked infantile spasm syndrome?

X-linked infantile spasm syndrome can have different inheritance patterns depending on the genetic cause.

When caused by mutations in the ARX gene, this condition is inherited in an X-linked recessive pattern. The ARX gene is located on the X chromosome, which is one of the two sex chromosomes. In males (who have only one X chromosome), one altered copy of the gene in each cell is sufficient to cause the condition. Usually in females (who have two X chromosomes), a mutation would have to occur in both copies of the gene to cause the disorder. However, in some instances, one altered copy of the ARX gene is sufficient because the X chromosome with the normal copy of the ARX gene is turned off through a process called X-inactivation. Early in embryonic development in females, one of the two X chromosomes is permanently inactivated in somatic cells (cells other than egg and sperm cells). X-inactivation ensures that females, like males, have only one active copy of the X chromosome in each body cell. Usually X-inactivation occurs randomly, such that each X chromosome is active in about half of the body cells. Sometimes X-inactivation is not random, and one X chromosome is active in more than half of cells. When X-inactivation does not occur randomly, it is called skewed X-inactivation. Some ARX gene mutations may be associated with skewed X-inactivation, which results in the inactivation of the X chromosome with the normal copy of the ARX gene in most cells of the body. This skewed X-inactivation causes the chromosome with the mutated ARX gene to be expressed in more than half of cells, causing X-linked infantile spasm syndrome.

When caused by mutations in the CDKL5 gene, this condition is thought to have an X-linked dominant inheritance pattern. The CDKL5 gene is also located on the X chromosome, making this condition X-linked. The inheritance is dominant because one copy of the altered gene in each cell is sufficient to cause the condition in both males and females.

X-linked infantile spasm syndrome caused by CDKL5 gene mutations usually occurs in individuals with no history of the disorder in their family. These mutations likely occur in early embryonic development (called de novo mutations). Because males have only one X chromosome, X-linked dominant disorders are often more severe in males than in females. Male fetuses with CDKL5-related X-linked infantile spasm syndrome may not survive to birth, so more females are diagnosed with the condition. In females, the distribution of active and inactive X chromosomes due to X-inactivation may affect whether a woman develops the condition or the severity of the signs and symptoms. Generally, the larger the proportion of active X chromosomes that contain the mutated CDKL5 gene, the more severe the signs and symptoms of the condition are.

A characteristic of X-linked inheritance is that fathers cannot pass X-linked traits to their sons.

Is there any treatment?

Treatment with corticosteroids such as prednisone is standard, although serious side effects can occur. Several newer antiepileptic medications, such as topiramate may ease some symptoms. Vigabatrin (Sabril©) has been approved by the U.S. Food and Drug Administration to treat infantile spasms in children ages one month to two years. Some children have spasms as the result of brain lesions, and surgical removal of these lesions may result in improvement.

What is the prognosis?

The prognosis for children with IS is dependent on the underlying causes of the seizures. The intellectual prognosis for children with IS is generally poor because many babies with IS have neurological impairment prior to the onset of spasms. Epileptic spasms usually reduce in number by mid-childhood, but more than half of the children with IS will develop other types of seizures. There appears to be a close relationship between IS and Lennox-Gastaut Syndrome, an epileptic disorder of later childhood.

Chapter 31

Lennox-Gastaut Syndrome

What is Lennox-Gastaut syndrome?

Lennox-Gastaut syndrome is a form of severe epilepsy that begins in childhood. It is characterized by multiple types of seizures and intellectual disability.

People with Lennox-Gastaut syndrome begin having frequent seizures in early childhood, usually between ages 3 and 5. More than three-quarters of affected individuals have tonic seizures, which cause the muscles to stiffen (contract) uncontrollably. These seizures occur most often during sleep. Also common are atypical absence seizures, which cause a partial or complete loss of consciousness. Additionally, many affected individuals have drop attacks, which are sudden episodes of weak muscle tone. Drop attacks can result in falls that cause serious or life-threatening injuries. Other types of seizures have been reported less frequently in people with Lennox-Gastaut syndrome.

Most of the seizures associated with Lennox-Gastaut syndrome are very brief. However, more than two-thirds of affected individuals experience at least one prolonged period of seizure activity known as nonconvulsive status epilepticus. These episodes can cause confusion and a loss of alertness lasting from hours to weeks.

This chapter includes excerpts from "Lennox-Gastaut Syndrome," Genetics Home Reference, March 10, 2015; and text from "Lennox-Gastaut Syndrome Information Page," National Institutes of Neurological Disorders and Stroke (NINDS), February 13, 2015.

Almost all children with Lennox-Gastaut syndrome develop learning problems and intellectual disability associated with their frequent seizures. Because the seizures associated with this condition are difficult to control with medication, the intellectual disability tends to worsen with time. Some affected children develop additional neurological abnormalities and behavioral problems. Many also have delayed development of motor skills such as sitting and crawling. As a result of their seizures and progressive intellectual disability, most people with Lennox-Gastaut syndrome require help with some or all of the usual activities of daily living. However, a small percentage of affected adults live independently.

People with Lennox-Gastaut syndrome have an increased risk of death compared to their peers of the same age. Although the increased risk is not fully understood, it is partly due to poorly controlled seizures and injuries from falls.

How common is Lennox-Gastaut syndrome?

Lennox-Gastaut syndrome affects an estimated 1 in 50,000 to 1 in 100,000 children. This condition accounts for about 4 percent of all cases of childhood epilepsy. For unknown reasons, it appears to be more common in males than in females.

What genes are related to Lennox-Gastaut syndrome?

Researchers have not identified any genes specific to Lennox-Gastaut syndrome, although the disorder likely has a genetic component. About two-thirds of cases are described as symptomatic, which means that they are related to an existing neurological problem. Symptomatic Lennox-Gastaut syndrome can be associated with brain injuries that occur before or during birth, problems with blood flow in the developing brain, brain infections, or other disorders affecting the nervous system. The condition can also result from a brain malformation known as cortical dysplasia or occur as part of a genetic disorder called tuberous sclerosis. Many people with Lennox-Gastaut syndrome have a history of recurrent seizures beginning in infancy (infantile spasms) or a related condition called West syndrome.

In about one-third of cases, the cause of Lennox-Gastaut syndrome is unknown. When the disorder occurs without an apparent underlying reason, it is described as cryptogenic. Individuals with cryptogenic Lennox-Gastaut syndrome have no history of epilepsy, neurological problems, or delayed development prior to the onset of the disorder.

How do people inherit Lennox-Gastaut syndrome?

Most cases of Lennox-Gastaut syndrome are sporadic, which means they occur in people with no history of the disorder in their family. However, 3 to 30 percent of people with this condition have a family history of some type of epilepsy. People with the cryptogenic form of Lennox-Gastaut syndrome are more likely than people with the symptomatic form to have a family history of epilepsy.

Is there any treatment?

Treatment for Lennox-Gastaut syndrome includes clobazam and anti-epileptic medications such as valproate, lamotrigine, felbamate, or topiramate. There is usually no single antiepileptic medication that will control seizures. Children who improve initially may later show tolerance to a drug or have uncontrollable seizures.

What is the prognosis?

The prognosis for individuals with Lennox-Gastaut syndrome varies. There is no cure for the disorder. Complete recovery, including freedom from seizures and normal development, is very unusual.

Part Eight

Other Brain Disorders

Chapter 32

Agnosia

Overview

Agnosia is characterized by an inability to recognize and identify objects and/or persons. Symptoms may vary, according to the area of the brain that is affected. It can be limited to one sensory modality such as vision or hearing; for example, a person may have difficulty in recognizing an object as a cup or identifying a sound as a cough. Agnosia can result from strokes, traumatic brain injury, dementia, a tumor, developmental disorders, overexposure to environmental toxins (e.g., carbon monoxide poisoning), or other neurological conditions. Visual agnosia may also occur in association with other underlying disorders. People with agnosia may retain their cognitive abilities in other areas. Treatment of primary agnosia is symptomatic and supportive; when it is caused by an underlying disorder, treatment of the disorder may reduce symptoms and help prevent further brain damage.

What are the signs and symptoms of agnosia?

People with primary visual agnosia may have one or several impairments in visual recognition without impairment of intelligence, motivation, and/or attention. Vision is almost always intact and the mind is clear. Some affected individuals do not have the ability to recognize

Text in this chapter is excerpted from "Agnosia," National Center for Advancing Translational Sciences at the National Institutes of Health (NIH), April 22, 2011.

familiar objects. They can see objects, but are unable to identify them by sight. However, objects may be identified by touch, sound, and/or smell. For example, affected individuals may not be able to identify a set of keys by sight, but can identify them upon holding them in their hands.

Some researchers separate visual agnosia into two broad categories: apperceptive agnosia and associative agnosia. Apperceptive agnosia refers to individuals who cannot properly process what they see, meaning they have difficult identifying shapes or differentiating between different objects (visual stimuli). Affected individuals may not be able to recognize that pictures of the same object from different angles are of the same object. Affected individuals may be unable to copy (e.g., draw a picture) of an object. Associative agnosia refers to people who cannot match an object with their memory. They can accurately describe an object and even draw a picture of the object, but are unable to state what the object is or is used for. However, if told verbally what the object is, an affected individual will be able to describe what it is used for.

In some cases, individuals with primary visual agnosia cannot identify familiar people (prosopagnosia). They can see the person clearly and can describe the person (e.g., hair and eye color), but cannot identify the person by name. People with prosopagnosia may identify people by touch, smell, speech, or the way that they walk (gait). In some rare cases, affected individuals cannot recognize their own face.

Some people have a form of primary visual agnosia associated with the loss of the ability to identify their surroundings (loss of environmental familiarity agnosia). Symptoms include the inability to recognize familiar places or buildings. Affected individuals may be able to describe a familiar environment from memory and point to it on a map.

Simultanagnosia is a characterized by the inability to read and the inability to view one's surroundings as a whole. The affected individual can see parts of the surrounding scene, but not the whole. There is an inability to comprehend more than one part of a visual scene at a time or to coordinate the parts.

In rare cases, people with primary visual agnosia may not be able to recognize or point to various parts of the body (autotopagnosia). Symptoms may also include loss of the ability to distinguish left from right.

What causes agnosia?

Primary visual agnosia occurs as a result of damage to the brain. Symptoms develop due to the inability to retrieve information from those damaged areas that are associated with visual memory. Lesions may occur as a result of traumatic brain injury, stroke, tumor, or over-exposure to dangerous environmental toxins (e.g., carbon monoxide poisoning). In some cases, the cause of the brain damage may not be known. Symptoms may vary, according to the area of the brain that is affected.

Visual agnosia may also occur in association with other underlying disorders (secondary visual agnosia) such as Alzheimer's disease, agenesis of the corpus callosum, MELAS, and other diseases that result in progressive dementia. Disorders that may precede the development of primary visual agnosia (and may be useful in identifying an underlying cause of some forms of this disorder) include Alzheimer's disease, Pick's disease, and a rare disorder called Balint's syndrome.

How might agnosia be diagnosed?

A variety of psychophysical tests can be conducted to pinpoint the nature of the visual process that is disrupted in an individual. Brain damage that causes visual agnosia may be identified through imaging techniques, including computed tomography (CT scan) and magnetic resonance imaging (MRI).

Chapter 33

Chiari Malformation

What are Chiari malformations?

Chiari malformations (CMs) are structural defects in the cerebellum, the part of the brain that controls balance. Normally the cerebellum and parts of the brain stem sit in an indented space at the lower rear of the skull, above the foramen magnum (a funnel-like opening to the spinal canal). When part of the cerebellum is located below the foramen magnum, it is called a Chiari malformation.

CMs may develop when the bony space is smaller than normal, causing the cerebellum and brain stem to be pushed downward into the foramen magnum and into the upper spinal canal. The resulting pressure on the cerebellum and brain stem may affect functions controlled by these areas and block the flow of cerebrospinal fluid (CSF)—the clear liquid that surrounds and cushions the brain and spinal cord—to and from the brain.

What causes these malformations?

CM has several different causes. It can be caused by structural defects in the brain and spinal cord that occur during fetal development, whether caused by genetic mutations or lack of proper vitamins or nutrients in the maternal diet. This is called primary or congenital

Text in this chapter is excerpted from "Chiari Malformation Fact Sheet," National Institute of Neurological Disorders and Stroke (NINDS), December 10, 2014.

CM. It can also be caused later in life if spinal fluid is drained excessively from the lumbar or thoracic areas of the spine either due to injury, exposure to harmful substances, or infection. This is called acquired or secondary CM. Primary CM is much more common than secondary CM.

How are they classified?

CMs are classified by the severity of the disorder and the parts of the brain that protrude into the spinal canal.

Type I involves the extension of the cerebellar tonsils (the lower part of the cerebellum) into the foramen magnum, without involving the brain stem. Normally, only the spinal cord passes through this opening. Type I—which may not cause symptoms—is the most common form of CM and is usually first noticed in adolescence or adulthood, often by accident during an examination for another condition. Type I is the only type of CM that can be acquired.

Type II, also called classic CM, involves the extension of both cerebellar and brain stem tissue into the foramen magnum. Also, the cerebellar vermis (the nerve tissue that connects the two halves of the cerebellum) may be only partially complete or absent. Type II is usually accompanied by a myelomeningocele—a form of spina bifida that occurs when the spinal canal and backbone do not close before birth, causing the spinal cord and its protective membrane to protrude through a sac-like opening in the back. A myelomeningocele usually results in partial or complete paralysis of the area below the spinal opening. The term Arnold-Chiari malformation (named after two pioneering researchers) is specific to Type II malformations.

Type III is the most serious form of CM. The cerebellum and brain stem protrude, or herniate, through the foramen magnum and into the spinal cord. Part of the brain's fourth ventricle, a cavity that connects with the upper parts of the brain and circulates CSF, may also protrude through the hole and into the spinal cord. In rare instances, the herniated cerebellar tissue can enter an occipital encephalocele, a pouch-like structure that protrudes out of the back of the head or the neck and contains brain matter. The covering of the brain or spinal cord can also protrude through an abnormal opening in the back or skull. Type III causes severe neurological defects.

Type IV involves an incomplete or underdeveloped cerebellum—a condition known as cerebellar hypoplasia. In this rare form of CM, the cerebellar tonsils are located in a normal position but parts of the cerebellum are missing, and portions of the skull and spinal cord may be visible.

Another form of the disorder, under debate by some scientists, is Type 0, in which there is no protrusion of the cerebellum through the foramen magnum but headache and other symptoms of CM are present.

What are the symptoms of a Chiari malformation?

Individuals with CM may complain of neck pain, balance problems, muscle weakness, numbness or other abnormal feelings in the arms or legs, dizziness, vision problems, difficulty swallowing, ringing or buzzing in the ears, hearing loss, vomiting, insomnia, depression, or headache made worse by coughing or straining. Hand coordination and fine motor skills may be affected. Symptoms may change for some individuals, depending on the buildup of CSF and resulting pressure on the tissues and nerves. Persons with a Type I CM may not have symptoms. Adolescents and adults who have CM but no symptoms initially may, later in life, develop signs of the disorder. Infants may have symptoms from any type of CM and may have difficulty swallowing, irritability when being fed, excessive drooling, a weak cry, gagging or vomiting, arm weakness, a stiff neck, breathing problems, developmental delays, and an inability to gain weight.

Are other conditions associated with Chiari malformations?

Individuals who have a CM often have these related conditions:

Hydrocephalus is an excessive buildup of CSF in the brain. A CM can block the normal flow of this fluid, resulting in pressure within the head that can cause mental defects and/or an enlarged or misshapen skull. Severe hydrocephalus, if left untreated, can be fatal. The disorder can occur with any type of CM, but is most commonly associated with Type II.

Spina bifida is the incomplete development of the spinal cord and/ or its protective covering. The bones around the spinal cord don't form properly, leaving part of the cord exposed and resulting in partial or complete paralysis. Individuals with Type II CM usually have a myelomeningocele, a form of spina bifida in which the bones in the back and lower spine don't form properly and extend out of the back in a sac-like opening.

Syringomyelia, or hydromyelia, is a disorder in which a CSF-filled tubular cyst, or syrinx, forms within the spinal cord's central canal.

The growing syrinx destroys the center of the spinal cord, resulting in pain, weakness, and stiffness in the back, shoulders, arms, or legs. Other symptoms may include headaches and a loss of the ability to feel extremes of hot or cold, especially in the hands. Some individuals also have severe arm and neck pain.

Tethered cord syndrome occurs when the spinal cord attaches itself to the bony spine. This progressive disorder causes abnormal stretching of the spinal cord and can result in permanent damage to the muscles and nerves in the lower body and legs. Children who have a myelomeningocele have an increased risk of developing a tethered cord later in life.

Spinal curvature is common among individuals with syringomyelia or CM Type I. Two types of spinal curvature can occur in conjunction with CMs: scoliosis, a bending of the spine to the left or right; and kyphosis, a forward bending of the spine. Spinal curvature is seen most often in children with CM, whose skeleton has not fully matured.

CMs may also be associated with certain hereditary syndromes that affect neurological and skeletal abnormalities, other disorders that affect bone formation and growth, fusion of segments of the bones in the neck, and extra folds in the brain.

How common are Chiari malformations?

In the past, it was estimated that the condition occurs in about one in every 1,000 births. However, the increased use of diagnostic imaging has shown that CM may be much more common. Complicating this estimation is the fact that some children who are born with the condition may not show symptoms until adolescence or adulthood, if at all. CMs occur more often in women than in men and Type II malformations are more prevalent in certain groups, including people of Celtic descent.

How are Chiari malformations diagnosed?

Many people with CMs have no symptoms and their malformations are discovered only during the course of diagnosis or treatment for another disorder. The doctor will perform a physical exam and check the person's memory, cognition, balance (a function controlled by the cerebellum), touch, reflexes, sensation, and motor skills (functions controlled by the spinal cord). The physician may also order one of the following diagnostic tests:

An *X-ray* uses electromagnetic energy to produce images of bones and certain tissues on film. An X-ray of the head and neck cannot reveal a CM but can identify bone abnormalities that are often associated with CM. This safe and painless procedure can be done in a doctor's office and takes only a few minutes.

Computed tomography (also called a CT scan) uses X-rays and a computer to produce two-dimensional pictures of bone and vascular irregularities, certain brain tumors and cysts, brain damage from head injury, and other disorders. Scanning takes about 3 to 5 minutes. This painless, noninvasive procedure is done at an imaging center or hospital on an outpatient basis and can identify hydrocephalus and bone abnormalities associated with CM.

Magnetic resonance imaging (MRI) is the imaging procedure most often used to diagnose a CM. Like CT, it is painless and noninvasive and is performed at an imaging center or hospital. MRI uses radio waves and a powerful magnetic field to produce either a detailed three-dimensional picture or a two-dimensional "slice" of body structures, including tissues, organs, bones, and nerves. Depending on the part(s) of the body to be scanned, MRI can take up to an hour to complete.

How are they treated?

Some CMs are asymptomatic and do not interfere with a person's activities of daily living. In other cases, medications may ease certain symptoms, such as pain.

Surgery is the only treatment available to correct functional disturbances or halt the progression of damage to the central nervous system. Most individuals who have surgery see a reduction in their symptoms and/or prolonged periods of relative stability. More than one surgery may be needed to treat the condition.

Posterior fossa decompression surgery is performed on adults with CM to create more space for the cerebellum and to relieve pressure on the spinal column. Surgery involves making an incision at the back of the head and removing a small portion of the bottom of the skull (and sometimes part of the spinal column) to correct the irregular bony structure. The neurosurgeon may use a procedure called electrocautery to shrink the cerebellar tonsils. This surgical technique involves destroying tissue with high-frequency electrical currents.

A related procedure, called a spinal laminectomy, involves the surgical removal of part of the arched, bony roof of the spinal canal (the lamina) to increase the size of the spinal canal and relieve pressure on the spinal cord and nerve roots.

The surgeon may also make an incision in the dura (the covering of the brain) to examine the brain and spinal cord. Additional tissue may be added to the dura to create more space for the flow of CSF.

Infants and children with myelomeningocele may require surgery to reposition the spinal cord and close the opening in the back.

Hydrocephalus may be treated with a shunt system that drains excess fluid and relieves pressure inside the head. A sturdy tube that is surgically inserted into the head is connected to a flexible tube that is placed under the skin, where it can drain the excess fluid into either the chest wall or the abdomen so it can be absorbed by the body. An alternative surgical treatment to relieve hydrocephalus is third ventriculostomy, a procedure that improves the flow of CSF. A small perforation is made in the floor of the third ventricle and the CSF is diverted into the subarachnoid space to relieve pressure.

Similarly, surgeons may open the spinal cord and insert a shunt to drain a syringomyelia or hydromyelia. A small tube or catheter may be inserted into the syrinx for continued drainage.

What research is being done?

Within the Federal government, the National Institute of Neurological Disorders and Stroke (NINDS), a component of the National Institutes of Health (NIH), supports and conducts research on brain and nervous system disorders, including Chiari malformations. The NINDS conducts research in its laboratories at the NIH, in Bethesda, Maryland, and supports research through grants to major medical research institutions across the country.

In one study, NINDS scientists are trying to better understand the genetic factors responsible for the malformation by examining individuals with CM who have a family member with either a CM or syringomyelia.

NINDS scientists are examining individuals who either have syringomyelia or are at risk of developing the disorder, including patients with Chiari I malformation. By recording more than 5 years of symptoms, muscle strength, general level of functioning, and MRI scan findings from individuals who receive standard treatment for syringomyelia, researchers can obtain more information about factors that influence its development, progression, and relief of symptoms. Study results may allow scientists to provide more accurate recommendations to future patients with syringomyelia regarding optimal surgical or non-surgical treatment of their condition.

AN NIH study is reviewing an alternative surgical treatment for syringomyelia. By examining people with syringomyelia, in which there is an obstruction in CSF flow, NIH scientists hope to learn whether a surgical procedure that relieves the obstruction in CSF flow can correct the problem without having to cut into the spinal cord itself. The NIH's Management of Myelomeningocele Study is comparing prenatal surgery to the conventional post-birth approach of closing the opening in the spine and back that is common to some forms of CM. The study will enroll 200 women whose fetuses have spina bifida and will compare the safety and efficacy of the different surgeries. Preliminary clinical evidence of intrauterine closure of the myelomeningocele suggests the procedure reduces the incidence of shunt dependent hydrocephalus and restores the cerebellum and brain stem to more normal configuration. At 1 year and 2½ years after surgery the children will be tested for motor function, developmental progress, and bladder, kidney, and brain development.

Chapter 34

Facts about Encephalocele

Encephalocele is a rare type of neural tube defect (NTD) present at birth that affects the brain. The neural tube is a narrow channel that folds and closes during the third and fouth weeks of pregnancy to form the brain and spinal cord. Encephalocele is described as a sac-like protrusion or projection of the brain and the membranes that cover it through an opening in the skull. Encephalocele happens when the neural tube does not close completely during pregnancy. The result is an opening in the midline of the upper part of the skull, the area between the forehead and nose, or the back of the skull.

Usually encephaloceles are found right after birth, but sometimes a small encephalocele in the nose and forehead region can go undetected.

What We Know About Encephalocele

How often does encephalocele occur?

CDC estimates that each year about 375 babies in the United States are born with encephalocele. In other words, about 1 out of every 10,000 babies born in the United States each year will have encephalocele.

Text in this chapter is excerpted from "Facts about Encephalocele," Centers for Disease Control and Prevention (CDC), October 20, 2014.

What problems do children with encephalocele have?

When located in the back of the skull, encephalocele often is linked to nervous system problems. Encephalocele usually is seen with other brain and face defects.

Signs of encephalocele can include:

- Buildup of too much fluid in the brain
- Complete loss of strength in the arms and legs
- An unusually small head
- Uncoordinated movement of the voluntary muscles, such as those involved in walking and reaching
- Developmental delay
- Vision problems
- Mental and growth retardation
- Seizures

What We Still Do Not Know About Encephalocele

What causes encephalocele?

Although the exact cause of encephalocele is unknown, scientists believe that many factors are involved.

There is a genetic component to the condition, meaning it often occurs among families with a history of spina bifida and anencephaly. Some researchers also believe that certain environmental exposures before or during pregnancy might be causes, but more research is needed. We at CDC work with many other researchers to study risk factors that can increase the chance of having a baby with encephalocele, as well as outcomes of babies with encephalocele.

Following is an example of what our research has found:

- Several factors appear to lead to lower survival rates for infants with encephalocele, including preterm birth, low birthweight, having multiple birth defects, and being Black or African American.

Can encephalocele be prevented?

Currently, there is no known way to prevent encephalocele, although steps can be taken to lower the risk. Recent studies have shown that the addition of a B vitamin called folic acid to the diet of women who might become pregnant can greatly reduce the number of babies born with NTDs. CDC has recommended that all women of childbearing age consume 400 micrograms of folic acid daily. A single daily serving of most multivitamins and fortified cereals contain 400 micrograms of folic acid.

In addition, mothers can take steps before and during pregnancy to be healthy, including not smoking and not drinking alcohol during pregnancy.

Chapter 35

Headache

Introduction

You're sitting at your desk, working on a difficult task, when it suddenly feels as if a belt or vice is being tightened around the top of your head. Or you have periodic headaches that occur with nausea and increased sensitivity to light or sound. Maybe you are involved in a routine, non-stressful task when you're struck by head or neck pain.

Sound familiar? If so, you've suffered one of the many types of headache that can occur on its own or as part of another disease or health condition.

Anyone can experience a headache. Nearly 2 out of 3 children will have a headache by age 15. More than 9 in 10 adults will experience a headache sometime in their life. Headache is our most common form of pain and a major reason cited for days missed at work or school as well as visits to the doctor. Without proper treatment, headaches can be severe and interfere with daily activities.

Certain types of headache run in families. Episodes of headache may ease or even disappear for a time and recur later in life. It's possible to have more than one type of headache at the same time.

Primary headaches occur independently and are not caused by another medical condition. It's uncertain what sets the process of a

---

Text in this chapter is excerpted from "Headache: Hope through Research," National Institute of Neurological Disorders and Stroke (NINDS), February 23, 2015.

primary headache in motion. A cascade of events that affect blood vessels and nerves inside and outside the head causes pain signals to be sent to the brain. Brain chemicals called neurotransmitters are involved in creating head pain, as are changes in nerve cell activity (called cortical spreading depression). Migraine, cluster, and tension-type headache are the more familiar types of primary headache.

Secondary headaches are symptoms of another health disorder that causes pain-sensitive nerve endings to be pressed on or pulled or pushed out of place. They may result from underlying conditions including fever, infection, medication overuse, stress or emotional conflict, high blood pressure, psychiatric disorders, head injury or trauma, stroke, tumors, and nerve disorders (particularly trigeminal neuralgia, a chronic pain condition that typically affects a major nerve on one side of the jaw or cheek).

Headaches can range in frequency and severity of pain. Some individuals may experience headaches once or twice a year, while others may experience headaches more than 15 days a month. Some headaches may recur or last for weeks at a time. Pain can range from mild to disabling and may be accompanied by symptoms such as nausea or increased sensitivity to noise or light, depending on the type of headache.

Why Headaches Hurt

Information about touch, pain, temperature, and vibration in the head and neck is sent to the brain by the trigeminal nerve, one of 12 pairs of cranial nerves that start at the base of the brain.

The nerve has three branches that conduct sensations from the scalp, the blood vessels inside and outside of the skull, the lining around the brain (the meninges), and the face, mouth, neck, ears, eyes, and throat.

Brain tissue itself lacks pain-sensitive nerves and does not feel pain. Headaches occur when pain-sensitive nerve endings called nociceptors react to headache triggers (such as stress, certain foods or odors, or use of medicines) and send messages through the trigeminal nerve to the thalamus, the brain's "relay station" for pain sensation from all over the body. The thalamus controls the body's sensitivity to light and noise and sends messages to parts of the brain that manage awareness of pain and emotional response to it. Other parts of the brain may also be part of the process, causing nausea, vomiting, diarrhea, trouble concentrating, and other neurological symptoms.

When to See a Doctor

Not all headaches require a physician's attention. But headaches can signal a more serious disorder that requires prompt medical care. Immediately call or see a physician if you or someone you're with experience any of these symptoms:

- Sudden, severe headache that may be accompanied by a stiff neck.

- Severe headache accompanied by fever, nausea, or vomiting that is not related to another illness.

- "First" or "worst" headache, often accompanied by confusion, weakness, double vision, or loss of consciousness.

- Headache that worsens over days or weeks or has changed in pattern or behavior.

- Recurring headache in children.

- Headache following a head injury.

- Headache and a loss of sensation or weakness in any part of the body, which could be a sign of a stroke.

- Headache associated with convulsions.

- Headache associated with shortness of breath.

- Two or more headaches a week.

- Persistent headache in someone who has been previously headache-free, particularly in someone over age 50.

- New headaches in someone with a history of cancer or HIV/AIDS.

Diagnosing Your Headache

How and under what circumstances a person experiences a headache can be key to diagnosing its cause. Keeping a headache journal can help a physician better diagnose your type of headache and determine the best treatment. After each headache, note the time of day when it occurred; its intensity and duration; any sensitivity to light, odors, or sound; activity immediately prior to the headache; use of prescription and nonprescription medicines; amount of sleep the previous night; any stressful or emotional conditions; any influence from weather or daily activity; foods and fluids consumed in the past

24 hours; and any known health conditions at that time. Women should record the days of their menstrual cycles. Include notes about other family members who have a history of headache or other disorder. A pattern may emerge that can be helpful to reducing or preventing headaches.

Once your doctor has reviewed your medical and headache history and conducted a physical and neurological exam, lab screening and diagnostic tests may be ordered to either rule out or identify conditions that might be the cause of your headaches. Blood tests and urinalysis can help diagnose brain or spinal cord infections, blood vessel damage, and toxins that affect the nervous system. Testing a sample of the fluid that surrounds the brain and spinal cord can detect infections, bleeding in the brain (called a brain hemorrhage), and measure any buildup of pressure within the skull. Diagnostic imaging, such as with Computed Tomography (CT) and Magnetic Resonance Imaging (MRI), can detect irregularities in blood vessels and bones, certain brain tumors and cysts, brain damage from head injury, brain hemorrhage, inflammation, infection, and other disorders. Neuroimaging also gives doctors a way to see what's happening in the brain during headache attacks. An electroencephalogram (EEG) measures brain wave activity and can help diagnose brain tumors, seizures, head injury, and inflammation that may lead to headaches.

Headache Types and Their Treatment

The International Classification of Headache Disorders, published by the International Headache Society, is used to classify more than 150 types of primary and secondary headache disorders.

Primary Headache Disorders, including Migraine

Primary headache disorders are divided into four main groups: migraine, tension-type headache, trigeminal autonomic cephalgias (a group of short-lasting but severe headaches), and a miscellaneous group.

MIGRAINE

If you suffer from migraine headaches, you're not alone. About 12 percent of the U.S. population experience migraines, one form of vascular headaches. Vascular headaches are characterized by throbbing and pulsating pain caused by the activation of nerve fibers that reside within the wall of brain blood vessels traveling within the meninges.

Blood vessels narrow, temporarily, which decreases the flow of blood and oxygen to the brain. This causes other blood vessels to open wider and increase blood flow.

Migraines involve recurrent attacks of moderate to severe pain that is throbbing or pulsing and often strikes one side of the head. Untreated attacks last from 4 to 72 hours. Other common symptoms are increased sensitivity to light, noise, and odors; and nausea and vomiting. Routine physical activity, movement, or even coughing or sneezing can worsen the headache pain.

Migraines occur most frequently in the morning, especially upon waking. Some people have migraines at predictable times, such as before menstruation or on weekends following a stressful week of work. Many people feel exhausted or weak following a migraine but are usually symptom-free between attacks.

A number of different factors can increase your risk of having a migraine. These factors, which trigger the headache process, vary from person to person and include sudden changes in weather or environment, too much or not enough sleep, strong odors or fumes, emotion, stress, overexertion, loud or sudden noises, motion sickness, low blood sugar, skipped meals, tobacco, depression, anxiety, head trauma, hangover, some medications, hormonal changes, and bright or flashing lights. Medication overuse or missed doses may also cause headaches. In some 50 percent of migraine sufferers, foods or ingredients can trigger headaches. These include aspartame, caffeine (or caffeine withdrawal), wine and other types of alcohol, chocolate, aged cheeses, monosodium glutamate, some fruits and nuts, fermented or pickled goods, yeast, and cured or processed meats. Keeping a diet journal will help identify food triggers.

Who Gets Migraines? Migraines occur in both children and adults, but affect adult women three times more often than men. There is evidence that migraines are genetic, with most migraine sufferers having a family history of the disorder. They also frequently occur in people who have other medical conditions. Depression, anxiety, bipolar disorder, sleep disorders, and epilepsy are more common in individuals with migraine than in the general population. Migraine sufferers—in particular those individuals who have pre-migraine symptoms referred to as aura—have a slightly increased risk of having a stroke.

Migraine in women often relates to changes in hormones. The headaches may begin at the start of the first menstrual cycle or during pregnancy. Most women see improvement after menopause, although surgical removal of the ovaries usually worsens migraines. Women with migraine who take oral contraceptives may experience changes in the frequency and severity of attacks, while women who do not suffer from headaches may develop migraines as a side effect of oral contraceptives.

Phases of Migraine. Migraine is divided into four phases, all of which may be present during the attack:

- Premonitory symptoms occur up to 24 hours prior to developing a migraine. These include food cravings, unexplained mood changes (depression or euphoria), uncontrollable yawning, fluid retention, or increased urination.

- Aura. Some people will see flashing or bright lights or what looks like heat waves immediately prior to or during the migraine, while others may experience muscle weakness or the sensation of being touched or grabbed.

- Headache. A migraine usually starts gradually and builds in intensity. It is possible to have migraine without a headache.

- Postdrome (following the headache). Individuals are often exhausted or confused following a migraine. The postdrome period may last up to a day before people feel healthy.

Types of Migraine. The two major types of migraine are:

- **Migraine with aura**, previously called classic migraine, includes visual disturbances and other neurological symptoms that appear about 10 to 60 minutes before the actual headache and usually last no more than an hour. Individuals may temporarily lose part or all of their vision. The aura may occur without headache pain, which can strike at any time. Other classic symptoms include trouble speaking; an abnormal sensation, numbness, or muscle weakness on one side of the body; a tingling sensation in the hands or face, and confusion. Nausea, loss of appetite, and increased sensitivity to light, sound, or noise may precede the headache.

- **Migraine without aura**, or common migraine, is the more frequent form of migraine. Symptoms include headache pain that occurs without warning and is usually felt on one side of the head, along with nausea, confusion, blurred vision, mood changes, fatigue, and increased sensitivity to light, sound, or noise.

Other types of migraine include:

- **Abdominal migraine** mostly affects young children and involves moderate to severe pain in the middle of the abdomen lasting 1 to 72 hours, with little or no headache. Additional symptoms include nausea, vomiting, and loss of appetite. Many children who develop abdominal migraine will have migraine headaches later in life.

- **Basilar-type migraine** mainly affects children and adolescents. It occurs most often in teenage girls and may be associated with their menstrual cycle. Symptoms include partial or total loss of vision or double vision, dizziness and loss of balance, poor muscle coordination, slurred speech, a ringing in the ears, and fainting. The throbbing pain may come on suddenly and is felt on both sides at the back of the head.

- **Hemiplegic migraine** is a rare but severe form of migraine that causes temporary paralysis-sometimes lasting several days-on one side of the body prior to or during a headache. Symptoms such as vertigo, a pricking or stabbing sensation, and problems seeing, speaking, or swallowing may begin prior to the headache pain and usually stop shortly thereafter. When it runs in families the disorder is called Familial Hemiplegic Migraine (FHM). Though rare, at least three distinct genetic forms of FHM have been identified. These genetic mutations make the brain more sensitive or excitable, most likely by increasing brain levels of a chemical called glutamate.

- **Menstrually-related migraine** affects women around the time of their period, although most women with menstrually-related migraine also have migraines at other times of the month. Symptoms may include migraine without aura (which is much more common during menses than migraine with aura), pulsing pain on one side of the head, nausea, vomiting, and increased sensitivity to sound and light.

- **Migraine without headache** is characterized by visual problems or other aura symptoms, nausea, vomiting, and constipation, but without head pain. Headache specialists have suggested that fever, dizziness, and/or unexplained pain in a particular part of the body could also be possible types of headache-free migraine.

- **Ophthalmoplegic migraine** an uncommon form of migraine with head pain, along with a droopy eyelid, large pupil, and double vision that may last for weeks, long after the pain is gone.

- **Retinal migraine** is a condition characterized by attacks of visual loss or disturbances in one eye. These attacks, like the more common visual auras, are usually associated with migraine headaches.

- **Status migrainosus** is a rare and severe type of acute migraine in which disabling pain and nausea can last 72 hours or longer. The pain and nausea may be so intense that sufferers need to be hospitalized.

Migraine Treatment. Migraine treatment is aimed at relieving symptoms and preventing additional attacks. Quick steps to ease symptoms may include napping or resting with eyes closed in a quiet, darkened room; placing a cool cloth or ice pack on the forehead, and drinking lots of fluid, particularly if the migraine is accompanied by vomiting. Small amounts of caffeine may help relieve symptoms during a migraine's early stages.

Drug therapy for migraine is divided into acute and preventive treatment. Acute or "abortive" medications are taken as soon as symptoms occur to relieve pain and restore function. Preventive treatment involves taking medicines daily to reduce the severity of future attacks or keep them from happening. The U.S. Food and Drug Administration (FDA) has approved a variety of drugs for these treatment methods. Headache drug use should be monitored by a physician, since some drugs may cause side effects.

Acute treatment for migraine may include any of the following drugs.

- Triptan drugs increase levels of the neurotransmitter serotonin in the brain. Serotonin causes blood vessels to constrict and lowers the pain threshold. Triptans—the preferred treatment for migraine—ease moderate to severe migraine pain and are available as tablets, nasal sprays, and injections.

- Ergot derivative drugs bind to serotonin receptors on nerve cells and decrease the transmission of pain messages along nerve fibers. They are most effective during the early stages of migraine and are available as nasal sprays and injections.

- Non-prescription analgesics or over-the-counter drugs such as ibuprofen, aspirin, or acetaminophen can ease the pain of less severe migraine headache.

- Combination analgesics involve a mix of drugs such as acetaminophen plus caffeine and/or a narcotic for migraine that may be resistant to simple analgesics.

- Nonsteroidal anti-inflammatory drugs can reduce inflammation and alleviate pain.

- Nausea relief drugs can ease queasiness brought on by various types of headache.

- Narcotics are prescribed briefly to relieve pain. These drugs should not be used to treat chronic headaches.

Taking headache relief drugs more than three times a week may lead to **medication overuse headache** (previously called rebound headache), in which the initial headache is relieved temporarily but reappears as the drug wears off. Taking more of the drug to treat the new headache leads to progressively shorter periods of pain relief and results in a pattern of recurrent chronic headache. Headache pain ranges from moderate to severe and may occur with nausea or irritability. It may take weeks for these headaches to end once the drug is stopped.

Everyone with migraine needs effective treatment at the time of the headaches. Some people with frequent and severe migraine need preventive medications. In general, prevention should be considered if migraines occur one or more times weekly, or if migraines are less frequent but disabling. Preventive medicines are also recommended for individuals who take symptomatic headache treatment more than three times a week. Physicians will also recommend that a migraine sufferer take one or more preventive medications two to three months to assess drug effectiveness, unless intolerable side effects occur.

Several preventive medicines for migraine were initially marketed for conditions other than migraine.

- Anticonvulsants may be helpful for people with other types of headaches in addition to migraine. Although they were originally developed for treating epilepsy, these drugs increase levels of certain neurotransmitters and dampen pain impulses.

- Beta-blockers are drugs for treating high blood pressure that are often effective for migraine.

- Calcium channel blockers are medications that are also used to treat high blood pressure treatment and help to stabilize blood vessel walls. These drugs appear to work by preventing the blood vessels from either narrowing or widening, which affects blood flow to the brain.

- Antidepressants are drugs that work on different chemicals in the brain; their effectiveness in treating migraine is not directly related to their effect on mood. Antidepressants may be helpful for individuals with other types of headaches because they increase the production of serotonin and may also affect levels of other chemicals, such as norepinephrine and dopamine. The types of antidepressants used for migraine treatment include selective serotonin reuptake inhibitors, serotonin and norepinephrine reuptake inhibitors, and tricyclic antidepressants (which are also used to treat tension-type headaches).

Natural treatments for migraine include riboflavin (vitamin B2), magnesium, coenzyme Q10, and butterbur.

Non-drug therapy for migraine includes biofeedback and relaxation training, both of which help individuals cope with or control the development of pain and the body's response to stress.

Lifestyle changes that reduce or prevent migraine attacks in some individuals include exercising, avoiding food and beverages that trigger headaches, eating regularly scheduled meals with adequate hydration, stopping certain medications, and establishing a consistent sleep schedule. Obesity increases the risk of developing chronic daily headache, so a weight loss program is recommended for obese individuals.

TENSION-TYPE

Tension-type headache, previously called muscle contraction headache, is the most common type of headache. Its name indicates the role of stress and mental or emotional conflict in triggering the pain and contracting muscles in the neck, face, scalp, and jaw. Tension-type headaches may also be caused by jaw clenching, intense work, missed meals, depression, anxiety, or too little sleep. Sleep apnea may also cause tension-type headaches, especially in the morning. The pain is usually mild to moderate and feels as if constant pressure is being applied to the front of the face or to the head or neck. It also may feel as if a belt is being tightened around the head. Most often the pain is felt on both sides of the head. People who suffer tension-type headaches may also feel overly sensitive to light and sound but there is no pre-headache aura as with migraine. Typically, tension-type headaches usually disappear once the period of stress or related cause has ended.

Tension-type headaches affect women slightly more often than men. The headaches usually begin in adolescence and reach peak activity in the 30s. They have not been linked to hormones and do not have a strong hereditary connection.

There are two forms of tension-type headache: Episodic tension-type headaches occur between 10 and 15 days per month, with each attack lasting from 30 minutes to several days. Although the pain is not disabling, the severity of pain typically increases with the frequency of attacks. Chronic tension-type attacks usually occur more than 15 days per month over a 3-month period. The pain, which can be constant over a period of days or months, strikes both sides of the head and is more severe and disabling than episodic headache pain. Chronic tension headaches can cause sore scalps-even combing your hair can be painful. Most individuals will have had some form of episodic tension-type headache prior to onset of chronic tension-type headache.

Depression and anxiety can cause tension-type headaches. Headaches may appear in the early morning or evening, when conflicts in the office or at home are anticipated. Other causes include physical postures that strain head and neck muscles (such as holding your chin down while reading or holding a phone between your shoulder and ear), degenerative arthritis of the neck, and temporomandibular joint dysfunction (a disorder of the joints between the temporal bone located above the ear and the mandible, or lower jaw bone).

The first step in caring for a tension-type headache involves treating any specific disorder or disease that may be causing it. For example, arthritis of the neck is treated with anti-inflammatory medication and temporomandibular joint dysfunction may be helped by corrective devices for the mouth and jaw. A sleep study may be needed to detect sleep apnea and should be considered when there is a history of snoring, daytime sleepiness, or obesity.

A physician may suggest using analgesics, nonsteroidal anti-inflammatory drugs, or antidepressants to treat a tension-type headache that is not associated with a disease. Triptan drugs, barbiturates (drugs that have a relaxing or sedative effect), and ergot derivatives may provide relief to people who suffer from both migraine and tension-type headache.

Alternative therapies for chronic tension-type headaches include biofeedback, relaxation training, meditation, and cognitive-behavioral therapy to reduce stress. A hot shower or moist heat applied to the back of the neck may ease symptoms of infrequent tension headaches. Physical therapy, massage, and gentle exercise of the neck may also be helpful.

TRIGEMINAL AUTONOMIC CEPHALGIAS

Some primary headaches are characterized by severe pain in or around the eye on one side of the face and autonomic (or involuntary) features on the same side, such as red and teary eye, drooping eyelid, and runny nose. These disorders, called trigeminal autonomic cephalgias (cephalgia meaning head pain), differ in attack duration and frequency, and have episodic and chronic forms. Episodic attacks occur on a daily or near-daily basis for weeks or months with pain-free remissions. Chronic attacks occur on a daily or near-daily basis for a year or more with only brief remissions.

Cluster headache—the most severe form of primary headache—involves sudden, extremely painful headaches that occur in "clusters," usually at the same time of the day and night for several weeks. They strike one side of the head, often behind or around one eye, and may be preceded by a migraine-like aura and nausea. The pain usually peaks 5 to 10 minutes after onset and continues at that intensity for up to 3 hours. The nose and the eye on the affected side of the face may get red, swollen, and teary. Some people will experience restlessness and agitation, changes in heart rate and blood pressure, and sensitivity to light, sound, or smell. Cluster headaches often wake people from sleep.

Cluster headaches generally begin between the ages of 20 and 50 but may start at any age, occur more often in men than in women, and are more common in smokers than in nonsmokers. The attacks are usually less frequent and shorter than migraines. It's common to have 1 to 3 cluster headaches a day with 2 cluster periods a year, separated by months of freedom from symptoms. The cluster periods often appear seasonally, usually in the spring and fall, and may be mistaken for allergies. A small group of people develop a chronic form of the disorder, which is characterized by bouts of headaches that can go on for years with only brief periods (1 month or less) of remission. Cluster headaches occur more often at night than during the day, suggesting they could be caused by irregularities in the body's sleep-wake cycle. Alcohol (especially red wine) and smoking can provoke attacks. Studies show a connection between cluster headache and prior head trauma. An increased familial risk of these headaches suggests that there may be a genetic cause.

Treatment options include oxygen therapy—in which pure oxygen is breathed through a mask to reduce blood flow to the brain—and triptan drugs. Certain antipsychotic drugs, calcium-channel blockers, and anticonvulsants can reduce pain severity and frequency of attacks. In extreme cases, electrical stimulation of the occipital nerve to prevent nerve signaling or surgical procedures that destroy or cut certain facial nerves may provide relief.

Paroxysmal hemicrania is a rare form of primary headache that usually begins in adulthood. Pain and related symptoms may be similar to those felt in cluster headaches, but with shorter duration. Attacks typically occur 5 to 40 times per day, with each attack lasting 2 to 45 minutes. Severe throbbing, claw-like, or piercing pain is felt on one side of the face-in, around, or behind the eye and occasionally reaching to the back of the neck. Other symptoms may include red and watery eyes, a drooping or swollen eyelid on the affected side of the face, and nasal congestion. Individuals may also feel dull pain, soreness, or tenderness between attacks or increased sensitivity to light on the affected side of the face. Paroxysmal hemicrania has two forms: chronic, in which individuals experience attacks on a daily basis for a year or more, and episodic, in which the headaches may stop for months or years before recurring. Certain movements of the head or neck, external pressure to the neck, and alcohol use may trigger these headaches. Attacks occur more often in women than in men and have no familial pattern.

The nonsteroidal anti-inflammatory drug indomethacin can quickly halt the pain and related symptoms of paroxysmal hemicrania, but symptoms recur once the drug treatment is stopped. Non-prescription analgesics and calcium-channel blockers can ease discomfort, particularly if taken when symptoms first appear.

SUNCT (Short-lasting, Unilateral, Neuralgiform headache attacks with Conjunctival injection and Tearing) is a very rare type of headache with bursts of moderate to severe burning, piercing, or throbbing pain that is usually felt in the forehead, eye, or temple on one side of the head. The pain usually peaks within seconds of onset and may follow a pattern of increasing and decreasing intensity. Attacks typically occur during the day and last from 5 seconds to 4 minutes per episode. Individuals generally have five to six attacks per hour and are pain-free between attacks. This primary headache is slightly more common in men than in women, with onset usually after age 50. SUNCT may be episodic, occurring once or twice annually with headaches that remit and recur, or chronic, lasting more than 1year.

Symptoms include reddish or bloodshot eyes (conjunctival injection), watery eyes, stuffy or runny nose, sweaty forehead, puffy eyelids, increased pressure within the eye on the affected side of the head, and increased blood pressure.

SUNCT is very difficult to treat. Anticonvulsants may relieve some of the symptoms, while anesthetics and corticosteroid drugs can treat some of the severe pain felt during these headaches. Surgery and glycerol injections to block nerve signaling along the trigeminal nerve have poor outcomes and provide only temporary relief in severe cases. Doctors are beginning to use deep brain stimulation (involving a surgically implanted battery-powered electrode that emits pulses of energy to surrounding brain tissue) to reduce the frequency of attacks in severely affected individuals.

MISCELLANEOUS PRIMARY HEADACHES

Other headaches that are not caused by other disorders include:

Chronic daily headache refers to a group of headache disorders that occur at least 15 days a month during a 3-month period. In addition to chronic tension-type headache, chronic migraine, and medication overuse headache (discussed above), these headaches include hemicrania continua and new daily persistent headache. Individuals feel constant, mostly moderate pain throughout the day on the sides or top of the head. They may also experience other types of headache. Adolescents and adults may experience chronic daily headaches. In children, stress from school and family activities may contribute to these headaches.

- **Hemicrania** continua is marked by continuous, fluctuating pain that always occurs on the same side of the face and head. The headache may last from minutes to days and is associated with symptoms including tearing, red and irritated eyes, sweating, stuffy or runny nose, and swollen and drooping eyelids. The pain may get worse as the headache progresses. Migraine-like symptoms include nausea, vomiting, and sensitivity to light and sound. Physical exertion and alcohol use may increase headache severity. The disorder is more common in women than in men and its cause is unknown. Hemicrania continua has two forms: chronic, with daily headaches, and remitting or episodic, in which headaches may occur over a period of 6 months and are followed by a pain-free period of weeks to months before recurring. Most individuals have attacks of increased pain three to five times per 24-hour cycle. The nonsteroidal anti-inflammatory drug indomethacin usually provides rapid relief from symptoms. Corticosteroids may also provide temporary relief from some symptoms.

- New Daily Persistent Headache (NDPH), previously called chronic benign daily headache, is known for its constant daily pain that ranges from mild to severe. Individuals can often recount the exact date and time that the headache began. Daily headaches can occur for more than 3 months (and sometimes years) without lessening or ending. Symptoms include an abnormal sensitivity to light or sound, nausea, lightheadedness, and a pressing, throbbing, or tightening pain felt on both sides of the head. NDPH occurs more often in women than in men. Most sufferers do not have a prior history of headache. NDPH may occur spontaneously or following infection, medication use, trauma, high spinal fluid pressure, or other condition. The disorder has two forms: one that usually ends on its own within several months and does not require treatment, and a longer-lasting form that is difficult to treat. Muscle relaxants, antidepressants, and anticonvulsants may provide some relief.

Primary stabbing headache, also known as "ice pick" or "jabs and jolts" headache, is characterized by intense piercing pain that strikes without warning and generally lasts 1 to 10 seconds. The stabbing pain usually occurs around the eye but may be felt in multiple sites along the trigeminal nerve. Onset typically occurs between 45 and 50 years of age. Some individuals may have only one headache per year while others may have multiple headaches daily. Most attacks are spontaneous but headaches may be triggered by sudden movement, bright lights, or emotional stress. Primary stabbing headache occurs most often in people who have migraine, hemicrania continua, tension-type, or cluster headaches. The disorder is hard to treat, because each attack is extremely short. Indomethacin and other headache preventive medications can relieve pain in people who have multiple episodes of primary stabbing headache.

Primary exertional headache may be brought on by fits of coughing or sneezing or intense physical activity such as running, basketball, lifting weights, or sexual activity. The headache begins at the onset of activity. Pain rarely lasts more than several minutes but can last up to 2 days. Symptoms may include nausea and vomiting. This type of headache is typically seen in individuals who have a family history of migraine. Warm-up exercises prior to the physical activity can help prevent the headache and indomethacin can relieve the headache pain.

Hypnic headache, previously called "alarm-clock" headache, awakens people mostly at night. Onset is usually after age 50. Hypnic headache may occur 15 or more times per month, with no known trigger. Bouts of mild to moderate throbbing pain usually last from 15 minutes to 3 hours after waking and are most often felt on both sides of the head. Other symptoms include nausea or increased sensitivity to sound or light. Hypnic headache may be a disorder of rapid eye movement (REM) sleep as the attacks occur most often during dreaming. Both men and women are affected by this disorder, which is usually treated with caffeine, indomethacin, or lithium.

If you've ever eaten or inhaled a cold substance very fast, you may have had what's called an ice cream headache(sometimes called "brain freeze"). This headache happens when cold materials such as cold drinks or ice cream hit the warm roof of your mouth. Local blood vessels constrict to reduce the loss of body heat and then relax and allow the blood flow to increase. The resulting burst of pain lasts for about 5 minutes. Ice cream headache is more common in individuals who have migraine. The pain stops once the body adapts to the temperature change.

Secondary Headache Disorders

Secondary headache disorders are caused by an underlying illness or condition that affects the brain. Secondary headaches are usually diagnosed based on other symptoms that occur concurrently and the characteristics of the headaches. Some of the more serious causes of secondary headache include:

Brain tumor. A tumor that is growing in the brain can press against nerve tissue and pain-sensitive blood vessel walls, disrupting communication between the brain and the nerves or restricting the supply of blood to the brain. Headaches may develop, worsen, become more frequent, or come and go, often at irregular periods. Headache pain may worsen when coughing, changing posture, or straining, and may be severe upon waking. Treatment options include surgery, radiation therapy, and chemotherapy. However, the vast majority of individuals with headache do not have brain tumors.

Disorders of blood vessels in the brain, including stroke. Several disorders associated with blood vessel formation and activity can cause headache. Most notable among these conditions is stroke. Headache itself can cause stroke or accompany a series of blood vessel disorders that can cause a stroke.

There are two forms of stroke. A hemorrhagic stroke occurs when an artery in the brain bursts, spilling blood into the surrounding tissue. An ischemic stroke occurs when an artery supplying the brain with blood becomes blocked, suddenly decreasing or stopping blood flow and causing brain cells to die.

Hemorrhagic stroke

A hemorrhagic stroke is usually associated with disturbed brain function and an extremely painful headache that develops suddenly and may worsen with physical activity, coughing, or straining. Headache conditions associated with hemorrhagic stroke include:

- A subarachnoid hemorrhage is the rupture of a blood vessel located within the subarachnoid space—a fluid-filled space between layers of connective tissue (meninges) that surround the brain. The first sign of a subarachnoid hemorrhage is typically a severe headache with a split-second onset and no known cause. Neurologists call this a thunderclap headache. Pain may also be felt in the neck and lower back. This sudden flood of blood can contaminate the cerebrospinal fluid that flows within the spaces of the brain and cause extensive damage throughout the brain.

- Intracerebral hemorrhage is usually associated with severe headache. Several conditions can render blood vessels in the brain prone to rupture and hemorrhaging. Chronic hypertension can weaken the blood vessel wall. Poor blood clotting ability due to blood disorders or blood-thinning medications like warfarin further increase the risk of bleeding. And some venous strokes (caused by clots in the brain's veins) often cause bleeding into the brain. At risk are mothers in the post-partum period and persons with dehydration, cancer, or infections.

- An aneurysm is the abnormal ballooning of an artery that causes the artery wall to weaken. A ruptured cerebral aneurysm can cause hemorrhagic stroke and a sudden, incredibly painful headache that is generally different in severity and intensity from other headaches individuals may have experienced. Individuals usually describe the thunderclap-like headache as "the worst headache of my life." There may be loss of consciousness and other neurological features. "Sentinel" or sudden warning headaches sometimes occur from an aneurysm that leaks prior to rupture. Cerebral aneurysms that have leaked or ruptured are life-threatening and require emergency medical attention. Not all aneurysms burst, and people with very small aneurysms may be monitored to detect any growth or onset of symptoms. Treatment options include blocking the flow of blood to the aneurysm surgically (intra-arterial) and catheter techniques to fill the aneurysm with coils or balloons.

- Arteriovenous malformation (AVM), an abnormal tangle of arteries and veins in the brain, causes headaches that vary in frequency, duration, and intensity as vascular malformations press on and displace normal tissue or leak blood into surrounding tissue. A headache consistently affecting one side of the head may be closely linked to the site of an AVM (although most one-sided headaches are caused by primary headache disorders). Symptoms may include seizures and hearing pulsating noises. Treatment options include decreasing blood flow to and from the malformation by injecting particles or glue, or through focused radiotherapy or surgery.

Ischemic stroke

Headache that accompanies ischemic stroke can be caused by several problems with the brain's vascular system. Headache is prominent in individuals with clots in the brain's veins. Head pain occurs on the side of the brain in which the clot blocks blood flow and is often felt in the eyes or on the side of the head. Conditions of ischemic stroke that can cause headache include:

- Arterial dissection is a tear within an artery that supplies the brain with blood flow. The most common dissection occurs in the carotid artery in the neck, with head pain on the same side of the body where the tear occurs. Vertebral artery dissection causes pain in the rear upper part of the neck. Cervical artery dissection can lead to stroke or transient ischemic attacks (strokes that last only a few minutes but signal a subsequent, more severe stroke). They are usually caused by neck strain, i.e., trauma, chiropractic manipulation, sports injuries, or even pronounced bending of the head backwards over a sink for hair washing ("beauty parlor stroke"). Immediate medical attention can be lifesaving.

- Vascular inflammation can cause the buildup of plaque, which can lead to ischemic stroke. Cerebral vasculitis, an inflammation of the brain's blood vessel system, may cause headache, stroke, and/

or progressive cognitive decline. Severe headache attributed to a chronic inflammatory disease of blood vessels on the outside of the head, called giant cell arteritis (previously known as temporal arteritis), usually affects people older than age 60. It also causes muscle pain and tenderness in the temple area. Individuals also may experience temporary, followed by permanent, loss of vision on one or both eyes, pain with chewing, a tender scalp, muscle aches, depression, and fatigue. Corticosteroids are typically used to treat vascular inflammation and can prevent blindness.

Exposure to a substance or its withdrawal. Headaches may result from toxic states such as drinking alcohol, following carbon monoxide poisoning, or from exposure to toxic chemicals and metals, cleaning products or solvents, and pesticides. In the most severe cases, rising toxin levels can cause a pulsing, throbbing headache that, if left untreated, can lead to systemic poisoning, organ failure, and permanent neurological damage. These headaches are usually treated by identifying and removing the cause of the toxic buildup. The withdrawal from certain medicines or caffeine after frequent or excessive use can also cause headaches.

Head injury. Headaches are often a symptom of a concussion or other head injury. The headache may develop either immediately or months after a blow to the head, with pain felt at the injury site or throughout the head. Emotional disturbances may worsen headache pain. In most cases, the cause of post-traumatic headache is unknown. Sometimes the cause is ruptured blood vessels, which result in an accumulation of blood called a hematoma. This mass of blood can displace brain tissue and cause headaches as well as weakness, confusion, memory loss, and seizures. Hematomas can be drained surgically to produce rapid relief of symptoms. Bleeding between the dura (the outermost layer of the protective covering of the brain) and the skull, called epidural hematoma, usually occurs minutes to hours after a skull fracture and is especially dangerous. Bleeding between the brain and the dura, called subdural hematoma, is frequently associated with a dull, persistent ache on one side of the head. Nausea, vomiting, and mild disturbance of brain function also occur. Subdural hematoma may occur after head trauma but also occurs spontaneously in elderly persons or in individuals taking anticoagulant medications.

Increased intracranial pressure. A growing tumor, infection, or hydrocephalus (an extensive buildup of cerebrospinal fluid in the brain) can raise pressure in the brain and compress nerves and blood vessels, causing headaches. Hydrocephalus is most often treated with the surgical placement of a shunt system that diverts the fluid to a site elsewhere in the body, where it can be absorbed as part of the circulatory process. Headache attributed to idiopathic intracranial hypertension, previously known as pseudotumor cerebri (meaning "false brain tumor"), is associated with severe headache. It can be caused by clotting in the major cerebral veins or certain medications (some antibiotics, withdrawal of corticosteroids, human growth hormone replacement, and vitamin A and related compounds). It is most commonly seen in young, overweight females. Diagnosis usually requires a spinal fluid examination to document the high pressure and the rapid resolution of headache after the spinal fluid is removed. Although called benign, the condition may lead to visual loss if left untreated. Weight loss, ending the use of the drug suspected of causing the problem, and diuretic treatment can help relieve the pressure.

Inflammation from meningitis, encephalitis, and other infections. Inflammation from infections can harm or destroy nerve cells and cause dull to severe headache pain, brain damage, or stroke, among other conditions. Inflammation of the brain and spinal cord (meningitis and encephalitis) requires urgent medical attention. Diagnosis and identification of the infection usually requires examination and culture of a sample of the cerebrospinal fluid. Treatment options include antibiotics, antiviral or antifungal drugs, corticosteroids, pain medications and sedatives, and anticonvulsants. Headaches may also occur with a fever or a flu-like infection. A headache may accompany a bacterial infection of the upper respiratory tract that spreads to and inflames the lining of the sinus cavities. When one or more of the cavities fills with fluid from the inflammation, the result is constant but dull facial pain and tenderness that worsens with straining or head movements. Treatment includes antibiotics, analgesics, and decongestants. Sinus infections do not generally cause chronic headaches.

Seizures. Migraine-like headache pain may occur during or after a seizure. Moderate to severe headache pain may last for several hours and worsen with sudden movements of the head or when sneezing, coughing, or bending. Other symptoms may include nausea, vomiting, fatigue, increased sensitivity to light or sound, and vision problems.

Spinal fluid leak. About one-fourth of people who undergo a lumbar puncture (which involves a small sampling of the spinal fluid being removed for testing) develop a headache due to a leak of cerebrospinal fluid following the procedure. Since the headache occurs only when the individual stands up, the "cure" is to lie down until the headache runs its course—anywhere from a few hours to several days. Severe post-dural headaches may be treated by injecting a small amount of the individual's own blood into the low back to stop the leak (called an epidural blood patch). Occasionally spinal fluid leaks spontaneously, causing this "low pressure headache."

Structural abnormalities of the head, neck and spine. Headache pain and loss of function may be triggered by structural abnormalities in the head or spine, restricted blood flow through the neck, irritation to nerves anywhere along the path from the spinal cord to the brain, or stressful or awkward positions of the head and neck. Surgery is the only treatment available to correct the condition or halt the progression of damage to the central nervous system. Medications may ease the pain. Cervicogenic headaches are caused by structural irregularities in either the head or neck. In a Chiari malformation, the back of the skull is too small for the brain. This forces a part of the brain to block the normal flow of spinal fluid and press on the brain stem. Chiari malformations are present at birth but may not cause symptoms until later in life. Common symptoms include dizziness, muscle weakness, vision problems, and headache that worsen with coughing or straining. Syringomyelia, a fluid-filled cyst within the spinal cord, can cause pain, numbness, weakness, and headaches.

Trigeminal neuralgia. The trigeminal nerve conducts sensations to the brain from the upper, middle, and lower portions of the face, as well as inside the mouth. The presumed cause of trigeminal neuralgia is a blood vessel pressing on the nerve as it exits the brain stem, but other causes have been described. Symptoms include headache and intense shock-like or stabbing pain that comes on suddenly and is typically felt on one side of the jaw or cheek. Muscle spasms may occur on the affected side of the face. The pain may occur spontaneously or be triggered by touching the cheek, as happens when shaving, washing, or applying makeup. The pain also may occur when eating, drinking, talking, smoking, or brushing teeth, or when the face is exposed to wind. Treatment options include anticonvulsants, antidepressants, and surgery to block pain signaling to the brain.

Children and Headache

Headaches are common in children. Headaches that begin early in life can develop into migraines as the child grows older. Migraines in children or adolescents can develop into tension-type headaches at any time. In contrast to adults with migraine, young children often feel migraine pain on both sides of the head and have headaches that usually last less than 2 hours. Children may look pale and appear restless or irritable before and during an attack. Other children may become nauseous, lose their appetite, or feel pain elsewhere in the body during the headache.

Headaches in children can be caused by a number of triggers, including emotional problems such as tension between family members, stress from school activities, weather changes, irregular eating and sleep, dehydration, and certain foods and drinks. Of special concern among children are headaches that occur after head injury or those accompanied by rash, fever, or sleepiness

It may be difficult to identify the type of headache because children often have problems describing where it hurts, how often the headaches occur, and how long they last. Asking a child with a headache to draw a picture of where the pain is and how it feels can make it easier for the doctor to determine the proper treatment.

Migraine in particular is often misdiagnosed in children. Parents and caretakers sometimes have to be detectives to help determine that a child has migraine. Clues to watch for include sensitivity to light and noise, which may be suspected when a child refuses to watch television or use the computer, or when the child stops playing to lie down in a dark room. Observe whether or not a child is able to eat during a headache. Very young children may seem cranky or irritable and complain of abdominal pain (abdominal migraine).

Headache treatment in children and teens usually includes rest, fluids, and over-the-counter pain relief medicines. Always consult with a physician before giving headache medicines to a child. Most tension-type headaches in children can be treated with over-the-counter medicines that are marked for children with usage guidelines based on the child's age and weight. Headaches in some children may also be treated effectively using relaxation/behavioral therapy. Children with cluster headache may be treated with oxygen therapy early in the initial phase of the attacks.

Headache and Sleep Disorders

Headaches are often a secondary symptom of a sleep disorder. For example, tension-type headache is regularly seen in persons with insomnia or sleep-wake cycle disorders. Nearly three-fourths of individuals who suffer from narcolepsy complain of either migraine or cluster headache. Migraines and cluster headaches appear to be related to the number of and transition between rapid eye movement (REM) and other sleep periods an individual has during sleep. Hypnic headache awakens individuals mainly at night but may also interrupt daytime naps. Reduced oxygen levels in people with sleep apnea may trigger early morning headaches.

Getting the proper amount of sleep can ease headache pain. Generally, too little or too much sleep can worsen headaches, as can overuse of sleep medicines. Daytime naps often reduce deep sleep at night and can produce headaches in some adults. Some sleep disorders and secondary headache are treated using antidepressants. Check with a doctor before using over-the-counter medicines to ease sleep-associated headaches.

Coping with Headache

Headache treatment is a partnership between you and your doctor, and honest communication is essential. Finding a quick fix to your headache may not be possible. It may take some time for your doctor or specialist to determine the best course of treatment. Avoid using over-the-counter medicines more than twice a week, as they may actually worsen headache pain and the frequency of attacks. Visit a local headache support group meeting (if available) to learn how others with headache cope with their pain and discomfort. Relax whenever possible to ease stress and related symptoms, get enough sleep, regularly perform aerobic exercises, and eat a regularly scheduled and healthy diet that avoids food triggers. Gaining more control over your headache, stress, and emotions will make you feel better and let you embrace daily activities as much as possible.

What Research is Being Done?

Several studies either conducted or supported by the National Institute of Neurological Disorders and Stroke (NINDS), a part of the National Institutes of Health, are revealing much about the headache process and may lead to new treatments or perhaps ways to block debilitating headache pain. Studies by other investigators are adding insight to headache etiology and treatment.

Understanding headache mechanisms and underlying causes

The molecular basis for migraine headaches and the aura associated with certain migraines is uncertain. One multi-faceted research study is examining how migraine with aura may affect metabolism and neurophysiological function. Investigators are also studying if particular regions of the visual cortex are unusually susceptible to the events in the brain that cause the aura. Another study component is investigating what happens at the beginning of a headache and how changes in the brain's meninges may lead to vascular and trigeminal nerve stimulation associated with the painful part of a migraine headache. Results may provide a greater understanding of migraine and assist the development of new therapies.

Mast cells, which are part of the immune system and are involved in the inflammatory allergic response, are activated in some chronic pain conditions, including headache. Researchers are examining the possibility of a relationship between the mast cells' anti-analgesic properties and their proximity to and enhanced activation of nerve fiber endings that receive and transmit pain signals (nociceptors). Mast cells may release substances that activate nociceptive nerve cells that transmit signals from the linings of the skull and its blood vessels. Findings that link mast cell activation to headache pain may identify drug targets that could lead to new analgesics for headache and other pain syndromes.

Cortical spreading depression (CSD) is a process in migraine with aura in which a wave of increased brain activity, followed by decreased activity, slowly spreads along the brain's surface. The wave of brain activity often travels across the part of the brain that processes vision and corresponds to the typical visual aura of migraine. Research has shown that migraines with aura may be associated with tiny areas of stroke-like brain damage caused by a short-term drop in oxygen levels (associated with the CSD) which prevents normal cell function and swelling in the brain's nerve cells. Animal studies have shown that CSD also irritates the trigeminal nerve, causing it to transmit pain signals and trigger inflammation in the membranes that surround the brain. CSD inhibiting drugs such as tonabersat are being tested in clinical trials for their usefulness in treating migraine and other neurological diseases. Other investigators hope to build on initial results showing that estrogen withdrawal makes it easier for CSD to occur in the brains of animals, which may explain the contribution of estrogen fluctuation to menstrual migraines. This research may result in a better understanding of how a migraine starts in the brain and offer new methods of treatment by interrupting this process and preventing the migraine.

Cutaneous allodynia is the feeling of pain or unpleasant sensations in response to normally nonpainful stimuli, such as light touch.

Researchers are investigating why it is present on the head or face in people with cluster headaches, to better understand neurological changes that occur with these headaches. Similar research is looking at why some people with migraines have more than the typical restricted allodynia that affects a particular area of the head predicted by the headache (for example, on the same side of the face as the migraine pain). Individuals with extended allodynia may experience unpleasant sensations on the side of the face opposite the headache pain or even on their feet. Previous studies have shown that sensitized nociceptors in the brain's coverings are involved in the throbbing pain of migraine and that other sensitized neurons found deeper in the brain are involved with restricted allodynia, but it is not certain which cells are responsible for extended allodynia. Future studies will explore whether nerve cells in the thalamus (which is involved in relaying signals between the brain and the body) become more sensitive a result of the headache pain and cause extended allodynia. Findings may offer a better understanding of how the nervous system changes and becomes more sensitive after repeated stimulation, resulting in chronic pain.

Social and other factors may impact headache. Researchers are examining how race and psychiatric conditions are related to headache severity, quality of life, the ability to reliably follow a treatment program, and treatment response in people with migraines, tension-type headache, substance abuse headache, or cluster headache.

Genetics of headache

Genetics may contribute to a predisposition for migraines. Most migraine sufferers have a family member with migraine. Researchers are studying the activity of different genes to see if they make some people more likely to have migraines. One strategy is to test for a gene in several families having members with migraine and then determine if the gene is related to migraine in a broader population.

In April 2008, researchers at the University of Helsinki reported significant evidence for linkage between a gene variant on a specific site on chromosome 10q22-q23 and susceptibility to common types of migraine. The findings were from a study of 1,675 migraine sufferers or their close relatives from 210 Finnish and Australian migraine families. Another study replicated the findings in the two populations and also showed that the site was particularly linked to female migraine sufferers. Although it has been known for some time that genetic factors shared by family members make people more susceptible to migraines, this study is the first to identify convincingly a specific gene locus for common forms of migraine.

Currently under investigation are gene expression patterns (signs of changes in gene activity) in the blood of individuals during migraine attacks and among individuals with chronic daily headaches. Preliminary studies show that children with acute migraines and chronic daily headaches have specific similar gene expression profiles in their blood that are different from healthy individuals and from children with other non-related neurological diseases. Researchers are exploring differences in gene expression profiles among individuals who respond to different types of headache drugs. Study results may indicate a molecular genomic approach using blood samples to detect genes that may be activated during headaches and identify which drugs are best used for each person with migraines.

Scientists are exploring the role of the calcitonin gene-related peptide (CGRP) in migraines. Levels of the CGRP molecule, which is involved in sending signals between neurons, increase during migraine attacks and revert to normal when the pain resolves. Researchers plan to use CGRP as a model and then to use functional magnetic resonance imaging to estimate the pain response in the central nervous system. Evidence from individuals with Familial Hemiplegic Migraine (FHM) with known mutations indicates that migraine pathways in FHM may be different from normal migraine. Investigators are also measuring levels of CGRP during the premonitory, mild, moderate, and severe phases of a single migraine compared to the baseline level when individuals are pain-free. The fluctuations of CGRP during the migraine process will help to define its role in migraine pain and may offer new opportunities for acute treatment.

Clinical studies in headache management

A major focus of headache research is the development of new drugs and other treatment options. Several drug studies seek to identify new drugs to treat various headache disorders and to find safer, more effective doses for medications already being used. Other research is aimed at identifying receptors or drug targets to stop the process of migraine aura in the brain.

Results of three randomized, placebo-controlled clinical trials show the drug topiramate is effective, safe, and generally well-tolerated for treating chronic migraine. Experts agree that treatment with combinations of preventive agents offers maximum relief for the majority of individuals with chronic migraine. An NINDS-funded clinical trial is examining the effectiveness and safety of the drug propranolol combined with topiramate in reducing the frequency of chronic migraine in 250 participants who will be randomly selected to receive treatment with both drugs or topiramate and placebo.

Sleep plays an important role in migraine. Migraine in older adults is sometimes triggered by sleep changes; regulating their sleep may lessen the frequency of migraine. Younger migraine sufferers often report migraine relief after sleep. Researchers are studying the use of the drug ramelteon, which is approved by the U.S. Food and Drug Administration for insomnia, in reducing the number of migraines over a 12-week period.

Headache is the most common symptom after a closed head injury, and it can last for more than 2 months in 60 percent of affected individuals. Unfortunately, individuals with chronic post-traumatic headaches also have cognitive and behavioral problems, and many drugs currently used to treat the headaches also have a negative influence on cognition. Scientists are testing different drugs, such as naratriptan (which acts like a neurotransmitter) and galantamine (used to treat Alzheimer's disease), to treat both the headache and cognitive disturbances in individuals with chronic post-traumatic headaches.

Non-pharmaceutical approaches to treatment and prevention

Historically, very little research has been done on children with headaches. A variety of headache education and drug and/or behavioral management techniques are aimed at improving headache treatment and prevention in children and adolescents. Scientists are testing the effectiveness of combined pain coping skills (including age appropriate biofeedback, muscle relaxation techniques, imagery, activity pacing, and the use of calming techniques) and the drug amitriptyline in reducing headache frequency, intensity, and depressive symptoms in youth ages 10 to 17 years. Additional studies include the use of alternative approaches such as yoga to decrease headache in adolescents, a modified diet to treat chronic daily headache in teenagers, and programs designed to teach very young children how to understand and self-manage their headaches.

Craniosacral therapy (CST) involves gentle massaging of the neck, head, and spine to release constraints in tissue in the head and around the spine. Limited preliminary data shows significant, sustained benefit of CST in a small group of individuals with migraine. Future research will gather data on the usefulness of CST in preventing migraines and examine the feasibility of a larger, randomized trial.

Electrical stimulation of the occipital nerve has effectively eased the symptoms of painful chronic headache conditions such as cluster headache as well as hard to treat migraine in small clinical studies. A tiny battery-powered rechargeable electrode, surgically implanted near the occipital nerve, sends continuous energy pulses to the nerve to ease pain. The use of this non-drug treatment in reducing migraine frequency, intensity, and effect on quality of life is being tested in larger clinical trials.

Chapter 36

Memory Loss

Differences between mild forgetfulness and more serious memory problems

What is mild forgetfulness?

It is true that some of us get more forgetful as we age. It may take longer to learn new things, remember certain words, or find our glasses. These changes are often signs of mild forgetfulness, not serious memory problems.

See your doctor if you're worried about your forgetfulness. Tell him or her about your concerns. Be sure to make a follow-up appointment to check your memory in the next 6 months to a year. If you think you might forget, ask a family member, friend, or the doctor's office to remind you.

What can I do about mild forgetfulness?

You can do many things to help keep your memory sharp and stay alert. Look at the list below for some helpful ideas.

Text in this chapter is excerpted from "Understanding Memory Loss: What To Do When You Have Trouble Remembering," National Institute of Aging at National Institutes of Health (NIH), January 22, 2015.

Here are some ways to help your memory:

- Learn a new skill.
- Volunteer in your community, at a school, or at your place of worship.
- Spend time with friends and family.
- Use memory tools such as big calendars, to-do lists, and notes to yourself.
- Put your wallet or purse, keys, and glasses in the same place each day.
- Get lots of rest.
- Exercise and eat well.
- Don't drink a lot of alcohol.
- Get help if you feel depressed for weeks at a time.

What is a serious memory problem?

Serious memory problems make it hard to do everyday things. For example, you may find it hard to drive, shop, or even talk with a friend. Signs of serious memory problems may include:

- asking the same questions over and over again
- getting lost in places you know well
- not being able to follow directions
- becoming more confused about time, people, and places
- not taking care of yourself—eating poorly, not bathing, or being unsafe

What can I do about serious memory problems?

See your doctor if you are having any of the problems listed above. It's important to find out what might be causing a serious memory problem. Once you know the cause, you can get the right treatment.

Serious memory problems—causes and treatments

Many things can cause serious memory problems, such as blood clots, depression, and Alzheimer's disease. Read below to learn more about causes and treatments of serious memory problems.

Medical conditions

Certain medical conditions can cause serious memory problems. These problems should go away once you get treatment. Some medical conditions that may cause memory problems are:

- bad reaction to certain medicines
- depression
- not eating enough healthy foods, or too few vitamins and minerals in your body
- drinking too much alcohol
- blood clots or tumors in the brain
- head injury, such as a concussion from a fall or accident
- thyroid, kidney, or liver problems

Treatment for medical conditions

These medical conditions are serious. See your doctor for treatment.

Emotional problems

Some emotional problems in older people can cause serious memory problems. Feeling sad, lonely, worried, or bored can cause you to be confused and forgetful.

Treatment for emotional problems

You may need to see a doctor or counselor for treatment. Once you get help, your memory problems should get better.

Being active, spending more time with family and friends, and learning new skills also can help you feel better and improve your memory.

Mild cognitive impairment

As some people grow older, they have more memory problems than other people their age. This condition is called mild cognitive impairment, or MCI. People with MCI can take care of themselves and do their normal activities. MCI memory problems may include:

- losing things often
- forgetting to go to events and appointments
- having more trouble coming up with words than other people of the same age

Your doctor can do thinking, memory, and language tests to see if you have MCI. He or she also may suggest that you see a specialist for more tests. Because MCI may be an early sign of Alzheimer's disease, it's really important to see your doctor or specialist every 6 to 12 months. See below for more about Alzheimer's disease.

Treatment for MCI

At this time, there is no proven treatment for MCI. Your doctor can check to see if you have any changes in your memory or thinking skills over time.

You may want to try to keep your memory sharp. The list in the previous section suggests some ways to help your memory.

Alzheimer's disease

Alzheimer's disease causes serious memory problems. The signs of Alzheimer's disease begin slowly and get worse over time. This is because changes in the brain cause large numbers of brain cells to die.

It may look like simple forgetfulness at first, but over time, people with Alzheimer's disease have trouble thinking clearly. They find it hard to do everyday things like shopping, driving, and cooking. As the illness gets worse, people with Alzheimer's disease may need someone to take care of all their needs at home or in a nursing home. These needs may include feeding, bathing, and dressing.

Treatment for Alzheimer's disease

Taking certain medicines can help a person in the early or middle stages of Alzheimer's disease. These medicines can keep symptoms, such as memory loss, from getting worse for a time. The medicines can have side effects and may not work for everyone. Talk with your doctor about side effects or other concerns you may have.

Other medicines can help if you are worried, depressed, or having problems sleeping.

Vascular dementia

Many people have never heard of vascular dementia. Like Alzheimer's disease, it is a medical condition that causes serious memory problems. Unlike Alzheimer's disease, signs of vascular dementia may appear suddenly. This is because the memory loss and confusion are caused by small strokes or changes in the blood supply to the brain. If the strokes stop, you may get better or stay the same for a long time. If you have more strokes, you may get worse.

Treatment for vascular dementia

You can take steps to lower your chances of having more strokes. These steps include:

- Control your high blood pressure.
- Treat your high cholesterol.
- Take care of your diabetes.
- Stop smoking.

Help for serious memory problems

What can I do if I'm worried about my memory?

See your doctor. If your doctor thinks your memory problems are serious, you may need to have a complete health check-up. The doctor will review your medicines and may test your blood and urine. You also may need to take tests that check your memory, problem solving, counting, and language skills.

In addition, the doctor may suggest a brain scan. Pictures from the scan can show normal and problem areas in the brain. Once the doctor finds out what is causing your memory problems, ask about the best treatment for you.

What can family members do to help?

If your family member or friend has a serious memory problem, you can help the person live as normal a life as possible. You can help the person stay active, go places, and keep up every day routines. You can remind the person of the time of day, where he or she lives, and what is happening at home and in the world. You also can help the person remember to take medicine or visit the doctor.

Some families use the following things to help with memory problems:

- big calendars to highlight important dates and events
- lists of the plans for each day
- notes about safety in the home
- written directions for using common household items
  (most people with Alzheimer's disease can still read)

Chapter 37

Multiple Sclerosis (MS)

Introduction

Multiple Sclerosis (MS) is the most common disabling neurological disease of young adults. It most often appears when people are between 20 to 40 years old. However, it can also affect children and older people.

The course of MS is unpredictable. A small number of those with MS will have a mild course with little to no disability, while another smaller group will have a steadily worsening disease that leads to increased disability over time. Most people with MS, however, will have short periods of symptoms followed by long stretches of relative relief, with partial or full recovery. There is no way to predict, at the beginning, how an individual person's disease will progress.

Researchers have spent decades trying to understand why some people get MS and others don't, and why some individuals with MS have symptoms that progress rapidly while others do not. How does the disease begin? Why is the course of MS so different from person to person? Is there anything we can do to prevent it? Can it be cured?

This chapter includes information about why MS develops, how it progresses, and what new therapies are being used to treat its symptoms and slow its progression. New treatments can reduce long-term disability for many people with MS. However, there are still no cures and no clear ways to prevent MS from developing.

Text in this chapter is excerpted from "Multiple Sclerosis: Hope through Research," National Institute of Neurological Disorders and Stroke (NINDS), March 3, 2015.

What is Multiple Sclerosis?

Multiple sclerosis (MS) is a neuroinflammatory disease that affects myelin, a substance that makes up the membrane (called the myelin sheath) that wraps around nerve fibers (axons). Myelinated axons are commonly called white matter. Researchers have learned that MS also damages the nerve cell bodies, which are found in the brain's gray matter, as well as the axons themselves in the brain, spinal cord, and optic nerve (the nerve that transmits visual information from the eye to the brain). As the disease progresses, the brain's cortex shrinks (cortical atrophy).

The term multiple sclerosis refers to the distinctive areas of scar tissue (sclerosis or plaques) that are visible in the white matter of people who have MS. Plaques can be as small as a pinhead or as large as the size of a golf ball. Doctors can see these areas by examining the brain and spinal cord using a type of brain scan called magnetic resonance imaging (MRI).

While MS sometimes causes severe disability, it is only rarely fatal and most people with MS have a normal life expectancy.

What are plaques made of and why do they develop?

Plaques, or lesions, are the result of an inflammatory process in the brain that causes immune system cells to attack myelin. The myelin sheath helps to speed nerve impulses traveling within the nervous system. Axons are also damaged in MS, although not as extensively, or as early in the disease, as myelin.

Under normal circumstances, cells of the immune system travel in and out of the brain patrolling for infectious agents (viruses, for example) or unhealthy cells. This is called the "surveillance" function of the immune system.

Surveillance cells usually won't spring into action unless they recognize an infectious agent or unhealthy cells. When they do, they produce substances to stop the infectious agent. If they encounter unhealthy cells, they either kill them directly or clean out the dying area and produce substances that promote healing and repair among the cells that are left.

Researchers have observed that immune cells behave differently in the brains of people with MS. They become active and attack what appears to be healthy myelin. It is unclear what triggers this attack. MS is one of many autoimmune disorders, such as rheumatoid arthritis and lupus, in which the immune system mistakenly attacks a person's healthy tissue as opposed to performing its normal role of attacking foreign invaders like viruses and bacteria. Whatever the reason, during these periods of immune system activity, most of the myelin within the affected area is damaged or destroyed. The axons also may be damaged. The symptoms of MS depend on the severity of the immune reaction as well as the location and extent of the plaques, which primarily appear in the brain stem, cerebellum, spinal cord, optic nerves, and the white matter of the brain around the brain ventricles (fluid-filled spaces inside of the brain).

What are the signs and symptoms of MS?

The symptoms of MS usually begin over one to several days, but in some forms, they may develop more slowly. They may be mild or severe and may go away quickly or last for months. Sometimes the initial symptoms of MS are overlooked because they disappear in a day or so and normal function returns. Because symptoms come and go in the majority of people with MS, the presence of symptoms is called an attack, or in medical terms, an exacerbation. Recovery from symptoms is referred to as remission, while a return of symptoms is called a relapse. This form of MS is therefore called relapsing-remitting MS, in contrast to a more slowly developing form called primary progressive MS. Progressive MS can also be a second stage of the illness that follows years of relapsing-remitting symptoms.

A diagnosis of MS is often delayed because MS shares symptoms with other neurological conditions and diseases.

The first symptoms of MS often include:

- vision problems such as blurred or double vision or optic neuritis, which causes pain in the eye and a rapid loss of vision
- weak, stiff muscles, often with painful muscle spasms
- tingling or numbness in the arms, legs, trunk of the body, or face
- clumsiness, particularly difficulty staying balanced when walking
- bladder control problems, either inability to control the bladder or urgency
- dizziness that doesn't go away

MS may also cause later symptoms such as:

- mental or physical fatigue which accompanies the above symptoms during an attack

- mood changes such as depression or euphoria

- changes in the ability to concentrate or to multitask effectively

- difficulty making decisions, planning, or prioritizing at work or in private life

Some people with MS develop transverse myelitis, a condition caused by inflammation in the spinal cord. Transverse myelitis causes loss of spinal cord function over a period of time lasting from several hours to several weeks. It usually begins as a sudden onset of lower back pain, muscle weakness, or abnormal sensations in the toes and feet, and can rapidly progress to more severe symptoms, including paralysis. In most cases of transverse myelitis, people recover at least some function within the first 12 weeks after an attack begins. Transverse myelitis can also result from viral infections, arteriovenous malformations, or neuroinflammatory problems unrelated to MS. In such instances, there are no plaques in the brain that suggest previous MS attacks.

Neuro-myelitis optica is a disorder associated with transverse myelitis as well as optic nerve inflammation. Patients with this disorder usually have antibodies against a particular protein in their spinal cord, called the aquaporin channel. These patients respond differently to treatment than most people with MS.

Most individuals with MS have muscle weakness, often in their hands and legs. Muscle stiffness and spasms can also be a problem. These symptoms may be severe enough to affect walking or standing. In some cases, MS leads to partial or complete paralysis. Many people with MS find that weakness and fatigue are worse when they have a fever or when they are exposed to heat. MS exacerbations may occur following common infections.

Tingling and burning sensations are common, as well as the opposite, numbness and loss of sensation. Moving the neck from side to side or flexing it back and forth may cause "Lhermitte's sign," a characteristic sensation of MS that feels like a sharp spike of electricity coursing down the spine.

While it is rare for pain to be the first sign of MS, pain often occurs with optic neuritis and trigeminal neuralgia, a neurological disorder that affects one of the nerves that runs across the jaw, cheek, and face. Painful spasms of the limbs and sharp pain shooting down the legs or around the abdomen can also be symptoms of MS.

Most individuals with MS experience difficulties with coordination and balance at some time during the course of the disease. Some may have a continuous trembling of the head, limbs, and body, especially during movement, although such trembling is more common with other disorders such as Parkinson's disease.

Fatigue is common, especially during exacerbations of MS. A person with MS may be tired all the time or may be easily fatigued from mental or physical exertion.

Urinary symptoms, including loss of bladder control and sudden attacks of urgency, are common as MS progresses. People with MS sometimes also develop constipation or sexual problems.

Depression is a common feature of MS. A small number of individuals with MS may develop more severe psychiatric disorders such as bipolar disorder and paranoia, or experience inappropriate episodes of high spirits, known as euphoria.

People with MS, especially those who have had the disease for a long time, can experience difficulty with thinking, learning, memory, and judgment. The first signs of what doctors call cognitive dysfunction may be subtle. The person may have problems finding the right word to say, or trouble remembering how to do routine tasks on the job or at home. Day-to-day decisions that once came easily may now be made more slowly and show poor judgment. Changes may be so small or happen so slowly that it takes a family member or friend to point them out.

How many people have MS?

No one knows exactly how many people have MS. Experts think there are currently 250,000 to 350,000 people in the United States diagnosed with MS. This estimate suggests that approximately 200 new cases are diagnosed every week. Studies of the prevalence (the proportion of individuals in a population having a particular disease) of MS indicate that the rate of the disease has increased steadily during the twentieth century.

As with most autoimmune disorders, twice as many women are affected by MS as men. MS is more common in colder climates. People of Northern European descent appear to be at the highest risk for the disease, regardless of where they live. Native Americans of North and South America, as well as Asian American populations, have relatively low rates of MS.

What causes MS?

The ultimate cause of MS is damage to myelin, nerve fibers, and neurons in the brain and spinal cord, which together make up the central nervous system (CNS). But how that happens, and why, are questions that challenge researchers. Evidence appears to show that MS is a disease caused by genetic vulnerabilities combined with environmental factors.

Although there is little doubt that the immune system contributes to the brain and spinal cord tissue destruction of MS, the exact target of the immune system attacks and which immune system cells cause the destruction isn't fully understood.

Researchers have several possible explanations for what might be going on. The immune system could be:

- fighting some kind of infectious agent (for example, a virus) that has components which mimic components of the brain (molecular mimicry)

- destroying brain cells because they are unhealthy

- mistakenly identifying normal brain cells as foreign

The last possibility has been the favored explanation for many years. Research now suggests that the first two activities might also play a role in the development of MS. There is a special barrier, called the blood-brain barrier, which separates the brain and spinal cord from the immune system. If there is a break in the barrier, it exposes the brain to the immune system for the first time. When this happens, the immune system may misinterpret the brain as "foreign."

Genetic susceptibility

Susceptibility to MS may be inherited. Studies of families indicate that relatives of an individual with MS have an increased risk for developing the disease. Experts estimate that about 15 percent of individuals with MS have one or more family members or relatives who also have MS. But even identical twins, whose DNA is exactly the same, have only a 1 in 3 chance of both having the disease. This suggests that MS is not entirely controlled by genes. Other factors must come into play.

Current research suggests that dozens of genes and possibly hundreds of variations in the genetic code (called gene variants) combine to create vulnerability to MS. Some of these genes have been identified. Most of the genes identified so far are associated with functions of the immune system. Additionally, many of the known genes are similar to those that have been identified in people with other autoimmune diseases as type 1 diabetes, rheumatoid arthritis or lupus. Researchers continue to look for additional genes and to study how they interact with each other to make an individual vulnerable to developing MS.

Sunlight and vitamin D

A number of studies have suggested that people who spend more time in the sun and those with relatively high levels of vitamin D are less likely to develop MS. Bright sunlight helps human skin produce vitamin D. Researchers believe that vitamin D may help regulate the immune system in ways that reduce the risk of MS. People from regions near the equator, where there is a great deal of bright sunlight, generally have a much lower risk of MS than people from temperate areas such as the United States and Canada. Other studies suggest that people with higher levels of vitamin D generally have less severe MS and fewer relapses.

Smoking

A number of studies have found that people who smoke are more likely to develop MS. People who smoke also tend to have more brain lesions and brain shrinkage than non-smokers. The reasons for this are currently unclear.

Infectious factors and viruses

A number of viruses have been found in people with MS, but the virus most consistently linked to the development of MS is Epstein Barr virus (EBV), the virus that causes mononucleosis.

Only about 5 percent of the population has not been infected by EBV. These individuals are at a lower risk for developing MS than those who have been infected. People who were infected with EBV in adolescence or adulthood and who therefore develop an exaggerated immune response to EBV are at a significantly higher risk for developing MS than those who were infected in early childhood. This suggests that it may be the type of immune response to EBV that predisposes to MS, rather than EBV infection itself. However, there is still no proof that EBV causes MS.

Autoimmune and inflammatory processes

Tissue inflammation and antibodies in the blood that fight normal components of the body and tissue in people with MS are similar to those found in other autoimmune diseases. Along with overlapping evidence from genetic studies, these findings suggest that MS results from some kind of disturbed regulation of the immune system.

How is MS diagnosed?

There is no single test used to diagnose MS. Doctors use a number of tests to rule out or confirm the diagnosis. There are many other disorders that can mimic MS. Some of these other disorders can be cured, while others require different treatments than those used for MS. Therefore it is very important to perform a thorough investigation before making a diagnosis.

In addition to a complete medical history, physical examination, and a detailed neurological examination, a doctor will order an MRI scan of the head and spine to look for the characteristic lesions of MS. MRI is used to generate images of the brain and/or spinal cord. Then a special dye or contrast agent is injected into a vein and the MRI is repeated. In regions with active inflammation in MS, there is disruption of the blood-brain barrier and the dye will leak into the active MS lesion.

Doctors may also order evoked potential tests, which use electrodes on the skin and painless electric signals to measure how quickly and accurately the nervous system responds to stimulation. In addition, they may request a lumbar puncture (sometimes called a "spinal tap") to obtain a sample of cerebrospinal fluid. This allows them to look for proteins and inflammatory cells associated with the disease and to rule out other diseases that may look similar to MS, including some infections and other illnesses. MS is confirmed when positive signs of the disease are found in different parts of the nervous system at more than one time interval and there is no alternative diagnosis.

What is the course of MS?

The course of MS is different for each individual, which makes it difficult to predict. For most people, it starts with a first attack, usually (but not always) followed by a full to almost-full recovery. Weeks, months, or even years may pass before another attack occurs, followed again by a period of relief from symptoms. This characteristic pattern is called relapsing-remitting MS.

Primary-progressive MS is characterized by a gradual physical decline with no noticeable remissions, although there may be temporary or minor relief from symptoms. This type of MS has a later onset, usually after age 40, and is just as common in men as in women.

Secondary-progressive MS begins with a relapsing-remitting course, followed by a later primary-progressive course. The majority of individuals with severe relapsing-remitting MS will develop secondary progressive MS if they are untreated.

Finally, there are some rare and unusual variants of MS. One of these is Marburg variant MS (also called malignant MS), which causes a swift and relentless decline resulting in significant disability or even death shortly after disease onset. Balo's concentric sclerosis, which causes concentric rings of demyelination that can be seen on an MRI, is another variant type of MS that can progress rapidly.

Determining the particular type of MS is important because the current disease modifying drugs have been proven beneficial only for the relapsing-remitting types of MS.

What is an exacerbation or attack of MS?

An exacerbation—which is also called a relapse, flare-up, or attack—is a sudden worsening of MS symptoms, or the appearance of new symptoms that lasts for at least 24 hours. MS relapses are thought to be associated with the development of new areas of damage in the brain. Exacerbations are characteristic of relapsing-remitting MS, in which attacks are followed by periods of complete or partial recovery with no apparent worsening of symptoms.

An attack may be mild or its symptoms may be severe enough to significantly interfere with life's daily activities. Most exacerbations last from several days to several weeks, although some have been known to last for months.

When the symptoms of the attack subside, an individual with MS is said to be in remission. However, MRI data have shown that this is somewhat misleading because MS lesions continue to appear during these remission periods. Patients do not experience symptoms during remission because the inflammation may not be severe or it may occur in areas of the brain that do not produce obvious symptoms. Research suggests that only about 1 out of every 10 MS lesions is perceived by a person with MS. Therefore, MRI examination plays a very important role in establishing an MS diagnosis, deciding when the disease should be treated, and determining whether treatments work effectively or not. It also has been a valuable tool to test whether an experimental new therapy is effective at reducing exacerbations.

Are there treatments available for MS?

There is still no cure for MS, but there are treatments for initial attacks, medications and therapies to improve symptoms, and recently developed drugs to slow the worsening of the disease. These new drugs have been shown to reduce the number and severity of relapses and to delay the long term progression of MS.

Treatments for attacks

The usual treatment for an initial MS attack is to inject high doses of a steroid drug, such as methylprednisolone, intravenously (into a vein) over the course of 3 to 5 days. It may sometimes be followed by a tapered dose of oral steroids. Intravenous steroids quickly and potently suppress the immune system, and reduce inflammation. Clinical trials have shown that these drugs hasten recovery.

The American Academy of Neurology recommends using plasma exchange as a secondary treatment for severe flare-ups in relapsing forms of MS when the patient does not have a good response to methylprednisolone. Plasma exchange, also known as plasmapheresis, involves taking blood out of the body and removing components in the blood's plasma that are thought to be harmful. The rest of the blood, plus replacement plasma, is then transfused back into the body. This treatment has not been shown to be effective for secondary progressive or chronic progressive forms of MS.

Treatments to help reduce disease activity and progression

During the past 20 years, researchers have made major breakthroughs in MS treatment due to new knowledge about the immune system and the ability to use MRI to monitor MS in patients. As a result, a number of medical therapies have been found to reduce relapses in persons with relapsing-remitting MS. These drugs are called disease modulating drugs.

There is debate among doctors about whether to start disease modulating drugs at the first signs of MS or to wait until the course of the disease is better defined before beginning treatment. On one hand, U.S. Food and Drug Administration (FDA)-approved medications to treat MS work best early in the course of the disease and work poorly, if at all, later in the progressive phase of the illness. Clinical trials have shown convincingly that delaying treatment, even for the 1 to 2 years that it may take for patients with MS to develop a second clinical attack, may lead to an irreversible increase in disability. In addition, people who begin treatment after their first attack have fewer brain lesions and fewer relapses over time.

On the other hand, initiating treatment in patients with a single attack and no signs of previous MS lesions, before MS is diagnosed, poses risks because all FDA-approved medications to treat MS are associated with some side effects. Therefore, the best strategy is to have a thorough diagnostic work-up at the time of first attack of MS. The work-up should exclude all other diseases that can mimic MS so that the diagnosis can be determined with a high probability. The diagnostic tests may include an evaluation of the cerebrospinal fluid and repeated MRI examinations. If such a thorough work-up cannot confirm the diagnosis of MS with certainty, it may be prudent to wait before starting treatment. However, each patient should have a scheduled follow-up evaluation by his or her neurologist 6 to 12 months after the initial diagnostic evaluation, even in the absence of any new attacks of the disease. Ideally, this evaluation should include an MRI examination to see if any new MS lesions have developed without causing symptoms.

Until recently, it appeared that a minority of people with MS had very mild disease or "benign MS" and would never get worse or become disabled. This group makes up 10 to 20 percent of those with MS. Doctors were concerned about exposing such benign MS patients to the side effects of MS drugs. However, recent data from the long-term follow-up of these patients indicate that after 10 to 20 years, some of these patients become disabled. Therefore, current evidence supports discussing the start of therapy early with all people who have MS, as long as the MS diagnosis has been thoroughly investigated and confirmed. There is an additional small group of individuals (approximately 1 percent) whose course will progress so rapidly that they will require aggressive and perhaps even experimental treatment.

The current FDA-approved therapies for MS are designed to modulate or suppress the inflammatory reactions of the disease. They are most effective for relapsing-remitting MS at early stages of the disease. These treatments include injectable beta interferon drugs. Interferons are signaling molecules that regulate immune cells. Potential side effects of beta interferon drugs include flu-like symptoms, such as fever, chills, muscle aches, and fatigue, which usually fade with continued therapy. A few individuals will notice a decrease in the effectiveness of the drugs after 18 to 24 months of treatment due to the development of antibodies that neutralize the drugs' effectiveness. If the person has flare-ups or worsening symptoms, doctors may switch treatment to alternative drugs.

Glatiramer acetate is another injectable immune-modulating drug used for MS. Exactly how it works is not entirely clear, but research has shown that it changes the balance of immune cells in the body. Side effects with glatiramer acetate are usually mild, but it can cause skin reactions and allergic reactions. It is approved only for relapsing forms of MS.

The drug mitoxantrone, which is administered intravenously four times a year, has been approved for especially severe forms of relapsing-remitting and secondary progressive MS. This drug has been associated with development of certain types of blood cancers in up to one percent of patients, as well as with heart damage. Therefore, this drug should be used as a last resort to treat patients with a form of MS that leads to rapid loss of function and for whom other treatments did not stop the disease.

Natalizumab works by preventing cells of the immune system from entering the brain and spinal cord. It is administered intravenously once a month. It is a very effective drug for many people, but it is associated with an increased risk of a potentially fatal viral infection of the brain called progressive multifocal encephalopathy (PML). People who take natalizumab must be carefully monitored for symptoms of PML, which include changes in vision, speech, and balance that do not remit like an MS attack. Therefore, natalizumab is generally recommended only for individuals who have not responded well to the other approved MS therapies or who are unable to tolerate them. Other side effects of natalizumab treatment include allergic and hypersensitivity reactions.

In 2010, the FDA approved fingolimod, the first MS drug that can be taken orally as a pill, to treat relapsing forms of MS. The drug prevents white blood cells called lymphocytes from leaving the lymph nodes and entering the blood and the brain and spinal cord. The decreased number of lymphocytes in the blood can make people taking fingolimod more susceptible to infections. The drug may also cause problems with eyes and with blood pressure and heart rate. Because of this, the drug must be administered in a doctor's office for the first time and the treating physician must evaluate the patient's vision and blood pressure during an early follow-up examination. The exact frequency of rare side effects (such as severe infections) of fingolimod is unknown.

Other FDA-approved drugs to treat relapsing forms of MS in adults include dimethyl fumarate and teriflunomide, both taken orally.

How do doctors treat the symptoms of MS?

MS causes a variety of symptoms that can interfere with daily activities but which can usually be treated or managed to reduce their

Table 37.1. Disease Modifying Drugs

Trade Name	Generic Name
Avonex	interferon beta-1a
Betaseron	interferon beta-1b
Rebif	interferon beta-1a
Copaxone	glatiramer acetate
Tysabri	natalizumab
Novantrone	mitoxantrone
Gilenya	fingolimod

impact. Many of these issues are best treated by neurologists who have advanced training in the treatment of MS and who can prescribe specific medications to treat the problems.

Vision problems

Eye and vision problems are common in people with MS but rarely result in permanent blindness. Inflammation of the optic nerve or damage to the myelin that covers the optic nerve and other nerve fibers can cause a number of symptoms, including blurring or graying of vision, blindness in one eye, loss of normal color vision, depth perception, or a dark spot in the center of the visual field (scotoma).

Uncontrolled horizontal or vertical eye movements (nystagmus) and "jumping vision" (opsoclonus) are common to MS, and can be either mild or severe enough to impair vision.

Double vision (diplopia) occurs when the two eyes are not perfectly aligned. This occurs commonly in MS when a pair of muscles that control a specific eye movement aren't coordinated due to weakness in one or both muscles. Double vision may increase with fatigue or as the result of spending too much time reading or on the computer. Periodically resting the eyes may be helpful.

Weak muscles, stiff muscles, painful muscle spasms, and weak reflexes

Muscle weakness is common in MS, along with muscle spasticity. Spasticity refers to muscles that are stiff or that go into spasms without any warning. Spasticity in MS can be as mild as a feeling of tightness in the muscles or so severe that it causes painful, uncontrolled spasms. It can also cause pain or tightness in and around the joints. It also frequently affects walking, reducing the normal flexibility or "bounce" involved in taking steps.

Tremor

People with MS sometimes develop tremor, or uncontrollable shaking, often triggered by movement. Tremor can be very disabling. Assistive devices and weights attached to limbs are sometimes helpful for people with tremor. Deep brain stimulation& and drugs such as clonazepam also may be useful.

Problems with walking and balance

Many people with MS experience difficulty walking. In fact, studies indicate that half of those with relapsing-remitting MS will need some kind of help walking within 15 years of their diagnosis if they remain untreated. The most common walking problem in people with MS experience is ataxia—unsteady, uncoordinated movements—due to damage with the areas of the brain that coordinate movement of muscles. People with severe ataxia generally benefit from the use of a cane, walker, or other assistive device. Physical therapy can also reduce walking problems in many cases.

In 2010, the FDA approved the drug dalfampridine to improve walking in patients with MS. It is the first drug approved for this use. Clinical trials showed that patients treated with dalfampridine had faster walking speeds than those treated with a placebo pill.

Fatigue

Fatigue is a common symptom of MS and may be both physical (for example, tiredness in the legs) and psychological (due to depression). Probably the most important measures people with MS can take to counter physical fatigue are to avoid excessive activity and to stay out of the heat, which often aggravates MS symptoms. On the other hand, daily physical activity programs of mild to moderate intensity can significantly reduce fatigue. An antidepressant such as fluoxetine may be prescribed if the fatigue is caused by depression. Other drugs that may reduce fatigue in some individuals include amantadine and modafinil.

Fatigue may be reduced if the person receives occupational therapy to simplify tasks and/or physical therapy to learn how to walk in a way that saves physical energy or that takes advantage of an assistive device. Some people benefit from stress management programs, relaxation training, membership in an MS support group, or individual psychotherapy. Treating sleep problems and MS symptoms that interfere with sleep (such as spastic muscles) may also help.

Pain

People with MS may experience several types of pain during the course of the disease.

Trigeminal neuralgia is a sharp, stabbing, facial pain caused by MS affecting the trigeminal nerve as it exits the brainstem on its way to the jaw and cheek. It can be treated with anticonvulsant or antispasmodic drugs, alcohol injections, or surgery.

People with MS occasionally develop central pain, a syndrome caused by damage to the brain and/or spinal cord. Drugs such as gabapentin and nortriptyline sometimes help to reduce central pain.

Burning, tingling, and prickling (commonly called "pins and needles") are sensations that happen in the absence of any stimulation. The medical term for them is dysesthesias" They are often chronic and hard to treat.

Chronic back or other musculoskeletal pain may be caused by walking problems or by using assistive aids incorrectly. Treatments may include heat, massage, ultrasound treatments, and physical therapy to correct faulty posture and strengthen and stretch muscles.

Problems with bladder control and constipation

The most common bladder control problems encountered by people with MS are urinary frequency, urgency, or the loss of bladder control. The same spasticity that causes spasms in legs can also affect the bladder. A small number of individuals will have the opposite problem—retaining large amounts of urine. Urologists can help with treatment of bladder-related problems. A number of medical treatments are available. Constipation is also common and can be treated with a high-fiber diet, laxatives, and other measures.

Sexual issues

People with MS sometimes experience sexual problems. Sexual arousal begins in the central nervous system, as the brain sends messages to the sex organs along nerves running through the spinal cord. If MS damages these nerve pathways, sexual response—including arousal and orgasm—can be directly affected. Sexual problems may also stem from MS symptoms such as fatigue, cramped or spastic muscles, and psychological factors related to lowered self-esteem or depression. Some of these problems can be corrected with medications. Psychological counseling also may be helpful.

Depression

Studies indicate that clinical depression is more frequent among people with MS than it is in the general population or in persons with many other chronic, disabling conditions. MS may cause depression as part of the disease process, since it damages myelin and nerve fibers inside the brain. If the plaques are in parts of the brain that are involved in emotional expression and control, a variety of behavioral changes can result, including depression. Depression can intensify symptoms of fatigue, pain, and sexual dysfunction. It is most often treated with selective serotonin reuptake inhibitor (SSRI) antidepressant medications, which are less likely than other antidepressant medications to cause fatigue.

Inappropriate laughing or crying

MS is sometimes associated with a condition called pseudobulbar affect that causes inappropriate and involuntary expressions of laughter, crying, or anger. These expressions are often unrelated to mood; for example, the person may cry when they are actually very happy, or laugh when they are not especially happy. In 2010 the FDA approved the first treatment specifically for pseudobulbar affect, a combination of the drugs dextromethorphan and quinidine. The condition can also be treated with other drugs such as amitriptyline or citalopram.

Cognitive changes

Half to three-quarters of people with MS experience cognitive impairment, which is a phrase doctors use to describe a decline in the ability to think quickly and clearly and to remember easily. These cognitive changes may appear at the same time as the physical symptoms or they may develop gradually over time. Some individuals with MS may feel as if they are thinking more slowly, are easily distracted, have trouble remembering, or are losing their way with words. The right word may often seem to be on the tip of their tongue.

Some experts believe that it is more likely to be cognitive decline, rather than physical impairment, that causes people with MS to eventually withdraw from the workforce. A number of neuropsychological tests have been developed to evaluate the cognitive status of individuals with MS. Based on the outcomes of these tests, a neuropsychologist can determine the extent of strengths and weaknesses in different cognitive areas. Drugs such as donepezil, which is usually used for Alzheimer's disease, may be helpful in some cases.

Complementary and Alternative Therapies

Many people with MS use some form of complementary or alternative medicine. These therapies come from many disciplines, cultures, and traditions and encompass techniques as different as acupuncture, aromatherapy, ayurvedic medicine, touch and energy therapies, physical movement disciplines such as yoga and tai chi, herbal supplements, and biofeedback.

Because of the risk of interactions between alternative and more conventional therapies, people with MS should discuss all the therapies they are using with their doctor, especially herbal supplements. Although herbal supplements are considered "natural," they have biologically-active ingredients that could have harmful effects on their own or interact harmfully with other medications.

What research is being done?

Although researchers haven't been able to identify the cause of MS with any certainty, there has been excellent progress in other areas of MS research—especially in development of new treatments to prevent exacerbations of the disease. New discoveries are constantly changing treatment options for patients.

Some researchers are investigating promising avenues for therapeutics, such as drugs that would protect myelin cells from damage or that could help them recover after an attack. Interfering with the inflammatory cells and substances involved in the development of MS lesions or keeping immune-system cells from crossing the blood-brain barrier could potentially thwart an attack.

There are many new treatments that have been shown to prevent the formation of new MS lesions in small studies. These treatments are now being tested in a large number of MS patients in Phase III clinical trials. These include injectable drugs called rituximab, ocrelizumab, daclizumab, and alemtuzumab and oral drugs such as cladribine, laquinimod, teriflunomide, and fumaric acid. NINDS is also sponsoring a clinical trial to determine whether combining two therapies, glatiramer acetate and beta-interferon, is beneficial for preventing relapses.

Several studies have shown that destroying the immune system with chemotherapy and then replacing it with immune system stem cells obtained from the patient's own blood can halt development of new MS lesions. This treatment appears to reset the immune system so that it no longer attacks the brain. This strategy is being tested in clinical trials. Other studies are investigating whether transplanting stem cells derived from bone marrow, called mesenchymal stem cells, may be helpful in MS.

A 2009 study suggested that a condition called chronic cerebrospinal venous insufficiency (CCSVI), which results from abnormalities in veins leading from the brain, may contribute to the symptoms of MS. However, studies exploring a link between CCSVI and MS have been inconclusive. In 2012, the U.S. Food and Drug Administration (FDA) issued a warning that procedures to relieve CCSVI have been linked to serious complications, including strokes, cranial nerve damage, and death. Because the surgery is risky and the potential for benefit is highly uncertain, patients should only undergo the procedure as part of a properly controlled clinical study with appropriate safeguards and follow-up evaluations.

Other studies are trying to find ways to stop progression of the disease in MS patients with primary progressive MS or secondary progressive MS, and to restore neurological function in these individuals. Researchers are investigating whether symptoms that do not respond to FDA-approved immunomodulatory treatments may be caused by problems with the energy-producing parts of neuronal cells, called mitochondria. Investigators also are trying to develop ways to help brain cells called oligodendrocytes produce new myelin in order to strengthen or repair damaged cells of the brain and spinal cord.

Some experimental drugs can protect brain cells from dying or help brain cells produce new myelin in test tubes or animal models. However, in order to test these drugs as potential treatments in humans, researchers need accurate indicators, or biomarkers, so that the amount of neuronal cell death and cell repair, including remyelination, can be measured. These biomarkers would help to show whether an experimental treatment is working as intended. As the number of available treatment options for MS continues to grow, researchers are also trying to identify biomarkers that could help doctors determine whether or not an individual will respond well to any particular therapy, or, ideally, to select the optimal treatment for each person with MS. Other studies aim to develop better imaging tools to diagnose MS and test drugs.

Some researchers are working to develop improved animal models that closely resemble MS in humans. Currently available animal models share many of the same disease mechanisms and symptoms as MS, but they do not fully mimic the disease. This means that drugs that work well in animal models are often less successful in human clinical trials. Having a more accurate animal model would reduce the time and expense of testing therapies that may not prove to be successful in treating the human disease.

Research funded by the NINDS is also exploring the roles of "susceptibility genes"—genes that are associated with an increased risk for MS. Several candidate genes have been identified and researchers are studying their function in the nervous system to discover how they may lead to the development of MS. This information may help to develop drugs that work specifically on those genes (or on collections of multiple genes that work together) that are specifically affected in MS.

Chapter 38

Narcolepsy

What is narcolepsy?

Narcolepsy is a chronic brain disorder that involves poor control of sleep-wake cycles. People with narcolepsy experience periods of extreme daytime sleepiness and sudden, irresistible bouts of sleep that can strike at any time. These "sleep attacks" usually last a few seconds to several minutes.

Narcolepsy can greatly affect daily activities. People may unwillingly fall asleep while at work or at school, when having a conversation, playing a game, eating a meal, or, most dangerously, when driving or operating other types of machinery. In addition to daytime sleepiness, other major symptoms may include *cataplexy* (a sudden loss of voluntary muscle tone while awake that makes a person go limp or unable to move), vivid dream-like images or hallucinations, as well as total paralysis just before falling asleep or just after waking-up.

Contrary to common beliefs, people with narcolepsy do not spend a substantially greater proportion of their time asleep during a 24-hour period than do normal sleepers. In addition to daytime drowsiness and uncontrollable sleep episodes, most individuals also experience poor sleep quality that can involve frequent waking during nighttime sleep, and other sleep disorders.

Text in this chapter is excerpted from "Narcolepsy Fact Sheet," National Institute of Neurological Disorders and Stroke (NINDS), January 5, 2015.

For most adults, a normal night's sleep lasts about 8 hours and is composed of four to six separate sleep cycles. A sleep cycle is defined by a segment of non-rapid eye movement (NREM) sleep followed by a period of rapid eye movement (REM) sleep. The NREM segment can be further divided into increasingly deeper stages of sleep according to the size and frequency of brain waves. REM sleep is accompanied by bursts of rapid eye movement along with sharply heightened brain activity and temporary paralysis of the muscles that control posture and body movement. When subjects are awakened, they report that they were "having a dream" more often if they had been in REM sleep than if they had been in NREM sleep. Transitions from NREM to REM sleep are controlled by interactions among groups of neurons (nerve cells) located in different parts of the brain.

For normal sleepers a typical sleep cycle is about 100 to 110 minutes long, beginning with NREM sleep and transitioning to REM sleep after 80 to 100 minutes. People with narcolepsy frequently enter REM sleep within a few minutes of falling asleep.

Who gets narcolepsy?

Narcolepsy affects both males and female equally and appears throughout the world. Symptoms often start in childhood or adolescence, but can occur later in life. The condition is life-long. Narcolepsy is not rare, but it is an under-recognized and underdiagnosed condition. Narcolepsy with cataplexy is estimated to affect about one in every 3,000 Americans. More cases without cataplexy are also likely to exist.

What are the symptoms?

People with narcolepsy experience various types of day and nighttime sleep problems that are associated with REM sleep disturbances that tend to begin subtly and may change dramatically over time. The most common major symptom, other than excessive daytime sleepiness (EDS), is cataplexy, which occurs in about 70 percent of all people with narcolepsy. Sleep paralysis and hallucinations are somewhat less common. Only 10 to 25 percent of affected individuals, however, display all four of these major symptoms during the course of their illness.

Excessive daytime sleepiness (EDS)

EDS, the symptom most consistently experienced by almost all individuals with narcolepsy, is usually the first to become clinically apparent. Generally, EDS interferes with normal activities on a daily basis, whether or not individuals had sufficient sleep at night. People with EDS describe it as a persistent sense of mental cloudiness, a lack of energy, a depressed mood, or extreme exhaustion. Some people experience memory lapses, and many have great difficulty maintaining their concentration while at school, work, or home. People tend to awaken from such unavoidable sleeps feeling refreshed and finding that their drowsiness and fatigue subsides for an hour or two.

Involuntary sleep episodes are sometimes very brief, lasting no more than seconds at a time. As many as 40 percent of people with narcolepsy are prone to *automatic behavior* during such "microsleeps." Automatic behavior involves performing a task during a short period of sleep but without any apparent interruption. During these episodes, people are usually engaged in habitual, essentially "second nature" activities such as taking notes in class, typing, or driving. They cannot recall their actions, and their performance is almost always impaired. Their handwriting may, for example, degenerate into an illegible scrawl, or they may store items in bizarre locations and then forget where they placed them. If an episode occurs while driving, individuals may get lost or have an accident.

EDS, the most common of all narcoleptic symptoms, can be the result of a wide range of medical conditions, including other sleep disorders such as sleep apnea, various viral or bacterial infections, mood disorders such as depression, and chronic illnesses such as anemia, congestive heart failure, and rheumatoid arthritis that disrupt normal sleep patterns. Some medications can also lead to EDS, as can consumption of caffeine, alcohol, and nicotine. Finally, sleep deprivation has become one of the most common causes of EDS among Americans.

Cataplexy

Cataplexy is a sudden loss of muscle tone while the person is awake that leads to feelings of weakness and a loss of voluntary muscle control. Attacks can occur at any time during the waking period, with individuals usually experiencing their first episodes several weeks or months after the onset of EDS. But in about 10 percent of all cases, cataplexy is the first symptom to appear and can be misdiagnosed as a seizure disorder. Cataplectic attacks vary in duration and severity. The loss of muscle tone can be barely perceptible, involving no more than a momentary sense of slight weakness in a limited number of muscles, such as mild drooping of the eyelids. The most severe attacks result in a complete loss of tone in all voluntary muscles, leading to physical collapse during which individuals are unable to move, speak, or keep their eyes open. But even during the most severe episodes, people remain fully conscious, a characteristic that distinguishes cataplexy from seizure disorders. Although cataplexy can occur spontaneously, it is more often triggered by sudden, strong emotions such as fear, anger, stress, excitement, or humor. Laughter is reportedly the most common trigger.

The loss of muscle tone during a cataplectic episode resembles the interruption of muscle activity that naturally occurs during REM sleep. A group of neurons in the brain stem halts activity during REM sleep, inhibiting muscle movement. Using an animal model, scientists have learned that this same group of neurons becomes inactive during cataplectic attacks, a discovery that provides a clue to at least one of the neurological abnormalities contributing to human narcoleptic symptoms.

Sleep paralysis

The temporary inability to move or speak while falling asleep or waking is similar to REM-induced inhibitions of voluntary muscle activity. This natural inhibition usually goes unnoticed by people who experience normal sleep because it occurs only when they are fully asleep and entering the REM stage at the appropriate time in the sleep cycle. The attacks usually last a few seconds or minutes. Experiencing sleep paralysis resembles undergoing a cataplectic attack affecting the entire body. As with cataplexy, people remain fully conscious. Even when severe, cataplexy and sleep paralysis do not result in permanent dysfunction—after episodes end—people rapidly recover their full capacity to move and speak.

Hallucinations

Hallucinations can accompany sleep paralysis and occur when people are falling asleep, waking, or during sleep. Referred to as *hypnagogic* hallucinations when occurring during sleep onset and as *hypnopompic* hallucinations when occurring during waking, these images are unusually vivid, seem real, and can be frightening. Most often, the content is primarily visual, but any of the other senses can be involved.

Disrupted nocturnal sleep

While individuals with narcolepsy have no difficulties falling asleep at night, most experience difficulties staying asleep. Sleep may be disrupted by insomnia, vivid dreaming, sleep talking, acting out while dreaming, and periodic leg movements.

Obesity

After developing narcolepsy, many individuals suddenly gain weight, a side effect that can be prevented by active treatment.

When do symptoms appear?

In most cases, symptoms first appear when people are between the ages of 7 and 25. In rare cases, however, narcolepsy may appear at younger age or in older adults. If left undiagnosed and untreated, early onset narcolepsy can interfere with psychological, social, and cognitive function and development and can undermine academic and social activities.

What causes narcolepsy?

Narcolepsy may have several causes. Most people with narcolepsy have low levels of the neurotransmitter *hypocretin*, which promotes wakefulness. Neurotransmitters are chemicals that neurons produce to communicate with each other and to regulate biological processes.

Most cases of narcolepsy are sporadic, meaning the disorder occurs in individuals with no known family history of the disorder. But clusters in families sometimes occur—up to 10 percent of individuals diagnosed with narcolepsy with cataplexy report having a close relative with the same symptoms. In extremely rare cases, narcolepsy is caused by a genetic defect that prevents normal production of hypocretin molecules. While close relatives of people with narcolepsy have a statistically higher risk of developing the disorder than do members of the general population, that risk remains low when compared to diseases that are purely genetic in origin.

When cataplexy is present, the cause is most often the discrete loss of brain cells that produce hypocretin. Although the reason for such cell loss remains unknown, it appears to be autoimmune in nature (an autoimmune disorder is when the body's immune system mistakenly attacks healthy cells or tissue). That is, the body's immune system selectively attacks hypocretin-containing brain cells.

Other factors appear to play important roles in the development of narcolepsy. Some rare cases are known to result from traumatic injuries to parts of the brain involved in REM sleep or from tumor growth and other disease processes in the same regions. Infections, exposure to toxins, dietary factors, stress, hormonal changes such as those occurring during puberty or menopause, and alterations in a person's sleep schedule are just a few of the many factors that may exert direct or indirect effects on the brain, thereby possibly contributing to disease development.

How is narcolepsy diagnosed?

A clinical examination and exhaustive medical history are essential for diagnosis and treatment. Your doctor may ask you to keep a sleep journal noting the times of sleep and symptoms over a one to two week period. Although none of the major symptoms is exclusive to narcolepsy, cataplexy is the most specific symptom and is rarely present outside of narcolepsy.

A physical exam can rule out or identify a condition that may be causing the symptoms. A battery of specialized tests, which can be performed in a sleep disorders clinic, is usually required before a diagnosis can be confirmed.

Two tests in particular are essential in confirming a diagnosis of narcolepsy: the polysomnogram (PSG) and the multiple sleep latency test (MSLT). The PSG is an overnight test that takes continuous multiple measurements while the individual is asleep to document abnormalities in the sleep cycle. It records heart and respiratory rates, electrical activity in the brain using electroencephalography, and nerve activity in muscles through electromyography. A PSG can help reveal whether REM sleep occurs at abnormal times in the sleep cycle and can rule out the possibility that an individual's symptoms result from another condition.

The MSLT is performed during the day to measure a person's tendency to fall asleep and to determine whether isolated elements of REM sleep intrude at inappropriate times during the waking hours. The sleep latency test measures the amount of time it takes for a person to fall asleep. As part of the test, an individual is asked to take four or five short naps usually scheduled 2 hours apart over the course of a day. Because sleep latency periods are normally 12 minutes or longer, a latency period of 8 minutes or less suggests a disorder of excessive daytime sleepiness. However, a sleep latency of 8 minutes or less can be due to many conditions other than narcolepsy. The MSLT also measures heart and respiratory rates, records nerve activity in muscles, and pinpoints the occurrence of abnormally timed REM episodes through EEG recordings. If a person enters REM sleep either at the beginning or within a few minutes of sleep onset during at least two of the scheduled naps, this is considered an indication of narcolepsy. Other reasons for REM sleep on the MSLT must be ruled out, such as the effects of medication and disrupted sleep from sleep apnea or an irregular work-rest schedule.

In some cases, human leukocyte antigen (HLA) typing (a marker of viral infection) may be helpful. Most HLA-associated disorders are autoimmune in nature. Certain alleles (genetic information found on a specific location on specific chromosomes) located on chromosome 6 are strongly associated with narcolepsy-cataplexy. To definitively identify a lack of hypocretin as the cause of narcolepsy, a sample of the cerebrospinal fluid (CSF) is removed by using a lumbar puncture and the level of hypocretin-1 is measured. When no other serious medical condition is present, low CSF hypocretin-1 can establish hypocretin deficiency as the cause of narcolepsy.

When cataplexy is not present, diagnosis must be made after excluding other possible causes of daytime sleepiness and fatigue, along with a positive MSLT.

What treatments are available?

Narcolepsy cannot yet be cured, but some of the symptoms can be treated with medicines and lifestyle changes. When cataplexy is present, the loss of hypocretin is believed to be irreversible and life-long. But EDS and cataplexy can be controlled in most individuals with drug treatment. Modafinil and sodium oxybate are two drugs that have been approved by the U.S. Food and Drug Administration for the treatment of narcolepsy.

Doctors prescribe central nervous system alerting agents such as modafinil and amphetamine-like stimulants such as methylphenidate to alleviate EDS and reduce the incidence of sleep attacks. For most people these medications are generally quite effective at reducing daytime drowsiness and improving levels of alertness. However, use of these medications may be associated with several undesirable side effects and must be carefully monitored. Common side effects include irritability and nervousness, shakiness, disturbances in heart rhythm, stomach upset, nighttime sleep disruption, and anorexia. Individuals may also develop tolerance with long-term use, leading to the need for increased dosages to maintain effectiveness. In addition, doctors should be careful when prescribing these drugs and people should be careful using them because the potential for abuse is high with any amphetamine.

Two classes of antidepressant drugs have proved effective in controlling cataplexy in many individuals: tricyclics (including imipramine, desipramine, clomipramine, and protriptyline) and selective serotonin and noradrenergic reuptake inhibitors (including venlafaxine, fluoxetine and atomoxetine). In general, antidepressants produce fewer adverse effects than do amphetamines. But troublesome side effects still occur in some individuals, including impotence, high blood pressure, and heart rhythm irregularities.

In addition to central nervous system alerting agents and antidepressants, sodium oxybate or gamma hydroxybutyrate, also known as GHB or Xyrem®, can be used to treat narcolepsy. Sodium oxybate is a strong sedative that must be taken during the night. Sodium oxybate induces sleep and reduces the symptoms of daytime sleepiness and cataplexy. Due to safety concerns associated with the use of this drug, the distribution of sodium oxybate is tightly restricted.

What behavioral strategies help people cope with symptoms?

Currently available medications do not enable all people with narcolepsy to consistently maintain a fully normal state of alertness. Drug therapy should accompany various behavioral strategies according to the needs of the affected individual.

Many individuals take short, regularly scheduled naps at times when they tend to feel sleepiest.

Improving the quality of nighttime sleep can combat EDS and help relieve persistent feelings of fatigue. Among the most important common-sense measures people can take to enhance sleep quality are:

- maintain a regular sleep schedule-go to bed and wake up at the same time every day
- avoid alcohol and caffeine-containing beverages for several hours before bedtime
- avoid large, heavy meals just before bedtime
- avoid smoking, especially at night
- maintain a comfortable, adequately warmed bedroom environment, and
- engage in relaxing activities such as a warm bath before bedtime

Exercising for at least 20 minutes per day at least 4 or 5 hours before bedtime also improves sleep quality and can help people with narcolepsy avoid gaining excess weight.

Safety precautions, particularly when driving, are particularly important for all persons with narcolepsy. EDS and cataplexy can lead to serious injury or death if left uncontrolled. Suddenly falling asleep or losing muscle control can transform actions that are ordinarily safe, such as walking down a long flight of stairs, into hazards. People with untreated narcoleptic symptoms are involved in automobile accidents roughly 10 times more frequently than the general population. However, accident rates are normal among individuals who have received appropriate medication.

Support groups frequently prove extremely beneficial because people with narcolepsy may become socially isolated due to embarrassment about or misunderstandings related to their symptoms. Many people also try to avoid strong emotions, since humor, excitement, and other intense feelings can trigger cataplectic attacks. Support groups also provide individuals with a network of social contacts who can offer practical help and emotional support.

The Americans with Disabilities Act requires employers to provide reasonable accommodations for all employees with disabilities. Adults can often negotiate with employers to modify their work schedules so they can take naps when necessary and perform their most demanding tasks when they are most alert. Similarly, children and adolescents with narcolepsy may be able to work with school administrators regarding special needs, including medication requirements during the school day, and to modify class schedules.

What is the state of the science involving narcolepsy?

During the past decade, scientists have made considerable progress in understanding narcolepsy-cataplexy pathogenesis and in identifying genes strongly associated with the disorder. The majority of people diagnosed with narcolepsy and cataplexy are known to have a specific HLA gene variant called DQB1*0602. They also frequently have specific alleles at a gene called the T-cell receptor alpha (TCRA), a protein on T cells that recognize HLA proteins. However, some people with narcolepsy-cataplexy do not have the variant genes, while many people in the general population without narcolepsy do possess these variant genes. Specific variations in HLA and TCRA genes increase an individual's predisposition to develop the disorders—possibly through a yet-undiscovered route involving changes in immune-system function—when other causative factors are present.

Many other genes besides those making up the HLA complex and the T-cell receptor may contribute to the development of narcolepsy.

Groups of neurons in several parts of the brain stem and the central brain, including the thalamus and hypothalamus, interact to control sleep. Large numbers of genes on different chromosomes control these neurons' activities, any of which could contribute to the development of the disease. Scientists studying narcolepsy in dogs have identified a mutation that appears to cause the disorder in Dobermans, Labradors, and Dachshunds. This mutated gene disrupts the ability to receive the signal from hypocretins (also known as orexins) that are produced by neurons located in the hypothalamus. The neurons that produce hypocretins are active during wakefulness, and research suggests that they keep the brain systems needed for wakefulness from shutting down unexpectedly. Mice born without functioning hypocretin genes develop symptoms of narcolepsy.

Except in rare cases, narcolepsy in humans is not associated with mutations of the hypocretin gene. However, scientists have found that brains from humans with narcolepsy often contain greatly reduced numbers of hypocretin-producing neurons. It is believed that certain HLA and TCR subtypes increase susceptibility to an immune attack on hypocretin neurons in the hypothalamus, leading to degeneration of these important cells. Other factors also may interfere with proper functioning of this system. The hypocretins regulate appetite and feeding behavior in addition to controlling sleep. Therefore, the loss of hypocretin-producing neurons may explain not only how narcolepsy develops in some people, but also why people with narcolepsy have higher rates of obesity compared to the general population.

Narcolepsy onset follows a seasonal pattern of higher rates in spring and early summer, following winter upper airway infection season. When studied close to disease onset, individuals with narcolepsy have high levels of antibodies to a marker called ASO, indicating response to a recent bacterial infection such as strep throat. In addition, there is growing evidence that exposure to H1N1 virus (also called swine flu), or a special form of H1N1 vaccine (administered in Europe) can act as a rare trigger for the disease. It is not yet known if these infectious agents are direct triggers for the disease, or whether they increase likelihood of disease indirectly.

What research is being done?

Within the Federal government, the National Institute of Neurological Disorders and Stroke (NINDS), a component of the National Institutes of Health (NIH), has primary responsibility for sponsoring research on neurological disorders. As part of its mission, the NINDS supports research on narcolepsy and other sleep disorders through grants to medical institutions across the country.

Within the National Heart, Lung, and Blood Institute, also a component of the NIH, the National Center on Sleep Disorders Research (NCSDR) coordinates Federal government sleep research activities, promotes doctoral and postdoctoral training programs, and educates the public and health care professionals about sleep disorders.

NINDS-sponsored researchers are conducting studies devoted to further clarifying the wide range of genetic factors—both HLA genes and non-HLA genes—that may cause narcolepsy. Other scientists are conducting investigations using animal models to identify neurotransmitters other than the hypocretins that may contribute to disease development. A greater understanding of the complex genetic and biochemical bases of narcolepsy will eventually lead to the formulation of new therapies to control symptoms and may lead to a cure. Researchers are also investigating the modes of action of wake-promoting compounds to widen the range of available therapeutic options.

Abnormal immunological processes may be an important element in the cause of narcolepsy. NINDS-sponsored scientists have demonstrated the presence of unusual, possibly pathological, forms of immunological activity in narcolepsy. Further, strep throat is now suggested to be involved as a trigger in some predisposed individuals. These researchers are now investigating whether drugs that suppress immunological processes may interrupt the development of narcolepsy.

Finally, the NINDS continues to support investigations into the basic biology of sleep, including the brain mechanisms involved in generating and regulating REM sleep. A more comprehensive understanding of the complex biology of sleep will undoubtedly further clarify the pathological processes that underlie narcolepsy and other sleep disorders.

Chapter 39

Peripheral Neuropathy

What is peripheral neuropathy?

An estimated 20 million people in the United States have some form of peripheral neuropathy, a condition that develops as a result of damage to the peripheral nervous system—the vast communications network that transmits information between the central nervous system (the brain and spinal cord) and every other part of the body. (Neuropathy means nerve disease or damage.) Symptoms can range from numbness or tingling, to pricking sensations (paresthesia), or muscle weakness. Areas of the body may become abnormally sensitive leading to an exaggeratedly intense or distorted experience of touch (allodynia). In such cases, pain may occur in response to a stimulus that does not normally provoke pain. Severe symptoms may include burning pain (especially at night), muscle wasting, paralysis, or organ or gland dysfunction. Damage to nerves that supply internal organs may impair digestion, sweating, sexual function, and urination. In the most extreme cases, breathing may become difficult, or organ failure may occur.

Peripheral nerves send sensory information back to the brain and spinal cord, such as a message that the feet are cold. Peripheral nerves also carry signals from the brain and spinal cord to the muscles to

---

Text in this chapter is excerpted from "Peripheral Neuropathy Fact Sheet," National Institute of Neurological Disorders and Stroke (NINDS), February 23, 2015.

generate movement. Damage to the peripheral nervous system interferes with these vital connections. Like static on a telephone line, peripheral neuropathy distorts and sometimes interrupts messages between the brain and spinal cord and the rest of the body.

Peripheral neuropathies can present in a variety of forms and follow different patterns. Symptoms may be experienced over a period of days, weeks, or years. They can be acute or chronic. In acute neuropathies such as Guillain-Barré syndrome (in which the body's immune system attacks part of the peripheral nervous system and impairs sending and receiving nerve signals), symptoms appear suddenly, progress rapidly, and resolve slowly as damaged nerves heal. In chronic forms, symptoms begin subtly and progress slowly. Some people may have periods of relief followed by relapse. Others may reach a plateau stage where symptoms stay the same for many months or years. Many chronic neuropathies worsen over time. Although neuropathy may be painful and potentially debilitating, very few forms are fatal.

In diabetic neuropathy, one of the most common forms of peripheral neuropathy, nerve damage occurs in an ascending pattern. The first nerve fibers to malfunction are the ones that travel the furthest from the brain and the spinal cord. Pain and numbness often are felt symmetrically in both feet followed by a gradual progression up both legs. Later, the fingers, hands, and arms may become affected.

How are the peripheral neuropathies classified?

More than 100 types of peripheral neuropathy have been identified, each with its own symptoms and prognosis. In general, peripheral neuropathies are classified according to the type of damage to the nerves. Some forms of neuropathy involve damage to only one nerve and are called mononeuropathies. More frequently, however, multiple nerves are affected, called polyneuropathy.

Some peripheral neuropathies are due to damage to the axons (the long, threadlike portion of the nerve cell), while others are due to damage to the myelin sheath, the fatty protein that coats and insulates the axon. Peripheral neuropathies may also be caused by a combination of both axonal damage and demyelination. Electrodiagnostic studies can help healthcare providers determine the type of damage involved.

What are the symptoms of peripheral nerve damage?

Symptoms vary depending on whether motor, sensory, or autonomic nerves are damaged. Motor nerves control voluntary movement of muscles such as those used for walking, grasping things, or talking. Sensory nerves transmit information such as the feeling of a light touch or the pain from a cut. Autonomic nerves control organ activities that are regulated automatically such as breathing, digesting food, and heart and gland functions. Some neuropathies may affect all three types of nerves; others primarily affect one or two types. Doctors may use terms such as predominantly motor neuropathy, predominantly sensory neuropathy, sensory-motor neuropathy, or autonomic neuropathy to describe the types of nerves involved in an individual's condition.

Motor nerve damage is most commonly associated with muscle weakness. Other symptoms may include painful cramps and fasciculations (uncontrolled muscle twitching visible under the skin), muscle atrophy (severe shrinkage of muscle size), and decreased reflexes.

Sensory nerve damage causes a variety of symptoms because sensory nerves have a broad range of functions. Larger sensory fibers enclosed in myelin register vibration, light touch, and position sense. Damage to large sensory fibers impairs touch, resulting in a general decrease in sensation. Since this is felt most in the hands and feet, people may feel as if they are wearing gloves and stockings even when they are not. This damage to larger sensory fibers may contribute to the loss of reflexes. Loss of position sense often makes people unable to coordinate complex movements like walking or fastening buttons, or to maintain their balance when their eyes are shut.

Smaller sensory fibers without myelin sheaths transmit pain and temperature sensations. Damage to these fibers can interfere with the ability to feel pain or changes in temperature. People may fail to sense that they have been injured from a cut or that a wound is becoming infected. Others may not detect pain that warns of impending heart attack or other acute conditions. Loss of pain sensation is a particularly serious problem for people with diabetes, contributing to the high rate of lower limb amputations among this population.

Neuropathic pain is a common, often difficult to control symptom of sensory nerve damage and can seriously affect emotional well-being and overall quality of life. Often worse at night, neuropathic pain seriously disrupts sleep and adds to the emotional burden of sensory nerve damage. Neuropathic pain can often be associated with an over-sensitization of pain receptors in the skin, so that people feel severe pain (allodynia) from stimuli that are normally painless. For example, some may experience pain from bed sheets draped lightly over the body. Over many years, sensory neuropathy may lead to changes in the skin, hair, as well as to joint and bone damage. Unrecognized injuries due to poor sensation contribute to these changes, so it is important for people with neuropathy to inspect numb areas for injury or damage.

Autonomic nerve damage symptoms are diverse since the parasympathetic and sympathetic nerves of the peripheral nervous system control nearly every organ in the body. Common symptoms of autonomic nerve damage include an inability to sweat normally, which may lead to heat intolerance; a loss of bladder control; and an inability to control muscles that expand or contract blood vessels to regulate blood pressure. A drop in blood pressure when a person moves suddenly from a seated to a standing position (a condition known as postural or orthostatic hypotension) may result in dizziness, lightheadedness, or fainting. Irregular heartbeats may also occur.

Gastrointestinal symptoms may accompany autonomic neuropathy. Malfunction of nerves controlling intestinal muscle contractions can lead to diarrhea, constipation, or incontinence. Many people also have problems eating or swallowing if autonomic nerves controlling these functions are affected.

What causes peripheral neuropathy?

Peripheral neuropathy may be either inherited or acquired through disease processes or trauma. In many cases, however, a specific cause cannot be identified. Doctors usually refer to neuropathies with no known cause as idiopathic.

Causes of acquired peripheral neuropathy include:

Physical injury (trauma) is the most common cause of acquired nerve injury.

- *Injury or sudden trauma,* such as from automobile accidents, falls, sports-related activities, and surgical procedures can cause nerves to be partially or completely severed, crushed, compressed, or stretched, sometimes so forcefully that they are partially or completely detached from the spinal cord. Less severe traumas also can cause serious nerve damage. Broken or dislocated bones can exert damaging pressure on neighboring nerves.

- *Repetitive stress* frequently leads to entrapment neuropathies, a form of compression injury. Cumulative damage can result from repetitive, awkward, and/or forceful activities that require movement of any group of joints for prolonged periods.

The resulting irritation may cause ligaments, tendons, and muscles to become inflamed and swollen, constricting the narrow passageways through which some nerves pass. Ulnar neuropathy and carpal tunnel syndrome are examples of the most common types of neuropathy from trapped or compressed nerves at the elbow or wrist.

Diseases or disorders and their related processes (such as inflammation) can be associated with peripheral neuropathy.

- *Metabolic and endocrine disorders* impair the body's ability to transform nutrients into energy and process waste products, and this can lead to nerve damage. Diabetes mellitus, characterized by chronically high blood glucose levels, is a leading cause of peripheral neuropathy in the United States. About 60 percent to 70 percent of people with diabetes have mild to severe forms of nervous system damage that can affect sensory, motor, and autonomic nerves and present with varied symptoms. Some metabolic liver diseases also lead to neuropathies as a result of chemical imbalances. Endocrine disorders that lead to hormonal imbalances can disturb normal metabolic processes and cause neuropathies. For example, an underproduction of thyroid hormones slows metabolism, leading to fluid retention and swollen tissues that can exert pressure on peripheral nerves. Overproduction of growth hormone can lead to acromegaly, a condition characterized by the abnormal enlargement of many parts of the skeleton, including the joints. Nerves running through these affected joints often become entrapped, causing pain.

- *Small vessel disease* can decrease oxygen supply to the peripheral nerves and lead to serious nerve tissue damage. Diabetes frequently leads to impaired blood flow to nerves. Various forms of vasculitis (blood vessel inflammation) frequently cause vessel walls to harden, thicken, and develop scar tissue, decreasing their diameter and impeding blood flow. Vasculitis is an example of nerve damage called mononeuritis multiplex or multifocal mononeuropathy, in which isolated nerves in two or more areas are damaged.

- *Autoimmune diseases,* in which the immune system attacks the body's own tissues, can lead to nerve damage. Sjogren's syndrome, lupus, and rheumatoid arthritis are among the autoimmune diseases that can be associated with peripheral neuropathy. When the tissue surrounding nerves becomes inflamed, the inflammation can spread directly into nerve fibers. Over time, these chronic autoimmune conditions can destroy joints, organs, and connective tissues, making nerve fibers more vulnerable to compression injuries and entrapment. Chronic conditions may alternate between remission and relapse. Acute inflammatory demyelinating neuropathy, better known as Guillain- Barré syndrome, can damage motor, sensory, and autonomic nerve fibers.

- Most people recover from this autoimmune syndrome although severe cases can be life threatening. Chronic inflammatory demyelinating polyneuropathy (CIDP) usually damages sensory and motor nerves, leaving autonomic nerves intact. Multifocal motor neuropathy is a form of inflammatory neuropathy that affects motor nerves exclusively. It may be chronic or acute.

- *Kidney disorders* may cause neuropathies. Kidney dysfunction can lead to abnormally high amounts of toxic substances in the blood that can damage nerve tissue. A majority of individuals who require dialysis because of kidney failure develop polyneuropathy.

- *Cancers* can infiltrate nerve fibers or exert damaging compression forces on nerve fibers. Tumors also can arise directly from nerve tissue cells. Paraneoplastic syndromes, a group of rare degenerative disorders that are triggered by a person's immune system response to a cancerous tumor, also can indirectly cause widespread nerve damage. Toxicity from the chemotherapeutic agents and radiation used to treat cancer also can cause peripheral neuropathy. An estimated 30 to 40 percent of people who undergo chemotherapy develop peripheral neuropathy and it is a leading reason why people with cancer stop chemotherapy early. The severity of chemotherapy-induced peripheral neuropathy (CIPN) varies from person to person. In some cases people may be able to ease their symptoms by lowering their chemotherapy dose or by stopping it temporarily. In others, CIPN may persist long after stopping chemotherapy.

- *Neuromas* are benign tumors that are caused by an overgrowth of nerve tissue that develops after a penetrating injury that severs nerve fibers. Neuromas are often associated with intense pain and sometimes they engulf neighboring nerves, leading to further damage and even greater pain. Neuroma formation can be one element of a more widespread neuropathic pain condition called complex regional pain syndrome or reflex sympathetic dystrophy syndrome, which can be caused by traumatic injuries or surgical trauma. Widespread polyneuropathy is often associated with neurofibromatosis, a genetic disorder in which multiple benign tumors grow on nerve tissue.

- *Infections* can cause peripheral neuropathy. Viruses and bacteria that can attack nerve tissues include herpes varicella zoster (shingles), Epstein-Barr virus, West Nile virus, cytomegalovirus, and herpes simplex members of the large family of human herpes viruses. These viruses can severely damage sensory nerves, causing attacks of sharp, lightning-like pain. Postherpetic neuralgia is long-lasting, particularly intense pain that often occurs after an attack of shingles. Lyme disease, diphtheria, and leprosy are bacterial diseases characterized by extensive peripheral nerve damage. Diphtheria and leprosy are rare in the United States, but the incidence of Lyme disease is on the rise.

- The tick-borne infection can involve a wide range of neuropathic disorders, including a rapidly developing, painful polyneuropathy, often within a few weeks of being infected. West Nile virus is spread by mosquitoes and is associated with a severe motor neuropathy. The inflammation triggered by infection sometimes results in various forms of inflammatory neuropathies that develop quickly or slowly.

- The human immunodeficiency virus (HIV) that causes AIDS is associated with several different forms of neuropathy, depending on the nerves affected and the specific stage of active immunodeficiency disease. A rapidly progressive, painful polyneuropathy affecting the feet and hands can be the first clinically apparent symptom of HIV infection. An estimated 30 percent of people who are HIV positive develop peripheral neuropathy; 20 percent develop distal neuropathic pain.

Exposure to toxins may damage nerves and cause peripheral neuropathy.

- *Medication toxicity* can be caused by many agents in addition to those for fighting cancer. Other agents that commonly cause peripheral neuropathy as a side effect include those used to fight infection such as antiretroviral agents for treating HIV. In addition, anticonvulsant agents and some heart and blood pressure medications can commonly cause peripheral neuropathy.

In most cases, the neuropathy resolves when these medications are discontinued or dosages are adjusted.

- *Environmental or industrial toxins* such as lead, mercury, and arsenic can cause peripheral neuropathy. In addition, certain insecticides and solvents have also been known to cause neuropathies.

- *Heavy alcohol consumption* is a common cause of peripheral neuropathy. Damage to the nerves associated with long-term alcohol abuse may not be reversible when a person stops drinking alcohol, however, doing so may provide some symptom relief and prevent further damage. Chronic alcohol abuse also frequently leads to nutritional deficiencies (including B12, thiamine, and folate) that contribute to the development of peripheral neuropathy.

Genetic mutations can either be inherited or arise de novo, meaning they are completely new mutations to an individual and are not passed along by either parent. Some genetic mutations lead to mild neuropathies with symptoms that begin in early adulthood and result in little, if any, significant impairment. More severe hereditary neuropathies often appear in infancy or childhood.

Advances in genetic testing in the last decade have led to significant strides in the ability to identify the genetic causes underlying peripheral neuropathies. For example, several genes have been found to play a role in different types of Charcot-Marie-Tooth, a group of disorders that are among the most common forms of inherited peripheral neuropathies. These neuropathies result from mutations in genes responsible for maintaining the health of the myelin sheath as well as the axons themselves. Key characteristics of Charcot-Marie-Tooth disorders include extreme weakening and wasting of muscles in the lower legs and feet, gait abnormalities, loss of tendon reflexes, and numbness in the lower limbs.

How is peripheral neuropathy diagnosed?

The symptoms of peripheral neuropathy are highly variable. A thorough neurological examination is required to sort out the cause of the symptoms and involves taking an extensive medical history (covering symptoms, work environment, social habits, exposure to toxins, alcohol use, risk of HIV or other infectious diseases, and family history of neurological diseases). In addition, tests are usually performed to identify the cause of the neuropathy as well as the extent and type of nerve damage.

A physical examination and various tests may reveal the presence of a systemic disease causing the nerve damage. Tests of muscle strength, as well as evidence of cramps or fasciculations, indicate motor fiber involvement. Evaluation of the person's ability to sense vibration, light touch, body position, temperature, and pain reveals any sensory nerve damage and may indicate whether small or large sensory nerve fibers are affected.

Blood tests can detect diabetes, vitamin deficiencies, liver or kidney dysfunction, other metabolic disorders, and signs of abnormal immune system activity. An examination of cerebrospinal fluid that surrounds the brain and spinal cord can reveal abnormal antibodies associated with some immune-mediated neuropathies. More specialized tests may reveal other blood or cardiovascular diseases, connective tissue disorders, or malignancies. Genetic tests are becoming available for a number of the inherited neuropathies.

Based on the results of the neurological exam, physical exam, patient history, and any previous screening or testing, the following additional tests may be ordered to help determine the nature and extent of the neuropathy:

- *Nerve conduction velocity (NCV)* tests can measure the degree of damage in large nerve fibers, revealing whether symptoms are caused by degeneration of the myelin sheath or the axon. The myelin covering is responsible for the very fast speed of nerve conduction. During this test, a probe electrically stimulates a nerve fiber, which responds by generating its own electrical impulse. An electrode placed further along the nerve's pathway measures the speed of impulse transmission along the axon. Slow transmission rates and impulse blockage tend to indicate damage to the myelin sheath, while a reduction in the strength of impulses at normal speeds is a sign of axonal degeneration.

- *Electromyography (EMG)* involves inserting a fine needle into a muscle to record electrical activity when muscles are at rest and when they contract. EMG tests detect abnormal electrical activity in motor neuropathy and can help differentiate between muscle and nerve disorders.

- *Magnetic resonance imaging (MRI)* can show muscle quality and size, detect fatty replacement of muscle tissue, and can help rule out tumors, herniated discs, or other abnormalities that may be causing the neuropathy.

- *Nerve biopsy* involves removing and examining a sample of nerve tissue, most often from the lower leg. Although this test can provide valuable information about the degree of nerve damage, it is an invasive procedure that is difficult to perform and may itself cause neuropathic side effects.

- *Skin biopsy* is a test in which doctors remove a thin skin sample and examine nerve fiber endings. This test offers some unique advantages over NCV tests and nerve biopsy. Unlike NCV, it can reveal damage present in smaller fibers; in contrast to conventional nerve biopsy, skin biopsy is less invasive, has fewer side effects, and is easier to perform.

What treatments are available?

Address underlying conditions

The first step in treating peripheral neuropathy is to address any contributing causes such as infection, toxin exposure, medication-related toxicity, vitamin deficiencies, hormonal deficiencies, autoimmune disorders, or compression that can lead to neuropathy. Peripheral nerves have the ability to regenerate axons, as long as the nerve cell itself has not died, which may lead to functional recovery over time. Correcting an underlying condition often can result in the neuropathy resolving on its own as the nerves recover or regenerate.

The adoption of healthy lifestyle habits such as maintaining optimal weight, avoiding exposure to toxins, exercising, eating a balanced diet, correcting vitamin deficiencies, and limiting or avoiding alcohol consumption can reduce the effects of peripheral neuropathy. Exercise can reduce cramps, improve muscle strength, and prevent muscle wasting. Various dietary strategies can improve gastrointestinal symptoms. Timely treatment of injuries can help prevent permanent damage. Smoking cessation is particularly important because smoking constricts the blood vessels that supply nutrients to the peripheral nerves and can worsen neuropathic symptoms. Self-care skills such as meticulous foot care and careful wound treatment in people with diabetes and others who have an impaired ability to feel pain can alleviate symptoms and improve quality of life. Such changes often create conditions that encourage nerve regeneration.

Systemic diseases frequently require more complex treatments. Strict control of blood glucose levels has been shown to reduce neuropathic symptoms and help people with diabetic neuropathy avoid further nerve damage.

Inflammatory and autoimmune conditions leading to neuropathy can be controlled in several ways. Immunosuppressive drugs such as prednisone, cyclosporine, or azathioprine may be beneficial. Plasmapheresis—a procedure in which blood is removed, cleansed of immune system cells and antibodies, and then returned to the body—can help reduce inflammation or suppress immune system activity. Large intravenously administered doses of immunoglobulins (antibodies that alter the immune system, and agents such as rituximab that target specific inflammatory cells) also can suppress abnormal immune system activity.

Symptom Management

Neuropathic pain, or pain caused by the injury to a nerve or nerves, is often difficult to control. Mild pain may sometimes be alleviated by over-the-counter analgesics such as nonsteroidal anti-inflammatory drugs (NSAIDs). More chronic and discomforting pain may need to be addressed through the care of a physician. Medications that are used for chronic neuropathic pain fall under several classes of drugs: antidepressants, anticonvulsant medications, antiarrhythmic medications, and narcotic agents. The antidepressant and anticonvulsant medications modulate pain through their mechanism of action on the peripheral nerves, spinal cord, or brain and tend to be the most effective types of medications to control neuropathic pain. Antidepressant medications include tricyclic antidepressants such as amitriptyline or newer serotonin-norepinephrine reuptake inhibitors such as duloxetine hydrochloride or venlafaxine. Anticonvulsant medications that are frequently used include gabapentin, pregabalin, topiramate, and carbamazepine, although other medications used for treating epilepsy may also be useful. Mexiletine is an antiarrhythmic medication that may be used for treatment of chronic painful neuropathies.

For pain that does not respond to the previously described medications, the addition of narcotic agents may be considered. Because the use of prescription-obtained pain relievers that contain opioids can lead to dependence and addiction, their use is recommended only after other means of controlling the pain have failed. One of the newest narcotic medications approved for the treatment of diabetic neuropathy is tapentadol, a drug with both opioid activity and norepinephrine-re-uptake inhibition activity of an antidepressant.

Topically administered medications are another option for neuropathic pain. Two agents are topical lidocaine, an anesthetic agent, and capsaicin, a substance found in hot peppers that modifies peripheral pain receptors. Topical agents are generally most appropriate for localized chronic pain such as herpes zoster neuralgia (shingles) pain. Their usefulness for treating diffuse chronic diabetic neuropathy is more limited.

Transcutaneous electrical nerve stimulation (TENS) is a non-invasive intervention used for pain relief in a range of conditions, and a number of studies have described its use for neuropathic pain. The therapy involves attaching electrodes to the skin at the site of pain or near associated nerves and then administering a gentle electrical current. Although data from controlled clinical trials are not available to broadly establish its efficacy for peripheral neuropathies, TENS has been shown in some studies to improve peripheral neuropathy symptoms associated with diabetes.

Other complementary approaches may provide additional support and pain relief. For example, mechanical aids such as hand or foot braces can help reduce pain and physical disability by compensating for muscle weakness or alleviating nerve compression. Orthopedic shoes can improve gait disturbances and help prevent foot injuries in people with a loss of pain sensation. Acupuncture, massage, and herbal medications also are considered in the treatment of neuropathic pain.

Surgical intervention can be considered for some types of neuropathies. Injuries to a single nerve caused by focal compression such as at the carpal tunnel of the wrist, or other entrapment neuropathies, may respond well to surgery that releases the nerve from the tissues compressing it. Some surgical procedures reduce pain by destroying the nerve; this approach is appropriate only for pain caused by a single nerve and when other forms of treatment have failed to provide relief. Peripheral neuropathies that involve more diffuse nerve damage, such as diabetic neuropathy, are not amenable to surgical intervention.

What research is being done?

The mission of the National Institute of Neurological Disorders and Stroke (NINDS) is to seek fundamental knowledge about the brain and nervous system and to use that knowledge to reduce the burden of neurological disease. The NINDS is a component of the National Institutes of Health (NIH), the leading supporter of biomedical research in the world.

NINDS-funded research on neuropathy ranges from clinical studies of the genetics and natural history of hereditary neuropathies to basic science investigations of the biological mechanisms responsible for chronic neuropathic pain. Other efforts are focused on understanding how immune system dysfunction contributes to peripheral nerve damage. Together, these diverse research areas will advance the development of new therapeutic and preventive strategies for peripheral neuropathies.

Specific genetic mutations have been identified for some of the known hereditary neuropathies. NINDS therefore supports studies to identify other genetic defects that may play roles in causing or modifying the course of disease. The Inherited Neuropathies Consortium, focused on Charcot-Marie-Tooth neuropathies, seeks to better characterize the natural history of several different forms and to identify genes that modify clinical features in these disorders. Better knowledge of genetic causes may help identify people who are at high risk for developing peripheral neuropathy before symptoms appear. Understanding the role of genetic mutations may also lead to the development of gene therapies that prevent or reduce cumulative nerve damage. In addition, advances from genetics research inform studies to understand disease mechanisms. For example, scientists are using animal models to study how inflammation and nerve damage result from mutations in the Autoimmune Regulator (AIRE) gene, the cause of chronic inflammatory demyelinating polyneuropathy (CIDP) in some people.

Several NINDS-funded studies aim to determine why nerve axons degenerate in different types of peripheral neuropathies. Rapid communication between the peripheral nervous system and the central nervous system depends on myelination, a process through which special cells called Schwann cells create an insulating sheath around axons. Research has shown that Schwann cells play a critical role in the regeneration of nerve cell axons in the peripheral nervous system. By better understanding myelination and Schwann cell function, researchers hope to find targets for new therapies to treat or prevent nerve damage associated with neuropathy.

One promising area of research focuses on a class of molecules called neurotrophic factors. These substances, produced naturally by the body, protect neurons from injury and enhance their survival. Neurotrophic factors also help maintain normal function in mature nerve cells, and some stimulate axon regeneration. Several NINDS-supported studies seek to learn more about the effects of these powerful chemicals on the peripheral nervous system.

Another area of research aims to better understand inflammatory peripheral neuropathies, such as Guillain-Barre syndrome (GBS), in which the body's immune system attacks peripheral nerves, damaging myelin and impairing signal conduction along affected nerves. NINDS-funded researchers are investigating the mechanisms by which the body's immune system stops recognizing peripheral nerves as "self" and starts attacking them. GBS is usually preceded by a microbial infection, some as common as food poisoning or the flu, and researchers hypothesize that antibodies generated by the immune system to fight bacteria also attack nervous system proteins. Studies to test this hypothesis may lead to treatments that prevent these antibodies from damaging nerves. As a different strategy, researchers are studying the blood-nerve barrier in inflammatory nervous system disorders and developing ways to reduce the movement of immune cells from the bloodstream into nerve tissue, which may reduce inflammation, demyelination and nerve injury.

Transcranial magnetic stimulation (TMS), which uses a coil either held above or placed on the scalp that delivers electromagnetic pulses to activate electrical currents in general or specific parts of the brain, has shown some analgesic effect in treating various pain conditions. Current studies are examining the effectiveness of TMS in treating peripheral and chronic neuropathies.

In addition to efforts to treat or prevent underlying nerve damage, other NINDS supported studies are informing new strategies for relieving neuropathic pain. Researchers are investigating the pathways that carry pain signals to the brain and are working to identify substances that will block this signaling.

Chapter 40

Restless Legs Syndrome

What is restless legs syndrome?

Restless legs syndrome (RLS) is a neurological disorder characterized by throbbing, pulling, creeping, or other unpleasant sensations in
the legs and an uncontrollable, and sometimes overwhelming, urge to
move them. Symptoms occur primarily at night when a person is relaxing or at rest and can increase in severity during the night. Moving
the legs relieves the discomfort. Often called paresthesias (abnormal
sensations) or dysesthesias (unpleasant abnormal sensations), the sensations range in severity from uncomfortable to irritating to painful.

The most distinctive or unusual aspect of the condition is that lying
down and trying to relax activates the symptoms. Most people with RLS
have difficulty falling asleep and staying asleep. Left untreated, the
condition causes exhaustion and daytime fatigue. Many people with RLS
report that their job, personal relations, and activities of daily living are
strongly affected as a result of their sleep deprivation. They are often
unable to concentrate, have impaired memory, or fail to accomplish daily
tasks. It also can make traveling difficult and can cause depression.

As many as 10 percent of the U.S. population may have RLS. Several studies have shown that moderate to severe RLS affects approximately 2-3 percent of adults (more than 5 million individuals). An
additional 5 percent appears to be affected by a milder form. Childhood

Text in this chapter is excerpted from "Restless Legs Syndrome Fact Sheet,"
National Institute of Neurological Disorders and Stroke (NINDS), February 23, 2015.

RLS is estimated to affect almost 1 million school-age children, with one-third having moderate to severe symptoms. Some people with RLS will not seek medical attention, believing that they will not be taken seriously, that their symptoms are too mild, or that their condition is not treatable. Some physicians wrongly attribute the symptoms to nervousness, insomnia, stress, arthritis, muscle cramps, or aging.

RLS occurs in both men and women, although the incidence is about twice as high in women. It may begin at any age. Many individuals who are severely affected are middle-aged or older, and the symptoms typically become more frequent and last longer with age.

RLS is classified as a movement disorder, as individuals are forced to move their legs in order to gain relief from symptoms.

More than 80 percent of people with RLS also experience a more common condition known as periodic limb movement of sleep (PLMS). PLMS is characterized by involuntary leg twitching or jerking movements during sleep that typically occur every 15 to 40 seconds, sometimes throughout the night. The symptoms cause repeated awakening and severely disrupted sleep. Although many individuals with RLS also develop PLMS, most people with PLMS do not experience RLS. People who have PLMS and do not have RLS or another cause for the PLMS may be diagnosed with periodic limb movement disorder (PLMD). PLMD may be a variant of RLS and thus respond to similar treatments.

What are common signs and symptoms of restless legs?

People with RLS feel uncomfortable sensations in their legs, especially when sitting or lying down, accompanied by an irresistible urge to move the affected limb. These sensations less commonly affect the arms, trunk, or head. Although the sensations can occur on just one side of the body, they most often affect both sides.

Because moving the legs (or other affected parts of the body) relieves the discomfort, people with RLS often keep their legs in motion to minimize or prevent the sensations. They may pace the floor, constantly move their legs while sitting, and toss and turn in bed.

A classic feature of RLS is that the symptoms are worse at night with a distinct symptom-free period in the early morning, allowing for more refreshing sleep at that time. Other triggering situations are periods of inactivity such as long car trips, sitting in a movie theater, long-distance flights, immobilization in a cast, or relaxation exercises. Many individuals also note a worsening of symptoms if their sleep is further reduced by events or activity.

RLS symptoms may vary from day to day and in severity and frequency from person to person. Individuals with mild RLS may have some disruption of sleep onset and minor interference in daytime activities. In moderately severe cases, symptoms occur only once or twice a week but result in significant delay of sleep onset, with some disruption of daytime function. In severe cases of RLS, the symptoms occur more than twice a week and result in burdensome interruption of sleep and impairment of daytime function.

Individuals with RLS can sometimes experience remissions—spontaneous improvement over a period of weeks or months before symptoms reappear—usually during the early stages of the disorder. In general, however, symptoms become more severe over time.

People who have both RLS and an associated medical condition tend to develop more severe symptoms rapidly. In contrast, those who have RLS that is not related to any other condition and experience onset at an early age show a very slow progression of the disorder; many years may pass before symptoms occur regularly.

What causes restless legs syndrome?

In most cases, the cause of RLS is unknown. However, it may have a genetic component; RLS is often found in families where the onset of symptoms is before age 40. Specific gene variants have been associated with RLS. Evidence indicates that low levels of iron in the brain also may be responsible for RLS.

Considerable evidence suggests that RLS is related to a dysfunction in the brain's basal ganglia circuits that use the neurotransmitter dopamine, which is needed to produce smooth, purposeful muscle activity and movement. Disruption of these pathways frequently results in involuntary movements. Individuals with Parkinson's disease, another disorder of the basal ganglia's dopamine pathways, often have RLS as well.

RLS also appears to be related to the following factors or conditions, although researchers do not yet know if these factors actually cause RLS:

- Chronic diseases such as kidney failure, diabetes, and peripheral neuropathy. Treating the underlying condition often provides relief from RLS symptoms.

- Certain medications that may aggravate symptoms. These medications include anti-nausea drugs (prochlorperazine or

metoclopramide), antipsychotic drugs (haloperidol or pheno-
thiazine derivatives), antidepressants that increase serotonin,
and some cold and allergy medications-that contain sedating
antihistamines.

- Pregnancy, especially in the last trimester. In most cases, symptoms usually disappear within 4 weeks after delivery.

Alcohol and sleep deprivation also may aggravate or trigger symptoms in some individuals. Reducing or completely eliminating these
factors may relieve symptoms, but it is unclear if this can prevent RLS
symptoms from occurring at all.

How is restless legs syndrome diagnosed?

There is no specific test for RLS. The four basic criteria for diagnosing
the disorder are:

- Symptoms that are worse at night and are absent or negligible
  in the morning;

- A strong and often overwhelming need or urge to move
  the affected limb(s), often associated with paresthesias or
  dysesthesias;

- Sensory symptoms that are triggered by rest, relaxation, or
  sleep; and

- Sensory symptoms that are relieved with movement and the
  relief persists as long as the movement continues.

Physicians should focus largely on the individual's descriptions of
symptoms, their triggers and relieving factors, as well as the presence
or absence of symptoms throughout the day. A neurological and physical exam, plus information from the individual's medical and family
history and list of current medications, may be helpful. Individuals
may be asked about frequency, duration, and intensity of symptoms as
well as their tendency toward daytime sleep patterns and sleepiness,
disturbance of sleep, or daytime function.

Laboratory tests may be performed to rule out other conditions.
Blood tests can identify iron and vitamin deficiencies as well as
other medical disorders associated with RLS. In some cases, sleep
studies such as polysomnography (a test that records the individual's brain waves, heartbeat, breathing, and leg movements during
an entire night) may identify the presence of other causes of sleep

disruption (e.g., sleep apnea), which may impact management of the disorder.

Diagnosing RLS in children may be especially difficult, since it may be hard for a child to describe where it hurts, when and how often the symptoms occur, and how long symptoms last. Pediatric RLS can sometimes be misdiagnosed as "growing pains" or attention deficit disorder.

How is restless legs syndrome treated?

RLS can be treated, with care directed toward relieving symptoms. Moving the affected limb(s) may provide temporary relief. Sometimes RLS symptoms can be controlled by finding and treating an associated medical condition, such as peripheral neuropathy or diabetes.

Certain lifestyle changes and activities that may reduce symptoms in persons with mild to moderate symptoms include decreased use of caffeine, alcohol, and tobacco; supplements to correct deficiencies in iron, folate, and magnesium; changing or maintaining a regular sleep pattern; a program of moderate exercise; and massaging the legs, taking a hot bath, or using a heating pad or ice pack. A trial of iron supplements is recommended only for individuals with low iron levels. Although many people find some relief with such measures, rarely do these efforts completely eliminate symptoms.

Medications are usually helpful but no single medication effectively manages RLS for all individuals. Trials of different drugs may be necessary. In addition, medications taken regularly may lose their effect over time, making it necessary to change medications periodically.

Common drugs prescribed to treat RLS include:

Dopaminergic agents (drugs that increase dopamine), largely used to treat Parkinson's disease, have been shown to reduce symptoms of RLS and PLMS when they are taken at bedtime and are considered the initial treatment of choice. The U.S. Food and Drug Administration (FDA) has approved ropinirole, pramipexole, and rotigotine to treat moderate to severe RLS. Both drugs are generally well tolerated but can cause nausea, dizziness, or other side effects. Good short-term results of treatment with levodopa plus carbidopa have been reported.

Although dopamine-related medications are effective in managing RLS, long-term use can lead to worsening of the symptoms in many individuals. This apparent progressive worsening is referred to as "augmentation." With chronic use, a person may begin to experience symptoms earlier in the evening than in the afternoon until finally the symptoms are present around the clock. The initial evening or bedtime dose becomes less effective, the symptoms at night become more intense, and symptoms begin to affect the arms or trunk. Fortunately, this apparent progression is reversible by removing the person from all dopamine-related medications. Another important adverse effect of dopamine medications that occurs in some people is the development of impulsive or obsessive behaviors such as obsessive gambling or shopping. Should they occur, these behaviors can be reversed by stopping the medication.

The FDA has approved gabapentin enacarbil, which metabolizes in the body to become gabapentin, for the treatment of moderate to severe RLS.

Other medications may be prescribed "off-label" (not specifically designed to treat RLS) to relieve some of the symptoms of the disorder.

Benzodiazepines can help individuals who have mild or intermittent symptoms obtain a more restful sleep. However, even if taken only at bedtime they can sometimes cause daytime sleepiness. Benzodiazepines such as clonazepam and diazepam are generally prescribed to treat anxiety, muscle spasms, and insomnia. Because these drugs also may induce or aggravate sleep apnea in some cases, they should not be used in people with this condition.

Opioids such as codeine, propoxyphene, or oxycodone may be prescribed at night to diminish pain and help to relax individuals with more severe symptoms. Side effects include dizziness, nausea, exacerbation of sleep apnea, and the risk of addiction.

Anticonvulsants such as gabapentin and pregabalin can decrease the sensory disturbances such as creeping and crawling sensations and nerve pain. Dizziness, fatigue, and sleepiness are among the possible side effects.

What is the prognosis of people with restless legs?

RLS is generally a lifelong condition for which there is no cure. Nevertheless, current therapies can control the disorder, minimizing symptoms and increasing periods of restful sleep. Symptoms may gradually worsen with age, although the decline may be somewhat faster for individuals who also suffer from an associated medical condition. In addition, some individuals have remissions—periods in which symptoms decrease or disappear for days, weeks, or months—although symptoms usually eventually reappear. A diagnosis of RLS does not indicate the onset of another neurological disease, such as Parkinson's disease.

What research is being done?

The National Institute of Neurological Disorders and Stroke (NINDS), a component of the National Institutes of Health, is the primary Federal sponsor of research on brain and nervous system disorders. The NINDS seeks to increase scientific understanding of RLS, find improved methods of diagnosing and treating the syndrome, and discover ways to prevent it.

NINDS-supported researchers are investigating the possible role of dopamine function in RLS. Researchers suspect that impaired transmission of dopamine signals may play a role in the disorder. Additional research should provide new information about how RLS occurs and may help investigators identify more successful treatment options.

Workshops and conferences sponsored by the NINDS as well as nongovernment organizations have emphasized the need for further research on animal models and the complex roles of dopamine interaction with iron levels. For example, serum ferritin, an index of iron deficiency, has been shown to predict the severity of RLS symptoms in older individuals.

In other related research, NINDS scientists are conducting studies to better understand the physiological mechanisms of PLMS associated with RLS.

Chapter 41

Wernicke-Korsakoff Syndrome

Overview

Wernicke-Korsakoff syndrome is a brain disorder due to thiamine deficiency that has been associated with both Wernicke's encephalopathy and Korsakoff syndrome. Wernicke's encephalopathy can result from alcohol abuse, dietary deficiencies, prolonged vomiting, eating disorders, or the effects of chemotherapy. Korsakoff's amnesic syndrome is a memory disorder that is associated with alcoholism and involvement of the heart, vascular, and nervous system. Although these conditions may appear to be two different disorders, they are generally considered to be different stages of Wernicke-Korsakoff syndrome. Wernicke's encephalopathy represents the "acute" phase and Korsakoff's amnesic syndrome represents the "chronic" phase.

What are the signs and symptoms of Wernicke-Korsakoff syndrome?

The symptoms of Wernicke encephalopathy include mental confusion, vision problems (including double vision, abnormal eye

Text in this chapter is excerpted from "Wernicke-Korsakoff Syndrome," National Center for Advancing Translational Sciences at the National Institutes of Health (NIH), October 20, 2011.

movements, and eyelid drooping), inability to think clearly, coma, hypothermia, hypotension, and loss of muscle coordination (ataxia). The symptoms of Korsakoff's amnesia include loss of memory, inability to form new memories, making of stories (confabulation), seeing or hearing things that are not really there (hallucinations), disorientation, and vision impairment. The main features of Korsakoff's amnesic syndrome are impairments in acquiring new information or establishing new memories, and in retrieving previous memories.

How might Wernicke-Korsakoff syndrome be treated?

The goals of treatment are to control symptoms as much as possible and to prevent progression of the disorder. Some people may need to be hospitalization initially to control the symptoms.

Treatment involves replacement of thiamine and providing proper nutrition and hydration. Intravenous thiamine is the treatment of choice. After the initial dose, daily doses of thiamine are usually recommended. Supplementation of electrolytes, particularly magnesium and potassium (often low in people with alcoholism), may be required in addition to thiamine. In those who are chronically malnourished, the remainder of the B vitamins also should be supplemented. Supplementation can be tapered as the patient resumes normal intake and shows improvement.

Because long-term alcohol use is the most common cause for Wernicke-Korsakoff syndrome, avoiding alcohol provides the best chance for recovery. Referral to an alcohol recovery program should be part of the treatment regimen.

Due to difficulties with movement, patients should be provided with assistance when walking during the initial phase of treatment. Patients may require physical therapy to assist with movement. Walking difficulties may be permanent, depending on the severity at initial presentation and the timeliness of therapy.

Part Nine

Additional Help and Information

Chapter 42

Recent Research in Brain Disorders

Chapter Contents

Section 42.1

Alzheimer's Disease Research

Text in this section is excerpted from "Study reveals how genetic changes lead to familial Alzheimer's disease," National Institute of Neurological Disorders and Stroke (NINDS), March 12, 2015.

Mutations in the presenilin-1 gene are the most common cause of inherited, early-onset forms of Alzheimer's disease. In a new study, published in Neuron, scientists replaced the normal mouse presenilin-1 gene with Alzheimer's-causing forms of the human gene to discover how these genetic changes may lead to the disorder. Their surprising results may transform the way scientists design drugs that target these mutations to treat inherited or familial Alzheimer's, a rare form of the disease that affects approximately 1 percent of people with the disorder. The study was partially funded by the National Institute of Neurological Disorders and Stroke (NINDS), part of the National Institutes of Health.

For decades, it has been unclear exactly how the presenilin mutations cause Alzheimer's disease. Presenilin is a component of an important enzyme, gamma secretase, which cuts up amyloid precursor protein into two protein fragments, Abeta40 and Abeta42. Abeta42 is found in plaques, the abnormal accumulations of protein in the brain which are a hallmark of Alzheimer's. Numerous studies suggested that presenilin-1 mutations increased activity of gamma-secretase. Investigators have developed drugs that block gamma-secretase, but they have so far failed in clinical trials to halt the disease.

The study led by Raymond Kelleher, M.D., Ph.D. and Jie Shen, Ph.D., professors of neurology at Harvard Medical School, Boston, provides a plot twist in the association of presenilin-1 mutations and inherited Alzheimer's disease. Using mice with altered forms of the presenilin gene, Drs. Kelleher and Shen discovered that the mutations may cause the disease by decreasing, rather than increasing, the activity of gamma-secretase.

One of the presenilin mutations also caused impairment of memory circuits in the mouse brain and age-dependent death of neurons.

"The findings by Drs. Shen and Kelleher are a significant departure from conventional thinking that should open up exciting and creative new possibilities at all levels of research, from basic molecular mechanisms all the way to clinical intervention," said Roderick Corriveau, Ph.D., program director at NINDS.

"This is a very striking example where we have mutations that inactivate gamma-secretase function and yet they trigger an array of features that resemble Alzheimer's disease, notably synaptic and cognitive deficits as well as neurodegeneration," said Dr. Kelleher.

Although plaques are the main biological indicator of Alzheimer's, neurodegenerative changes are also an important feature of the disease. These changes include loss of brain cells, accumulations of a protein called tau inside remaining neurons, cognitive deficits such as problems with memory, changes in the brain's electrical activity and inflammation. Commonly used mouse models of the disease exhibit excessive plaque deposition, but do not show symptoms of neurodegeneration. According to Dr. Kelleher, this may be one reason that treatments developed in mice have not been successful in patients.

"This study is the first example of a mouse model in which a familial Alzheimer's mutation is sufficient to cause neurodegeneration. The new model provides an opportunity that we hope will help with the development of therapies focusing on the devastating neurodegenerative changes that occur in the disease," Dr. Kelleher said.

Dr. Shen's previous work demonstrated that presenilins and gamma-secretase play an important role in learning and memory, communication between brain cells and neuronal survival, and cautioned against the use of gamma-secretase inhibitors for Alzheimer's disease therapy. Later, a large phase III trial was stopped because treatment with a gamma-secretase inhibitor worsened the cognitive ability of patients.

Although the majority of cases are not inherited, familial Alzheimer's disease is associated with early onset of the disorder, with symptoms often appearing before age 60. Drs. Shen and Kelleher hope that the mechanisms uncovered in this study may provide insight into the common forms of the disorder that affect more than five million people in the United States.

The results in this paper suggest a new approach for drug development. "We believe that restoring gamma-secretase would be a better, more effective therapeutic strategy for Alzheimer's patients," said Dr. Shen.

This work was supported by grants from the NINDS (NS041783, NS042818, NS075346), the Alzheimer's Association, and the Pew Scholars Program in the Biomedical Sciences.

References:

Xia et al. "Presenilin-1 Knockin Mice Reveal Loss-of-Function Mechanism for Familial Alzheimer's Disease," Neuron, March 4, 2015. DOI: 10.1016/j.neuron.2015.02.010

Section 42.2

Brain Cancer Research

Text in this section is excerpted from "Strengthening the immune
system's fight against brain cancer," National Institute of
Neurological Disorders and Stroke (NINDS), March 18, 2015.

When cancer strikes, it may be possible for patients to fight back with their own defenses, using a strategy known as immunotherapy. According to a new study published in Nature, researchers have found a way to enhance the effects of this therapeutic approach in glioblastoma, a deadly type of brain cancer, and possibly improve patient outcomes. The research was funded by the National Institute of Neurological Disorders and Stroke (NINDS) as well as the National Cancer Institute (NCI), which are part of the National Institutes of Health.

"The promise of dendritic cell-based therapy and other immunotherapies for brain cancer has been upheld for some time, but an important implication of this work is a demonstrated capacity to significantly improve the clinical impact of immunotherapy for patients with this very difficult disease," said Duane A. Mitchell, M.D., Ph.D., director of the Brain Tumor Immunotherapy Program at the University of Florida in Gainesville and co-lead author of the study.

Dendritic cells are specialized immune cells that normally capture microorganisms, and then migrate to the lymph nodes to prepare other immune players, such as T cells, to fight off the invaders.

Dendritic cells have been used for immunotherapy to target a variety of tumor types, including those that affect the brain. These cells are taken from the patient, engineered to express antigens from the tumor to create a vaccine, and then injected back into the patient. Once in the patient, the engineered dendritic cells activate T cells, which can fight the tumor and also prevent it from coming back, via an immune memory response.

Dr. Mitchell and his colleagues wanted to know if increasing dendritic cell migration to lymph nodes would improve the effects of the vaccine. To test this idea, a group of glioblastoma patients was randomized to receive a tetanus booster shot before getting the tumor-antigen expressing dendritic cell vaccine. The booster was designed to set off an inflammatory response at the site of the vaccination, prepping the immune system for a larger battle. The other group of patients were injected with their own native dendritic cells instead of a tetanus shot, and then treated with the tumor-antigen expressing dendritic cell vaccine. Both sets of patients were treated with the vaccine which was being tested for effectiveness against glioblastoma.

The vaccine used in this study was targeted against cytomegalovirus (CMV). Studies have shown that CMV is found in glioblastoma tumors, but it is unclear if the virus causes tumors or contributes to disease progression. Glioblastomas are a devastating form of brain cancer with five year survival rates under 10 percent. From the time of diagnosis, average survival time is less than two years.

"The role of CMV in glioblastoma has been a controversial area of research for several years. These new findings, and especially the dramatic survival rates, suggest that the virus may be an effective target for immune therapy. The results presented by Dr. Mitchell and his colleagues should stimulate more basic research on CMV and its potential therapeutic role in brain tumors and possibly other cancers," said Jane Fountain, Ph.D., program director at the NINDS.

The results showed that administering a tetanus booster before the vaccine increased dendritic cell migration to lymph nodes and also had a significant effect on clinical outcomes. The patients who received the tetanus booster lived more than 36.6 months after diagnosis compared to an average survival time of 18.5 months in those who received dendritic cells alone.

"We did not expect that enhancing dendritic cell migration would be associated with such a dramatic improvement on clinical outcomes in our patients," said Dr. Mitchell.

Next, the investigators used a mouse model to determine how the tetanus booster increased dendritic cell migration to the lymph nodes. The results suggested that giving a booster shot to mice that have received the tetanus vaccine activated a recall response in the exposed T cells. Acting through a chemical messenger known as CCL3, those T cells increased dendritic cell migration to the lymph nodes, which ultimately enhanced the effect of the dendritic cell vaccine on tumor growth suppression.

"Dendritic cell vaccines targeting glioblastoma can be very effective by enhancing migration of dendritic cells. We now understand how we may improve outcomes for patients receiving this type of therapy," said Dr. Mitchell. He added that larger clinical studies need to be conducted to confirm these results.

In addition, more research is necessary to define the role of CMV in glioblastoma and further determine mechanisms to enhance efficacy of vaccines in cancer therapy.

This work was supported by grants from the NINDS (NS20023, NS067037) and the National Cancer Institute (CA108786, CA177476, CA134844).

References:

Mitchell et al. "Tetanus toxoid and CCL3 improve dendritic cell vaccines in mice and glioblastoma patients," Nature, March 11, 2015.

Section 42.3

Multiple Sclerosis Research

Text in this section is excerpted from "Drugs that activate brain stem cells may reverse multiple sclerosis," National Institute of Neurological Disorders and Stroke (NINDS), April 22, 2015.

Two drugs already on the market—an antifungal and a steroid—may potentially take on new roles as treatments for multiple sclerosis. According to a study published in Nature today, researchers discovered that these drugs may activate stem cells in the brain to stimulate myelin producing cells and repair white matter, which is damaged in multiple sclerosis. The study was partially funded by the National Institute of Neurological Disorders and Stroke (NINDS), part of the National Institutes of Health.

Specialized cells called oligodendrocytes lay down multiple layers of a fatty white substance known as myelin around axons, the long "wires" that connect brain cells. Myelin acts as an insulator and enables fast communication between brain cells. In multiple sclerosis there is breakdown of myelin and this deterioration leads to muscle weakness, numbness and problems with vision, coordination and balance.

"To replace damaged cells, the scientific field has focused on direct transplantation of stem cell-derived tissues for regenerative medicine, and that approach is likely to provide enormous benefit down the road. We asked if we could find a faster and less invasive approach by using drugs to activate native nervous system stem cells and direct them to form new myelin. Our ultimate goal was to enhance the body's ability to repair itself," said Paul J. Tesar, Ph.D., associate professor at Case Western Reserve School of Medicine in Cleveland, and senior author of the study.

It is unknown how myelin-producing cells are damaged, but research suggests they may be targeted by malfunctioning immune cells and that multiple sclerosis may start as an autoimmune disorder. Current therapies for multiple sclerosis include anti-inflammatory drugs, which help prevent the episodic relapses common in multiple sclerosis, but are less effective at preventing long-term disability. Scientists believe that therapies that promote myelin repair might improve neurologic disability in people with multiple sclerosis.

Adult brains contain oligodendrocyte progenitor cells (OPCs), which are stem cells that generate myelin-producing cells. OPCs are found to multiply in the brains of multiple sclerosis patients as if to respond to myelin damage, but for unknown reasons they are not effective in restoring white matter. In the current study, Dr. Tesar wanted to see if drugs already approved for other uses were able to stimulate OPCs to increase myelination.

OPCs have been difficult to isolate and study, but Dr. Tesar and his colleagues, in collaboration with Robert Miller, Ph.D., professor at George Washington University School of Medicine and Health Sciences in Washington, D.C., developed a novel method to investigate these cells in a petri dish. Using this technique, they were able to quickly test the effects of hundreds of drugs on the stem cells.

The compounds screened in this study were obtained from a drug library maintained by NIH's National Center for Advancing Translational Sciences (NCATS). All are approved for use in humans. NCATS and Dr. Tesar have an ongoing collaboration and plan to expand the library of drugs screened against OPCs in the near future to identify other promising compounds.

Dr. Tesar's team found that two compounds in particular, miconazole (an antifungal) and clobetasol (a steroid), stimulated mouse and human OPCs into generating myelin-producing cells.

Next, they examined whether the drugs, when injected into a mouse model of multiple sclerosis, could improve re-myelination. They found that both drugs were effective in activating OPCs to enhance myelination and reverse paralysis. As a result, almost all of the animals regained the use of their hind limbs. They also found that the drugs acted through two very different molecular mechanisms.

"The ability to activate white matter cells in the brain, as shown in this study, opens up an exciting new avenue of therapy development for myelin disorders such as multiple sclerosis," said Ursula Utz, Ph.D., program director at the NINDS.

Dr. Tesar and his colleagues caution that more research is needed before miconazole and clobetasol can be tested in multiple sclerosis clinical trials. They are currently approved for use as creams or powders on the surfaces of the body but their safety administered in other forms, such as injections, in humans is unknown.

"Off-label use of the current forms of these drugs is more likely to increase other health concerns than alleviate multiple sclerosis symptoms. We are working tirelessly to ready a safe and effective drug for clinical use," Dr. Tesar said.

This work was supported by the NINDS (NS085246, NS030800, NS026543), the New York Stem Cell Foundation and the Myelin Repair Foundation, New York City.

Reference:

Najm et al. "Drug-based modulation of endogenous stem cells promotes functional remyelination in vivo," Nature, April 20, 2015.

Section 42.4

Parkinson's Disease Research

Text in this section is excerpted from "NIH scientists find six new genetic risk factors for Parkinson's," National Institute of Neurological Disorders and Stroke (NINDS), July 28, 2014.

Using data from over 18,000 patients, scientists have identified more than two dozen genetic risk factors involved in Parkinson's disease, including six that had not been previously reported. The study, published in Nature Genetics, was partially funded by the National Institutes of Health (NIH) and led by scientists working in NIH laboratories.

"Unraveling the genetic underpinnings of Parkinson's is vital to understanding the multiple mechanisms involved in this complex disease, and hopefully, may one day lead to effective therapies," said Andrew Singleton, Ph.D., a scientist at the NIH's National Institute on Aging (NIA) and senior author of the study.

Dr. Singleton and his colleagues collected and combined data from existing genome-wide association studies (GWAS), which allow scientists to find common variants, or subtle differences, in the genetic codes of large groups of individuals. The combined data included approximately 13,708 Parkinson's disease cases and 95,282 controls, all of European ancestry.

The investigators identified potential genetic risk variants, which increase the chances that a person may develop Parkinson's disease. Their results suggested that the more variants a person has, the greater the risk, up to three times higher, for developing the disorder in some cases.

"The study brought together a large international group of investigators from both public and private institutions who were interested in sharing data to accelerate the discovery of genetic risk factors for Parkinson's disease," said Margaret Sutherland, Ph.D., a program director at the National Institute of Neurological Disorders and Stroke (NINDS), part of NIH. "The advantage of this collaborative approach is highlighted in the identification of pathways and gene networks that may significantly increase our understanding of Parkinson's disease."

To obtain the data, the researchers collaborated with multiple public and private organizations, including the U.S. Department of Defense, the Michael J. Fox Foundation, 23andMe and many international investigators.

Affecting millions of people worldwide, Parkinson's disease is a degenerative disorder that causes movement problems, including trembling of the hands, arms, or legs, stiffness of limbs and trunk, slowed movements and problems with posture. Over time, patients may have difficulty walking, talking, or completing other simple tasks. Although nine genes have been shown to cause rare forms of Parkinson's disease, scientists continue to search for genetic risk factors to provide a complete genetic picture of the disorder.

The researchers confirmed the results in another sample of subjects, including 5,353 patients and 5,551 controls. By comparing the genetic regions to sequences on a state-of-the-art gene chip called NeuroX, the researchers confirmed that 24 variants represent genetic risk factors for Parkinson's disease, including six variants that had not been previously identified. The NeuroX gene chip contains the codes of approximately 24,000 common genetic variants thought to be associated with a broad spectrum of neurodegenerative disorders.

"The replication phase of the study demonstrates the utility of the NeuroX chip for unlocking the secrets of neurodegenerative disorders," said Dr. Sutherland. "The power of these high tech, data-driven genomic methods allows scientists to find the needle in the haystack that may ultimately lead to new treatments."

Some of the newly identified genetic risk factors are thought to be involved with Gaucher's disease, regulating inflammation and the nerve cell chemical messenger dopamine as well as alpha-synuclein, a protein that has been shown to accumulate in the brains of some cases of Parkinson's disease. Further research is needed to determine the roles of the variants identified in this study.

This work was supported by NIA Intramural Research Program and grants from the NINDS (NS037167, NS071674, NS060113, NS036630, NS17950, NS070867, NS36960), the NIA (AG000949, AG000932, AG008122, AG016495, AG033193, AG031287, AG013846, AG025259, AG023629, AG024826) and the National Institute of Environmental Health Sciences NIEHS (ES101986).

Reference:

Nalls et al. "Large-scale meta-analysis of genome-wide association data identifies six new risk loci for Parkinson's disease" Nat. Genetics, July 27, 2014. DOI: 10.1038/ng3043

Chapter 43

Glossary of Terms Related to Brain Disorders

abdominal migraine: a type of migraine that mostly affects young children and involves moderate to severe abdominal pain, with little or no headache.

acetylcholine: a neurotransmitter that plays an important role in many neurological functions, including learning and memory.

acquired cerebral palsy: cerebral palsy that occurs as a result of injury to the brain after birth or during early childhood.

action potential: the temporary change in charge across a membrane caused by a stimulus.

Terms in this chapter are excerpted from: "Alzheimer's Disease: Unraveling the Mystery," National Institute on Aging (NIA), January 22, 2015; "The Brain's Inner Workings: A Guide for Students" National Institute of Mental Health; "Cerebral Palsy: Hope Through Research," National Institute of Neurological Disorders and Stroke (NINDS), February 2, 2015; "Dementia: Hope Through Research," National Institute of Neurological Disorders and Stroke, February 23, 2015; "Headache: Hope Through Research," National Institute of Neurological Disorders and Stroke, February 23, 2015; "Huntington's Disease: Hope Through Research," National Institute of Neurological Disorders and Stroke, April 19, 2015; "Multiple Sclerosis: Hope Through Research," National Institute of Neurological Disorders and Stroke, March 3, 2015; "Shingles: Hope Through Research," National Institute of Neurological Disorders and Stroke, April 1, 2015; "Stroke: Hope Through Research," National Institute of Neurological Disorders and Stroke, April 7, 2015; "Traumatic Brain Injury: Hope Through Research," National Institute of Neurological Disorders and Stroke, February 3, 2015.

acute stroke: a stage of stroke starting at the onset of symptoms and last for a few hours thereafter.

acyclovir: one of three available antiviral drugs that can reduce the severity and duration of a shingles attack if given soon after onset.

agnosia: a cognitive disability characterized by ignorance of or inability to acknowledge one side of the body or one side of the visual field.

akinesia: decreased body movements.

alpha-synuclein: a protein that is implicated in abnormal clumps called Lewy bodies, which are seen in the brains of people with Parkinson's disease and some dementias. Disorders in which alpha-synuclein accumulates inside nerve cells are called synucleinopathies.

Alzheimer's disease: the most common cause of dementia in people aged 65 and older. Nearly all brain functions, including memory, movement, language, judgment, and behavior, are eventually affected.

amygdala: an almond-shaped structure involved in processing and remembering strong emotions such as fear. It is part of the limbic system and located deep inside the brain.

amyloid: a protein found in the characteristic clumps of tissue (called plaques) that appear in the brains of people with Alzheimer's disease; *see* also, plaques.

amyloid precursor protein (APP): the larger protein from which beta-amyloid is formed.

aneurysm: a weak or thin spot on an artery wall that has stretched or ballooned out from the wall and filled with blood, or damage to an artery leading to pooling of blood between the layers of the blood vessel walls.

anoxia: a state of almost no oxygen delivery to a cell, resulting in low energy production and possible death of the cell; *see* hypoxia.

antibodies: proteins made by the immune system that bind to structures (antigens) they recognize as foreign to the body.

anticoagulants: a drug therapy used to prevent the formation of blood clots that can become lodged in cerebral arteries and cause strokes.

antiplatelet agents: a type of anticoagulant drug therapy that prevents the formation of blood clots by preventing the accumulation of platelets that form the basis of blood clots; some common antiplatelets include aspirin and ticlopidine; *see* anticoagulants.

antithrombotics: a type of anticoagulant drug therapy that prevents the formation of blood clots by inhibiting the coagulating actions of the blood protein thrombin; some common antithrombotics include warfarin and heparin; *see* anticoagulants.

Apgar score: a numbered scoring system doctors use to assess a baby's physical state at the time of birth.

aphasia: difficulty understanding and/or producing spoken and written language; *see* also non-fluent aphasia.

apolipoprotein E: a protein that carries cholesterol in blood and that appears to play some role in brain function. The gene that produces this protein comes in several forms, or alleles: ε2, ε3, and ε4. The APOE ε2 allele is relatively rare and may provide some protection against AD (but it may increase risk of early heart disease). APOE ε3 is the most common allele and appears to play a neutral role in AD. APOE ε4 occurs in about 40 percent of all people with AD who develop the disease in later life; it increases the risk of developing AD.

apoplexy: a historical, but obsolete term for a cerebral stroke, most often intracerebral hemorrhage, that was applied to any condition that involved disorientation and/or paralysis.

apoptosis: cell death that occurs naturally as part of normal development, maintenance, and renewal of tissues within an organism.

apraxia: a movement disorder characterized by the inability to perform skilled or purposeful voluntary movements, generally caused by damage to the areas of the brain responsible for voluntary movement.

arachnoid membrane: one of the three membranes that cover the brain; it is between the pia mater and the dura. Collectively, these three membranes form the meninges.

arteriography: an x-ray of the artery taken when a special dye is injected into the artery.

arteriovenous malformation (AVM): a congenital disorder characterized by a complex tangled web of arteries and veins.

asphyxia: a lack of oxygen due to trouble with breathing or poor oxygen supply in the air.

ataxia: a condition in which the muscles fail to function in a coordinated manner.

atherosclerosis: a blood vessel disease characterized by deposits of lipid material on the inside of the walls of large to medium-sized arteries which make the artery walls thick, hard, brittle, and prone to breaking.

athetoid: making slow, sinuous, involuntary, writhing movements, especially with the hands.

atrial fibrillation: irregular beating of the left atrium, or left upper chamber, of the heart.

aura: a warning of a migraine headache. Usually visual, it may appear as flashing lights, zigzag lines, or a temporary loss of vision, along with numbness or trouble speaking.

autoimmune disease: a disease in which the body's defense system malfunctions and attacks a part of the body itself rather than foreign matter.

autonomic: occurring involuntary. Autonomic nervous system dysfunction is frequently associated with various types of migraine.

autosomal dominant disorder: a non-sex-linked disorder that can be inherited even if only one parent passes on the defective gene.

axon: the long extension from a neuron that transmits outgoing signals to other cells.

basal ganglia: a region located at the base of the brain composed of four clusters of neurons, or nerve cells. This area is responsible for body movement and coordination. The neuron groups most prominently and consistently affected by HD—the pallidum and striatum—are located here; *see* neuron, pallidum, striatum.

basilar-type migraine: a type of migraine, occurring primarily in young women, causing symptoms of abnormal brain stem functioning such as double vision, loss of peripheral vision, numbness, imbalance, or loss of consciousness.

benign intracranial hypertension: increased pressure within the brain that causes severe headaches. It can be caused by clotting in the major cerebral veins or from certain medications (including some antibiotics, human growth hormone replacement, and vitamin A and related compounds).

beta-amyloid: a part of the amyloid precursor protein found in plaques, the insoluble deposits outside neurons.

bilirubin: a bile pigment produced by the liver of the human body as a byproduct of digestion.

biofeedback: a process that increases an individual's voluntary control of physiologic states such as blood pressure and pain response.

bisphosphonates: a family of drugs that strengthen bones and reduce the risk of bone fracture in elderly adults.

blood-brain barrier: a network of blood vessels with closely spaced cells that controls the passage of substances from the blood into the central nervous system; *see* also, glia.

botulinum toxin: a drug commonly used to relax spastic muscles; it blocks the release of acetylcholine, a neurotransmitter that energizes muscle tissue.

brain death: an irreversible cessation of measurable brain function.

brain stem: the portion of the brain that connects to the spinal cord and controls automatic body functions, such as breathing, heart rate, and blood pressure.

brain-derived neurotrophic factor (BDNF): a growth factor that stimulates survival, growth, and adaptability of some neurons.

Broca's aphasia: *see* non-fluent aphasia.

Broca's area: part of the cerebral cortex on the left frontal lobe, which helps transform thoughts into words.

capillary: a tiny blood vessel. The brain has billions of capillaries that carry oxygen, glucose (the brain's principal source of energy), nutrients, and hormones to brain cells so they can do their work. Capillaries also carry away carbon dioxide and cell waste products.

capsaicin: an active ingredient in hot chili peppers used in topical ointments to relieve pain. It appears to work by reducing a chemical substance found at nerve endings and involved in transmitting pain signals to the brain. While somewhat effective for postherpetic neuralgia, it can cause severe burning in some patients.

carbamazepine: a drug that works both as an anticonvulsant and a pain reliever.

carotid artery: an artery, located on either side of the neck, that supplies the brain with blood.

carotid endarterectomy: surgery used to remove fatty deposits from the carotid arteries.

caudate nuclei: part of the striatum in the basal ganglia; *see* basal ganglia, striatum.

cell membrane: an essential part of every cell, composed of a double layer of lipids with pores and specialized receptors, that controls the cell's internal environment and its responses to outside stimuli.

central stroke pain (central pain syndrome): pain caused by damage to an area in the thalamus. The pain is a mixture of sensations, including heat and cold, burning, tingling, numbness, and sharp stabbing and underlying aching pain.

cephalgia: head pain.

cerebellum: the part of the brain responsible for maintaining the body's balance and coordination.

cerebral: relating to the two hemispheres of the human brain.

cerebral blood flow (CBF): the flow of blood through the arteries that lead to the brain, called the cerebrovascular system.

Cerebral cortex: the outer layer of nerve cells surrounding the cerebral hemispheres.

cerebral dysgenesis: defective brain development.

Cerebral hemispheres: the largest portion of the brain, composed of billions of nerve cells in two structures connected by the corpus callosum. The cerebral hemispheres control conscious thought, language, decision making, emotions, movement, and sensory functions.

Cerebrospinal fluid: the fluid found in and around the brain and spinal cord. It protects these organs by acting like a liquid cushion and by providing nutrients.

cerebrospinal fluid (CSF): the fluid that bathes and protects the brain and spinal cord.

cerebrovascular disease: a reduction in the supply of blood to the brain either by narrowing of the arteries through the buildup of plaque on the inside walls of the arteries, called stenosis, or through blockage of an artery due to a blood clot.

cerebrum: the portion of the forebrain involved in conscious thought, memory and analysis of sensory signals.

cervical arterial dissection: a tear in an artery wall that can lead to stroke or transient ischemic attacks.

cervicogenic headache: a type of headache caused by structural irregularities in either the neck or head.

chemoreceptor: receptors on membranes that receive chemical signals.

chickenpox: an acute contagious disease that usually occurs in children and is caused by the varicella-zoster virus.

cholesterol: a waxy substance, produced naturally by the liver and also found in foods, that circulates in the blood and helps maintain tissues and cell membranes. Excess cholesterol in the body can contribute to atherosclerosis and high blood pressure.

chorea: uncontrolled body movements. Chorea is derived from the Greek word for dance.

choreoathetoid: a condition characterized by aimless muscle movements and involuntary motions.

chromosome: the structures in cells that contain genes. They are composed of deoxyribonucleic acid (DNA) and proteins and, under a microscope, appear as rod-like structures.

chronic headache: headache that occurs 15 or more days a month over a 3-month period.

chronic traumatic encephalopathy: a form of dementia caused by repeated traumatic brain injury.

clinical trial: a research study involving humans that rigorously tests safety, side effects, and how well a medication or behavioral treatment works.

clipping: surgical procedure for treatment of brain aneurysms, involving clamping an aneurysm from a blood vessel, surgically removing this ballooned part of the blood vessel, and closing the opening in the artery wall.

closed head injury: an injury that occurs when the head suddenly and violently hits an object but the object does not break through the skull.

cluster headache: sudden, extremely painful headaches that occur in a closely grouped pattern several times a day and at the same times over a period of weeks.

cognitive functions: all aspects of conscious thought and mental activity, including learning, perceiving, making decisions, and remembering.

coma: a state of profound unconsciousness caused by disease, injury, or poison.

compressive cranial neuropathies: degeneration of nerves in the brain caused by pressure on those nerves.

computed tomography (CT): a type of diagnostic imaging that uses x-rays and computer technology to produce two-dimensional images of organs, bones, and tissues.

concussion: injury to the brain caused by a hard blow or violent shaking, causing a sudden and temporary impairment of brain function, such as a short loss of consciousness or disturbance of vision and equilibrium.

congenital cerebral palsy: cerebral palsy that is present at birth from causes that have occurred during fetal development.

contracture: a condition in which muscles become fixed in a rigid, abnormal position, which causes distortion or deformity.

contrecoup: a contusion caused by the shaking of the brain back and forth within the confines of the skull.

contusion: distinct area of swollen brain tissue mixed with blood released from broken blood vessels.

corpus callosum: thick bundles of nerve cell fibers that connect the two cerebral hemispheres.

cortex: part of the brain responsible for thought, perception, and memory. HD affects the basal ganglia and cortex; *see* basal ganglia.

cortical spreading depression: a wave of increased brain activity that slowly spreads from the back toward the front of the brain's surface and may be the basis for migraine aura.

corticobasal degeneration: a progressive disorder characterized by nerve cell loss and atrophy in multiple areas of the brain.

Coumadin®: a commonly used anticoagulant, also known as warfarin.

CSF fistula: a tear between two of the three membranes—the dura and arachnoid membranes—that encase the brain

cytokines: small, hormone-like proteins released by leukocytes, endothelial cells, and other cells to promote an inflammatory immune response to an injury.

cytotoxic edema: a state of cell compromise involving influx of fluids and toxic chemicals into a cell causing subsequent swelling of the cell.

deep brain stimulation: therapy that uses a surgically implanted, battery-operated medical device called a neurostimulator to deliver electrical stimulation to targeted areas in the brain that control movement, blocking the abnormal nerve signals that cause tremor and other movement symptoms.

deep vein thrombosis: formation of a blood clot deep within a vein.

dementia: a broad term referring to a decline in cognitive function to the extent that it interferes with daily life and activities.

dementia pugilistica: brain damage caused by cumulative and repetitive head trauma; common in career boxers.

demyelination: damage caused to myelin by recurrent attacks of inflammation. Demyelination ultimately results in nervous system scars, called plaques, which interrupt communications between the nerves and the rest of the body.

dendrite: a branch-like extension of a neuron that receives messages from other neurons.

deoxyribonucleic acid (DNA): the substance of heredity containing the genetic information necessary for cells to divide and produce proteins. DNA carries the code for every inherited characteristic of an organism; *see* gene.

depressed skull fracture: a fracture occurring when pieces of broken skull press into the tissues of the brain.

desipramine: an antidepressant often prescribed to help reduce the pain from postherpetic neuralgia. Doctors often prescribe it because it has fewer side effects than some other antidepressants.

detachable coil: a platinum coil that is inserted into an artery in the thigh and strung through the arteries to the site of an aneurysm. The coil is released into the aneurysm creating an immune response from the body. The body produces a blood clot inside the aneurysm, strengthening the artery walls and reducing the risk of rupture.

developmental delay: behind schedule in reaching the milestones of early childhood development.

differentiation: changes in cells to make them more specialized.

diffuse axonal injury: *see* shearing.

dominant: a trait that is apparent even when the gene for that disorder is inherited from only one parent; *see* autosomal dominant disorder, recessive, gene.

dopamine: a neurotransmitter that affects mood and helps control complex movements.

duplex Doppler ultrasound: a diagnostic imaging technique in which an image of an artery can be formed by bouncing sound waves off the moving blood in the artery and measuring the frequency changes of the echoes.

dura: a tough, fibrous membrane lining the brain; the outermost of the three membranes collectively called the meninges.

dysarthria: inability or difficulty articulating words due to emotional stress, brain injury, paralysis, or spasticity of the muscles needed for speech.

dysesthesias: abnormal sensations such as numbness, prickling, or "pins and needles."

dyskinetic: the impairment of the ability to perform voluntary movements, which results in awkward or incomplete movements.

dysphagia: trouble swallowing.

dystonia (dystonic): a condition of abnormal muscle tone.

early seizures: seizures that occur within 1 week after a traumatic brain injury.

early-onset Alzheimer's disease: a rare form of AD that usually affects people between ages 30 and 60. It is called familial AD (FAD) if it runs in the family.

edema: the swelling of a cell that results from the influx of large amounts of water or fluid into the cell.

embolic stroke: a stroke caused by an embolus.

embolus: a free-roaming clot that usually forms in the heart.

endocrine system: the system comprised of glands that secrete hormones as chemical messages to other parts of the body.

endoplasmic reticulum: a cell organelle that looks like a channel, isolating and transporting materials.

endothelial wall: a flat layer of cells that make up the innermost lining of a blood vessel.

entorhinal cortex: an area deep within the brain where damage from AD often begins.

enzyme: a protein that causes or speeds up a biochemical reaction.

epidural hematoma: bleeding between the brain's protective coating and the skull.

episodic: comes and goes.

ergot derivative drugs: drugs that bind to the neurotransmitter serotonin and help to decrease the transmission of pain messages along nerve fibers.

erosive gastritis: inflammation and degeneration of the tissues of the stomach.

exacerbation: a sudden worsening of symptoms or the appearance of new symptoms that lasts for at least 24 hours.

excitatory amino acids: a subset of neurotransmitters; proteins released by one neuron into the space between two neurons to promote an excitatory state in the other neuron.

extracranial/intracranial (EC/IC) bypass: a type of surgery that restores blood flow to a blood-deprived area of brain tissue by rerouting a healthy artery in the scalp to the area of brain tissue affected by a blocked artery.

famciclovir: one of three available antiviral drugs that can reduce the severity and duration of a shingles attack if given soon after onset.

fatigue: tiredness that may accompany activity or may persist even without exertion.

fluent aphasia: a condition in which patients display little meaning in their speech even though they speak in complete sentences. Also called Wernicke's or motor aphasia.

forebrain: the largest part of the human brain, composed primarily of the cerebrum.

free radical: a highly reactive molecule (typically oxygen or nitrogen) that combines easily with other molecules because it contains an unpaired electron. The combination with other molecules sometimes damages cells.

frontotemporal disorders: a group of dementias characterized by degeneration of nerve cells, especially those in the frontal and temporal lobes of the brain.

functional magnetic resonance imaging (fMRI): a type of imaging that measures increases in blood flow within the brain.

GABA: gamma-aminobutyric acid, a neurotransmitter with mostly inhibitory effects.

gabapentin: an anti-seizure medicine that is also used as a pain reliever.

gait analysis: a technique that uses cameras, force plates, electromyography, and computer analysis to objectively measure an individual's pattern of walking.

gene: the basic unit of heredity, composed of a segment of DNA containing the code for a specific trait; *see* deoxyribonucleic acid (DNA).

genetic risk factor: a variant in a cell's DNA that does not cause a disease by itself but may increase the chance that a person will develop a disease.

gestation: the period of fetal development from the time of conception until birth.

Glasgow Coma Scale: a clinical tool used to assess the degree of consciousness and neurological functioning—and therefore severity of brain injury—by testing motor responsiveness, verbal acuity, and eye opening.

glia: also called neuroglia; supportive cells of the nervous system that make up the blood-brain barrier, provide nutrients and oxygen to the vital neurons, and protect the neurons from infection, toxicity, and trauma. Some examples of glia are oligodendroglia, astrocytes, and microglia.

global aphasia: a condition in which patients suffer severe communication disabilities as a result of extensive damage to portions of the brain responsible for language.

glutamate: also known as glutamic acid, an amino acid that acts as an excitatory neurotransmitter in the brain.

Golgi body: a cell organelle that packages cell products for transport.

gray matter: part of the brain that contains nerve cells and has a gray color.

hematoma: heavy bleeding into or around the brain caused by damage to a major blood vessel in the head.

hemicrania continua: one-sided headaches that are chronic or continuous and respond to indomethacin treatment.

hemiparesis: paralysis affecting only one side of the body.

hemiplegia: complete paralysis on one side of the body.

hemiplegic migraine: a type of migraine causing temporary paralysis on one side of the body.

hemorrhagic stroke: stroke caused by bleeding out of one of the major arteries leading to the brain.

heparin: a type of anticoagulant.

herpes simplex: the medical term for a related but different virus that causes repeated mild blisters of the skin or mucous membrane. Herpes simplex rashes can return many times, whereas shingles usually appears no more than once or twice in a person's lifetime.

herpes viruses: a large family of viruses that cause a number of related conditions including, but not limited to, oral and genital herpes simplex, varicella (chickenpox), and herpes-zoster (shingles).

herpes zoster: the medical term for shingles; an infection caused by the varicella-zoster virus, one of the herpesviruses family of viruses.

high-density lipoprotein (HDL): also known as the good cholesterol; a compound consisting of a lipid and a protein that carries a small percentage of the total cholesterol in the blood and deposits it in the liver.

hindbrain: the most primitive part of the brain, which controls the body's most basic functions such as respiration and heart rate.

hippocampus: a structure in the brain that plays a major role in learning and memory and is involved in converting short-term to long-term memory.

histamines: a chemical signal in the body that causes a reaction to a foreign substance.

HIV-associated dementia: a dementia that results from infection with the human immunodeficiency virus that causes AIDS.

homeostasis: a state of equilibrium or balance among various fluids and chemicals in a cell, in tissues, or in the body as a whole.

hormone: A chemical message produced by an endocrine gland which travels through the bloodstream to a target organ.

huntingtin: the protein encoded by the gene that carries the HD defect. The repeated CAG sequence in the gene causes an abnormal form of huntingtin to be formed. The function of the normal form of huntingtin is not yet known.

hypermetabolism: a condition in which the body produces too much heat energy.

hypertension (high blood pressure): characterized by persistently high arterial blood pressure defined as a measurement greater than or equal to 140 mm/Hg systolic pressure over 90 mm/Hg diastolic pressure.

hypertonia: increased muscle tone.

hypnic headache: a rare form of headache that awakens individuals at night (also called "alarm-clock headache").

hypothalamus: a structure in the brain under the thalamus that monitors activities such as body temperature and food intake.

hypothyroidism: decreased production of thyroid hormone leading to low metabolic rate, weight gain, chronic drowsiness, dry skin and hair, and/or fluid accumulation and retention in connective tissues.

hypotonia: decreased muscle tone.

hypoxia: a state of decreased oxygen delivery to a cell so that the oxygen falls below normal levels; *see* anoxia.

hypoxic-ischemic encephalopathy: brain damage caused by poor blood flow or insufficient oxygen supply to the brain.

ice cream headache: a painful headache brought on by changes in blood flow that result from a sudden chilling of the roof of the mouth.

immediate seizures: seizures that occur within 24 hours of a traumatic brain injury.

immunosuppressed: having a weakened immune system. Common causes are certain illnesses (HIV, some cancers) or use of certain drugs such as prednisone.

incidence: the extent or frequency of an occurrence; the number of specific new events in a given period of time.

infarct: an area of tissue that is dead or dying because of a loss of blood supply.

infarction: a sudden loss of blood supply to tissue, causing the formation of an infarct.

interferons: signaling molecules that regulate immune cells.

interleukins: a group of cytokine-related proteins secreted by leukocytes and involved in the inflammatory immune response of the ischemic cascade.

intracerebral hematoma: bleeding within the brain caused by damage to a major blood vessel.

intracerebral hemorrhage: occurs when a vessel within the brain leaks blood into the brain.

intracranial pressure: buildup of pressure in the brain as a result of injury.

intrathecal baclofen: baclofen that is injected into the cerebrospinal fluid of the spinal cord to reduce spasticity.

ion pump: mechanisms in the cell membrane that use energy and enzymes to move ions across the cell membrane, establishing voltage (charge) across a membrane.

ions: charged atoms or stable groups of atoms.

ischemia: a loss of blood flow to tissue, caused by an obstruction of the blood vessel, usually in the form of plaque stenosis or a blood clot.

ischemic cascade: a series of events lasting for several hours to several days following initial ischemia that results in extensive cell death and tissue damage beyond the area of tissue originally affected by the initial lack of blood flow.

ischemic penumbra: areas of damaged, but still living, brain cells arranged in a patchwork pattern around areas of dead brain cells.

ischemic stroke: stroke caused by the formation of a clot that blocks blood flow through an artery to the brain.

jaundice: a blood disorder caused by the abnormal buildup of bilirubin in the bloodstream.

kindred: a group of related persons, such as a family or clan.

lacunar infarction: occlusion of a small artery in the brain resulting in a small area of dead brain tissue, called a lacunar infarct; often caused by stenosis of the small arteries, called small vessel disease.

large vessel disease: stenosis in large arteries of the cerebrovascular system.

latent: hidden, dormant, inactive. The virus that causes chickenpox remains hidden in the nervous system after the initial attack of chickenpox is over. When it becomes reactivated, usually many years later, the virus can cause shingles.

late-onset Alzheimer's disease: the most common form of AD. It occurs in people aged 60 and older.

lesion: an abnormal change in the structure of an organ due to disease or injury.

leukocytes: blood proteins involved in the inflammatory immune response of the ischemic cascade.

Lewy body dementia: one of the most common types of progressive dementia, characterized by the presence of abnormal structures called Lewy bodies in the brain.

lidocaine: a pain-killing drug sometimes used for treating postherpetic neuralgia. It is available in an adhesive fabric patch that can be placed on the skin directly over the site of the pain.

limbic system: a brain region that links the brain stem with the higher reasoning elements of the cerebral cortex. It controls emotions, instinctive behavior, and the sense of smell.

lipoprotein: small globules of cholesterol covered by a layer of protein; produced by the liver.

locked-in syndrome: a condition in which a patient is aware and awake, but cannot move or communicate due to complete paralysis of the body.

lordosis: an increased inward curvature of the lower spine.

low-density lipoprotein (LDL): also known as the bad cholesterol; a compound consisting of a lipid and a protein that carries the majority of the total cholesterol in the blood and deposits the excess along the inside of arterial walls.

magnetic resonance angiography (MRA): an imaging technique involving injection of a contrast dye into a blood vessel and using magnetic resonance techniques to create an image of the flowing blood through the vessel; often used to detect stenosis of the brain arteries inside the skull.

magnetic resonance imaging (MRI): an imaging technique that uses radio waves, magnetic fields, and computer analysis to create a picture of body tissues and structures.

marker: a piece of DNA that lies on the chromosome so close to a gene that the two are inherited together. Like a signpost, markers are used during genetic testing and research to locate the nearby presence of a gene. *See* chromosome, deoxyribonucleic acid (DNA).

medication overuse headache: caused by the overuse of drugs (more than 3 times weekly) to treat headache. While the medication may help to relieve the headaches temporarily, over time the underlying headache becomes worse and occurs more frequently, creating a vicious cycle of medication use and head pain. The pain improves when the medication is stopped.

meninges: the three layers of membrane that cover the brain and spinal cord.

meningitis: inflammation of the three membranes that envelop the brain and spinal cord, collectively known as the meninges; the meninges include the dura, pia mater, and arachnoid.

menstrually related migraine: a migraine that affects women around the time of their period.

metabolism: all of the chemical processes that take place inside the body. In some metabolic reactions, complex molecules are broken down to release energy. In others, the cells use energy to make complex compounds out of simpler ones (like making proteins from amino acids).

microtubule: an internal support structure for a neuron that guides nutrients and molecules from the body of the cell to the end of the axon.

midbrain: the upper part of the brainstem, which controls some reflexes and eye movements.

migraine: headaches that are usually pulsing or throbbing and occur on one or both sides of the head. They are moderate to severe in intensity, associated with nausea, vomiting, sensitivity to light and noise, and worsen with routine physical activity.

mild cognitive impairment (MCI): a condition in which a person has memory problems greater than those expected for his or her age, but not the personality or cognitive problems that characterize AD.

mitochondria: microscopic, energy-producing bodies within cells that are the cells' "power plants."

mitral annular calcification: a disease of the mitral valve of the heart.

mitral valve stenosis: a disease of the mitral heart valve involving the buildup of plaque-like material on and around the valve.

mixed dementia: dementia in which one form of dementia and another condition or dementia cause damage to the brain, for example, Alzheimer's disease and small vessel disease or vascular dementia.

motor aphasia: *see* non-fluent aphasia.

motor neuron: a nerve that causes a muscle to contract.

multi-infarct dementia: a type of vascular dementia caused by numerous small strokes in the brain.

mutation: a permanent change in a cell's DNA that can cause a disease.

myelin: a whitish, fatty layer surrounding an axon that helps the axon rapidly transmit electrical messages from the cell body to the synapse.

myoclonus: a condition in which muscles or portions of muscles contract involuntarily in a jerky fashion.

necrosis: a form of cell death resulting from anoxia, trauma, or any other form of irreversible damage to the cell; involves the release of toxic cellular material into the intercellular space, poisoning surrounding cells.

nerve: a bundle of axons in the nervous system.

nerve growth factor (NGF): a substance that maintains the health of nerve cells. NGF also promotes the growth of axons and dendrites, the parts of the nerve cell that are essential to its ability to communicate with other nerve cells.

nervous system: the system that coordinates an organism's response to the environment.

neural stem cells: cells found only in adult neural tissue that can develop into several different cell types in the central nervous system.

neurodegenerative disease: a disease characterized by a progressive decline in the structure, activity, and function of brain tissue. These diseases include AD, Parkinson's disease, frontotemporal lobar degeneration, and dementia with Lewy bodies. They are usually more common in older people.

neuroexcitation: the electrical activation of cells in the brain; neuroexcitation is part of the normal functioning of the brain or can also be the result of abnormal activity related to an injury.

neurofibrillary tangles: bundles of twisted filaments found in nerve cells in the brains of people with Alzheimer's disease. These tangles are largely made up of a protein called tau.

neuron: the main functional cell of the brain and nervous system, consisting of a cell body, an axon, and dendrites.

neuroprotective agents: medications that protect the brain from secondary injury caused by stroke.

neurotransmitters: special chemicals that transmit nerve impulses from one cell to another.

new daily persistent headache: a type of treatment-resistant chronic headache marked by daily pain that can last for years.

Nissl Body: an organelle in a cell that responds to Nissl stain, primarily comprised of rough endoplasmic reticulum.

nociceptors: nerve fiber endings that receive and transmit pain signals.

non-fluent aphasia: a condition in which patients have trouble recalling words and speaking in complete sentences. Also called Broca's or motor aphasia.

norepinephrine: a neurotransmitter that increases the rate of metabolism and helps an organism respond to threats.

nortriptyline: an antidepressant often prescribed to help reduce the pain from postherpetic neuralgia. Doctors often prescribe it because it has fewer side effects than some other antidepressants.

nucleus: the structure within a cell that contains the chromosomes and controls many of its activities.

occipital lobe: part of the cerebral cortex at the back of the brain, which processes images from the eyes and links it to memory.

oligodendrocytes: a type of support cell in the brain that produces myelin, the fatty sheath that surrounds and insulates axons.

ophthalmoplegic migraine: an uncommon form of migraine featuring a droopy eyelid, large pupil, and double vision that may last for weeks after the headache pain is gone.

oppositional defiant disorder (ODD): a psychiatric disorder characterized by two different sets of problems, one of which includes aggressiveness and the other a tendency to purposefully bother and irritate others.

optic neuritis: an inflammatory disorder of the optic nerve that usually occurs in only one eye and causes visual loss and sometimes blindness. It is generally temporary.

orthotic devices: special devices, such as splints or braces, used to treat posture problems involving the muscles, ligaments, or bones.

osteopenia: reduced density and mass of the bones.

oxidative damage: damage that can occur to cells when they are exposed to too many free radicals.

oxygen-free radicals: toxic chemicals released during the process of cellular respiration and released in excessive amounts during necrosis of a cell; involved in secondary cell death associated with the ischemic cascade.

pallidum: part of the basal ganglia of the brain. The pallidum is composed of the globus pallidus and the ventral pallidum; *see* basal ganglia.

palsy: paralysis, or the lack of control over voluntary movement.

paresis: *see* plegia.

parietal lobe: the topmost part of the cerebral cortex behind the frontal lobes which receives information about temperature, taste, touch and movement.

Parkinson's disease dementia: a secondary dementia that sometimes occurs in people with advanced Parkinson's disease. Many people with Parkinson's have the amyloid plaques and neurofibrillary tangles found in Alzheimer's disease, but it is not clear if the diseases are linked.

paroxysmal hemicrania: a rare form of headache that usually begins in adulthood and is marked by one-sided attacks that typically occur 5 to 40 times a day.

penetrating head injury: a brain injury in which an object pierces the skull and enters the brain tissue.

periventricular leukomalacia (PVL): "peri" means near; "ventricular" refers to the ventricles or fluid spaces of the brain; and "leukomalacia" refers to softening of the white matter of the brain. PVL is a condition in which the cells that make up white matter die near the ventricles. Under a microscope, the tissue looks soft and sponge.

persistent vegetative state: an ongoing state of severely impaired consciousness, in which the patient is incapable of voluntary motion.

placenta: an organ that joins a mother with her unborn baby and provides nourishment and sustenance.

plaque: fatty cholesterol deposits found along the inside of artery walls that lead to atherosclerosis and stenosis of the arteries.

plasma: the liquid portion of the blood that is involved in controlling infection.

plasmapheresis: the process of taking blood out of the body and removing components in the blood's plasma that are thought to be harmful before transfusing the blood back into the body (also called plasma exchange).

plasticity: the ability to be formed or molded; in reference to the brain, the ability to adapt to deficits and injury.

platelets: structures found in blood that are known primarily for their role in blood coagulation.

plegia: Also known as paresis. Weakness or paralysis. In cerebral palsy, these terms are typically combined with other phrases that describe the distribution of paralysis and weakness; for example, quadriplegia means paralysis of all four limbs.

pneumocephalus: a condition in which air or gas is trapped within the intracranial cavity.

positron emission tomography (PET): a tool used to diagnose brain functions and disorders. PET produces three-dimensional, colored images of chemicals or substances functioning within the body. These images are called PET scans. PET shows brain function, in contrast to CT or MRI, which show brain structure.

post-concussion syndrome (PCS): a complex, poorly understood problem that may cause headache after head injury; in most cases, patients cannot remember the event that caused the concussion and a variable period of time prior to the injury.

postdrome: the period following the headache.

postherpetic itch: severe, painful, and difficult to treat itching that sometimes accompanies postherpetic neuralgia. Topical local anesthetics provide relief to some patients.

postherpetic neuralgia: a condition characterized by pain that persists more than 3 months after healing of a shingles rash; caused by damage to the nervous system.

post-traumatic amnesia (PTA): a state of acute confusion due to a traumatic brain injury, marked by difficulty with perception, thinking, remembering, and concentration; during this acute stage, patients often cannot form new memories.

post-traumatic dementia: a condition marked by mental deterioration and emotional apathy following trauma.

post-traumatic epilepsy: recurrent seizures occurring more than 1 week after a traumatic brain injury.

potential: a voltage or difference in electrical charge.

prednisone: an anti-inflammatory corticosteroid drug routinely given to shingles patients when an eye or other facial nerve is involved.

premonitory: meaning before. Some individuals with migraine experience premonitory symptoms up to 24 hours prior to headache pain.

prevalence: the number of cases of a disease that are present in a particular population at a given time.

primary exertional headache: headache brought on by fits of coughing or sneezing, or by intense physical activity such as running or lifting.

primary headaches: headaches that occurs on their own with no detectable underlying cause, such as migraine, tension-type headache, and the trigeminal autonomic cephalgias.

primary stabbing headache: also called "ice pick headache" or "jabs and jolts" headache for its extremely intense pain that develops suddenly and generally lasts 1 to 10 seconds.

prompt: a verbal or physical support that helps a child get through an action.

prosodic dysfunction: problems with speech intonation or inflection.

pruning: process whereby an injury destroys an important neural network in children, and another less useful neural network that would have eventually died takes over the responsibilities of the damaged network.

putamen: an area of the brain that decreases in size as a result of the damage produced by HD.

quadriplegia: paralysis of both the arms and legs.

receptor: proteins that serve as recognition sites on cells and cause a response in the body when stimulated by chemicals called neurotransmitters. They act as on-and-off switches for the next nerve cell; *see* neuron, neurotransmitters.

recessive: a trait that is apparent only when the gene or genes for it are inherited from both parents; *see* dominant, gene.

recombinant tissue plasminogen activator (rt-PA): a genetically engineered form of t-PA, a thrombolytic, anti-clotting substance made naturally by the body.

reflex (simple): a direct response to a stimulus like that controlled by the spinal cord.

relapsing-remitting MS: a form of MS in which an episode of symptoms occurs and is followed by a recovery period before another attack occurs.

retinal migraine: a type of migraine that is characterized by attacks of visual loss or disturbances in one eye.

reversible vasoconstriction syndrome: a narrowing of the arteries in the brain that can cause sudden, "thunderclap" headache that may be brought on by bleeding in or around the brain.

Rh incompatibility: a blood condition in which antibodies in a pregnant woman's blood attack fetal blood cells and impair an unborn baby's supply of oxygen and nutrients.

rubella: also known as German measles, a viral infection that can damage the nervous system of an unborn baby if a mother contracts the disease during pregnancy.

schizophrenia: a brain disease caused by defects in neurotransmitters (especially dopamine), characterized by delusions and severe behavioral changes.

scoliosis: a disease of the spine in which the spinal column tilts or curves to one side of the body.

secondary headaches: headaches that are caused by an underlying condition or disease.

seizure: abnormal activity of nerve cells in the brain causing strange sensations, emotions, and behavior, or sometimes convulsions, muscle spasms, and loss of consciousness.

selective dorsal rhizotomy: a surgical procedure in which selected nerves are severed to reduce spasticity in the legs.

senile chorea: a relatively mild and rare disorder found in elderly adults and characterized by choreic movements. It is believed by some scientists to be caused by a different gene mutation than that causing HD.

sensory aphasia: *see* fluent aphasia.

sensory neuron: a neuron that receives a message from the environment.

serotonin: a neurotransmitter present throughout the body and brain that plays an important role in headache and migraine, mood disorders, regulating body temperature, sleep, vomiting, sexuality, and appetite.

shaken baby syndrome: a severe form of head injury that occurs when an infant or small child is shaken forcibly enough to cause the brain to bounce against the skull; the degree of brain damage depends on the extent and duration of the shaking. Minor symptoms include irritability, lethargy, tremors, or vomiting; major symptoms include seizures, coma, stupor, or death.

shearing (or diffuse axonal injury): damage to individual neurons resulting in disruption of neural networks and the breakdown of overall communication among neurons in the brain.

short-lasting, unilateral, neuralgiform headache attacks with conjunctival injection and tearing (SUNCT): a rare form of headache marked by brief recurrent bursts of moderate to severe burning, stabbing, or throbbing pain, usually on one side of the head and around the eye or temple, accompanied by symptoms including watery, reddish eyes, and runny nose.

single photon emission computed tomography (SPECT): an imaging technique that allows researchers to monitor blood flow to different parts of the brain.

small vessel disease: a cerebrovascular disease defined by stenosis in small arteries of the brain.

sodium-potassium pump: a mechanism in the membranes of neurons that can separate ions and create a voltage (charge) across a membrane.

spastic (or spasticity): describes stiff muscles and awkward movements.

spastic diplegia (or diparesis): a form of cerebral palsy in which spasticity affects both legs, but the arms are relatively or completely spared.

spastic hemiplegia (or hemiparesis): a form of cerebral palsy in which spasticity affects an arm and leg on one side of the body.

spastic quadriplegia (or quadriparesis): a form of cerebral palsy in which all four limbs are paralyzed or weakened equally.

spasticity: involuntary muscle contractions leading to spasms and stiffness or rigidity. In MS, this condition primarily affects the lower limbs.

spinal cord: the mass of nervous tissue along the axis of an animal (within the backbone of vertebrates).

status migrainosus: migraine lasting more than 72 hours.

stenosis: narrowing of an artery due to the buildup of plaque on the inside wall of the artery.

striatum: part of the basal ganglia of the brain. The striatum is composed of the caudate nucleus, putamen, and ventral striatum; *see* basal ganglia, caudate nuclei.

stroke buckle: three southeastern states, North Carolina, South Carolina, and Georgia, that have an extremely high stroke mortality rate.

stupor: a state of impaired consciousness in which the patient is unresponsive but can be aroused briefly by a strong stimulus.

subarachnoid hemorrhage: bleeding within the meninges, or outer membranes, of the brain into the clear fluid that surrounds the brain.

subdural hematoma: bleeding confined to the area between the dura and the arachnoid membranes.

subdural hygroma: a buildup of protein rich fluid in the area between the dura and the arachnoid membranes, usually caused by a tear in the arachnoid membrane.

synapse: the tiny gap between nerve cells across which neurotransmitters pass.

synaptic vesicle: a structure in the membrane at the end of an axon that releases a neurotransmitter. **syndrome of inappropriate secretion of antidiuretic hormone (SIADH):** a condition in which excessive secretion of antidiuretic hormone leads to a sodium deficiency in the blood and abnormally concentrated urine; symptoms include weakness, lethargy, confusion, coma, seizures, or death if left untreated.

tau: a protein that helps to maintain the structure of microtubules in normal nerve cells. Abnormal tau is a principal component of the paired helical filaments in neurofibrillary tangles.

tension-type headache: a primary headache that is band-like or squeezing and does not worsen with routine activity. It may be brought on by stress.

thalamus: a small structure in the front of the cerebral hemispheres that serves as a way station that receives sensory information of all kinds and relays it to the cortex; it also receives information from the cortex.

thrombolytics: drugs used to treat an ongoing, acute ischemic stroke by dissolving the blood clot causing the stroke and thereby restoring blood flow through the artery.

thrombosis: the formation of a blood clot in one of the cerebral arteries of the head or neck that stays attached to the artery wall until it grows large enough to block blood flow.

thrombotic stroke: a stroke caused by thrombosis.

tissue necrosis factors: chemicals released by leukocytes and other cells that cause secondary cell death during the inflammatory immune response associated with the ischemic cascade.

total serum cholesterol: a combined measurement of a person's high-density lipoprotein (HDL) and low-density lipoprotein (LDL).

t-PA: *see* recombinant tissue plasminogen activator.

trait: any genetically determined characteristic. *See* dominant, gene, recessive.

transcranial magnetic stimulation (TMS): a small magnetic current delivered to an area of the brain to promote plasticity and healing.

transgenic: an animal that has had a gene (like human APP) inserted into its chromosomes. Mice carrying the mutated human APP gene often develop plaques in their brains as they age.

transient ischemic attack (TIA): a short-lived stroke that lasts from a few minutes up to 24 hours; often called a mini-stroke.

transverse myelitis: an acute spinal cord disorder causing sudden low back pain and muscle weakness and abnormal sensory sensations in the lower extremities. Transverse myelitis often remits spontaneously; however, severe or long-lasting cases may lead to permanent disability.

tremor: an involuntary trembling or quivering.

trigger: something that brings about a disease or condition.

triptans: a family of drugs used to treat migraines and cluster headaches by preventing or stopping nerve tissue inflammation and resulting changes in blood vessels.

valacyclovir: one of three available antiviral drugs that can reduce the severity and duration of a shingles attack if given soon after onset.

varicella-zoster virus: a virus that causes two distinct diseases, chickenpox and shingles. It is a member of the herpesvirus family. "Varicella" is Latin for little pox; "zoster" is the Greek word for girdle. Medically, zoster is sometimes used as a synonym for shingles.

vascular: refers to blood vessels or the flow of blood.

vascular dementia: a type of dementia caused by brain damage from cerebrovascular or cardiovascular problems, usually strokes.

vasodilators: medications that increase blood flow to the brain by expanding or dilating blood vessels.

vasospasm: a dangerous side effect of subarachnoid hemorrhage in which the blood vessels in the subarachnoid space constrict erratically, cutting off blood flow.

vegetative state: a condition in which patients are unconscious and unaware of their surroundings, but continue to have a sleep/wake cycle and can have periods of alertness.

venous sinus thrombosis: a form of stroke caused by a clot that blocks blood flow in the brain's veins.

ventricles: cavities within the brain that are filled with cerebrospinal fluid. In HD, tissue loss causes enlargement of the ventricles.

ventriculostomy: a surgical procedure that drains cerebrospinal fluid from the brain by creating an opening in one of the small cavities called ventricles.

vertebral artery: an artery on either side of the neck; *see* carotid artery.

vesicle: a small container for transporting neurotransmitters and other molecules from one part of the neuron to another.

warfarin: a commonly used anticoagulant, also known as Coumadin®.

Wernicke's aphasia: *see* fluent aphasia.

white matter: nerve fibers that are the site of many MS lesions and that connect areas of gray matter in the brain and spinal cord.

zoster sine herpete: a case of shingles in which there are no blisters or other signs of the illness on the skin.

Chapter 44

Directory of Organizations with Information about Brain Disorders

**Acoustic Neuroma
Association**
600 Peachtree Pkwy.
Ste. 108
Cumming, GA 30041
877-200-8211; Fax: 877-202-0239
http://www.anausa.org
info@anausa.org

**Agency for Healthcare
Research and Quality
(AHRQ)**
540 Gaither Rd., Ste. 2000
Rockville, MD 20850
301-427-1104
http://www.ahrq.gov

**Agency for Toxic Substances
and Disease Registry**
4770 BufoRd. Hwy. NE
Atlanta, GA 30341
800-232-4636
http://www.atsdr.cdc.gov

**AIDSInfo (AIDS Information
Service)**
P.O. Box 4780
Rockville, MD 20849-6303
800-448-0440; Fax: 301-315-2818
http://aidsinfo.nih.gov
ContactUs@aidsinfo.nih.gov

Resources in this chapter were compiled from several sources deemed reliable. Inclusion does not imply endorsement. This list is not comprehensive; it is intended as a starting point for gathering of information.

651

ALS Association
27001 Agoura Rd., Ste. 250
Calabasas Hills, CA 91301-5104
1-800-782-4747
http://www.alsa.org
alsinfo@alsa-national.org

ALS Therapy Development Institute
300 Technology Sq.
Ste. 400
Cambridge, MA 02139
617-441-7200; Fax: 617-441-7299
http://www.als.net

Alzheimer's Association
225 North Michigan Ave., Fl. 17
Chicago, IL 60601-7633
1-800-272-3900
http://www.alz.org
info@alz.org

Alzheimer's Disease Education and Referral Center (ADEAR)
P.O. Box 8250
Silver Spring, MD 20907-8250
800-438-4380; Fax: 301-495-3334
http://www.nia.nih.gov/
alzheimers
adear@nia.nih.gov

Alzheimer's Drug Discovery Foundation
57 W. 57th St.
Ste. 904
New York, NY 10019
212-901-8000; Fax: 212-901-8010
http://www.alzdiscovery.org
info@alzdiscovery.org

Alzheimer's Foundation of America
322 Eighth Ave., 7th Fl.
New York, NY 10001
866-232-8484; Fax: 646-638-1546
http://www.alzfdn.org

American Association of Neurological Surgeons
5550 Meadowbrook Dr.
Rolling Meadows, IL 60008-3852
888-566- 2267; Fax:
847-378-0600
http://www.aans.org
info@aans.org

American Autoimmune Related Diseases Association
22100 Gratiot Ave.
Eastpointe, MI 48021
800-598-4668; Fax: 586-776-3903
http://www.aaRd.a.org
aaRd.a@aaRd.a.org

American Brain Tumor Association
8550 W. Bryn Mawr Ave.
Ste. 550
Chicago, IL 60631
800-866-2282; Fax: 773-577-8738
http://www.abta.org
E-mail: info@abta.org

American Chronic Pain Association (ACPA)
P.O. Box 850
Rocklin, CA 95677
800-533-3231; Fax:
916- 632-3208
http://www.theacpa.org
ACPA@theacpa.org

*American College of
Radiology*
1891 Preston White Dr.
Reston, VA 20191
800-227-5463
http://www.acr.org
info@acr.org

*American Diabetes
Association*
1701 North BeauregaRd. St.
Alexandria, VA 22311
800- 342-2383
http://www.diabetes.org
askada@diabetes.org

*American Headache Society
Committee for Headache
Education (ACHE)*
19 Mantua Rd.
Mt. Royal, NJ 08061
856-423-0043; Fax: 856-423-0082
http://www.achenet.org
achehq@talley.com

American Heart Association
7272 Greenville Ave.
Dallas, TX 75231
800- 242-8721
http://www.heart.org
inquiries@heart.org

*American Stroke Association:
A Division of American
Heart Association*
7272 Greenville Ave.
Dallas, TX 75231
1-888-478-7653; Fax:
214-706-5231
http://www.strokeassociation.org

*American Syringomyelia
& Chiari Alliance Project
(ASAP)*
P.O. Box 1586
Longview, TX 75606-1586
800- 272-7282); Fax:
903-757-7456
http://www.asap.org
info@asap.org

Angioma Alliance
520 W. 21st St.
Ste. G2-411
Norfolk, VA 23517 -1950
Fax: 757-623-0616
http://www. angiomaalliance.org
info@angioma.org

*Antiepileptic Drug
Pregnancy Registry*
Massachusetts General Hospital
121 Innerbelt Rd.
Rm. 220
Somerville, MA 02143
888- 233-2334; Fax:
617-724-8307
http://www2.massgeneral.org/aed/
info@aedpregnancyregistry.org

*ARCH National Respite
Network and Resource
Center*
4016 Oxford. St.
Annandale, VA 22003
703.256.2084; Fax: 703.256.0541
http://www.archrespite.org
jkagan@archrespite.org

Association for Frontotemporal Degeneration (AFTD)
Radnor Station Bldg. 2
Ste. 320
290 King of Prussia Rd.
Radnor, PA 19087
866-507-7222
http://www.theaftd.org
info@theaftd.org

Batten Disease Support and Research Association
1175 Dublin Rd.
Columbus, OH 43215
800-448-4570; Fax: 866-648-8718
http://www.bdsra.org
bdsra1@bdsra.org

Birth Defect Research for Children, Inc.
976 Lake Baldwin Ln.
Ste. 104
Orlando, FL 32814
407-895-0802
http://www.birthdefects.org
staff@birthdefects.org

Brain Aneurysm Foundation
269 Hanover St., Bldg. 3
Hanover, MA 02339
888-272-4602; Fax: 781-826-5566
http://www.bafound.org
office@bafound.org

Brain Attack Coalition
Bldg. 31, Rm. 8A-16
31 Center Dr., MSC 2540
Bethesda, MD 20892
301-496-5751; Fax: 301-468-5981
http://www.brainattackcoalition.org/

Brain Injury Association of America, Inc.
1608 Spring Hill Rd.
Ste. 110
Vienna, VA 22182
800-444-6443; Fax: 703-761-0755
http://www.biausa.org
braininjuryinfo@biausa.org

Brain Injury Resource Center
Phone: 206-621-8558
http://www.headinjury.com
brain@headinjury.com

Brain Resources and Information Network (BRAIN)
National Institute of Neurological Disorders & Stroke
P.O. Box 5801
Bethesda, MD 20824
800-352-9424; Fax: 301-402-2186
http://www.ninds.nih.gov
braininfo@ninds.nih.gov

Brain Trauma Foundation
7 World Trade Center
34th Fl.
250 Greenwich St.
New York, NY 10017
212-772-0608; Fax: 212-772-0357
http://www.braintrauma.org

BrightFocus Foundation
22512 Gateway Center Dr.
Clarksburg, MD 20871
1- 800-437-2423; Fax:
301-258-9454
http://www.brightfocus.org/alzheimers/
info@brightfocus.org

Caregiver Action Network
1130 Connecticut Ave. NW
Ste. 300
Washington, DC 20036
Phone: (202) 454-3970
http://www.caregiveraction.org/
info@caregiveraction.org

Centers for Disease Control and Prevention (CDC)
U.S. Department of Health and Human Services
1600 Clifton Rd., N.E.
Atlanta, GA 30333 -4027
800 -232-4636
http://www.cdc.gov

Center for Parent Information and Resources
c/o Statewide Parent Advocacy Network
35 Halsey St., Fourth Fl.
Newark, NJ 07102
http://www.parentcenterhub.org/
contact-us/
malizo@spannj.org

Cerebral Palsy International Research Foundation
3 Columbus Cir., 15th Fl.
New York, NY 10019
212-520-1686;
http://www.cpirf.org
info@cpirf.org

Charcot-Marie-Tooth Association (CMTA)
PO Box 105
Glenolden, PA 19036
800-606- 2682; Fax:
610-499-9267
http://www.cmtausa.org/
info@cmtausa.org

Chiari & Syringomyelia Foundation
29 Crest Loop
Staten Island, NY 10312
718-966-2593
http://www.csfinfo.org
info@CSFinfo.org

Children's Hemiplegia and Stroke Assocn. (CHASA)
4101 W. Green Oaks, Ste.. 305
PMB 149
Arlington, TX 76016
http://www.chasa.org

Citizens United for Research in Epilepsy (CURE)
430 W. Erie
Ste. 210
Chicago, IL 60654
312-255-1801; Fax: 312-255-1809
http://www.CUREepilepsy.org
info@CUREepilepsy.org

CJD Aware!
2527 South Carrollton Ave.
New Orleans, LA 70118-3013
504-861-4627
http://www.cjdaware.com
cjdaware@iwon.com; info@
cjdaware.com

Columbia-Presbyterian Medical Center
Lucy G. Moses Center for Memory and Behavioral Disorders
Neurological Institute
710 W. 168th St., 3Rd. Fl.4
New York, NY
212-305-6939
http://cumc.columbia.edu/dept/
neurology/memory

Creutzfeldt-Jakob Disease (CJD) Foundation Inc.
341 W. 38th St., Ste. 501
New York, NY 10018
800-659-1991; Fax: 212-256-0359
http://www.cjdfoundation.org
help@cjdfoundation.org

CurePSP
30 East Padonia Rd., Ste. 201
Timonium, MD 21093
800-457-4777
http://www.curepsp.org

Dana Alliance for Brain Initiatives
505 Fifth Ave., 6th Fl.
New York, NY 10017
212-223-4040
http://www.dana.org/
danaalliances
dabiinfo@dana.org

EaSte.r Seals
233 South Wacker Dr.
Ste. 2400
Chicago, IL 60606
800-221-6827; Fax: 312-726-1494
http://www.eaSte.rseals.com

Eldercare Locator
1-800-677-1116
http://www.eldercare.gov

Elizabeth Glaser Pediatric AIDS Foundation
1140 Connecticut Ave., NW
Ste. 200
Washington, DC 20036
888-499- 4673; Fax:
202-296-9185
http://www.pedaids.org
info@pedaids.org

Epilepsy Foundation
8301 Professional Place East,
Ste. 200
Landover, MD 20785-7223
800- 332-1000; Fax:
301- 459-1569
http://www.epilepsy.com
ContactUs@efa.org

Family Caregiver Alliance
785 Market St., Ste. 750
San Francisco, CA 94103
1-800-445-8106
http://www.caregiver.org

Center on Technology and Disability
1825 Connecticut Ave. NW
Washington DC 20009
202-884-8588
http:// www.ctdinstitute.org
E-mail: ctd@fhi360.org

Fibromuscular Dysplasia Society of America (FMDSA)
20325 Center Ridge Rd.
Ste. 360
Rocky River, OH 44116
888-709-7089
http://www.fmdsa.org/
admin@fmdsa.org

U.S. Food and Drug Administration (FDA)
10903 New Hampshire Ave.
Silver Spring, MD 20993
888-463-6332
http://www.fda.gov

**The Foundation for
Peripheral Neuropathy**
485 Half Day Rd.
Ste. 350
Buffalo Grove, IL 60089
877-883-9942; Fax: 847-883-9960
http://www.foundationforpn.org
info@tffpn.org

**Friedreich's Ataxia Research
Alliance (FARA)**
533 W. Uwchlan Ave.
Downingtown, PA 19335
484-879-6160; Fax: 484-872-1402
http://www.CureFA.org
info@CureFA.org

FTD Support Forum
www.ftdsupportforum.com

Genetic Alliance, Inc.
4301 Connecticut Ave., N.W.
Ste. 404
Washington, DC 20008-2369
800 336- 4363; Fax:
202-966-8553
http://www.geneticalliance.org
info@geneticalliance.org

**Hazel K. Goddess Fund for
Stroke Research in Women**
785 Park Ave. #3E
New York, NY 10021
561-623-0504; Fax: 561.623.0502
http://www.thegoddessfund.org
anne@thegoddessfund.org

Heart Rhythm Society
1325 G St., NW
Ste. 400
Washington, DC 20005
202-464-3400; Fax: 202-464-3401
http://www.hrsonline.org/
info@HRSonline.org

**Hereditary Disease
Foundation**
3960 Broadway
6th Fl.
New York, NY 10032
212-928-2121; Fax: 212-928-2172
http://www.hdfoundation.org/
home.php
cures@hdfoundation.org

**Hide and Seek Foundation
for Lysosomal Disease
Research**
http://www.hideandseek.org

**Hope for Hypothalamic
Hamartomas (Hope for HH)**
P. O. Box 721
Waddell, AZ 85355
http://hopeforhh.org/
admin@hopeforhh.org

**Huntington's Disease Society
of America**
505 Eighth Ave.
Ste. 902
New York, NY 10018
800-345- 4372
http://hdsa.org
hdsainfo@hdsa.org

Hydrocephalus Association
4340 East W. Hwy.
Ste. 905
Bethesda, MD 20814-4447
888-598-3789; Fax: 301-202-3813
http://www.hydroassoc.org
E-mail: info@hydroassoc.org

*Indiana University School of
Medicine*
Indiana Alzheimer's Disease
Center
355 W. 16th St., Ste. 4100
Indianapolis, IN 46202
317-963-5500; Fax: 317-963-7547
http://iadc.iupui.edu

*International RadioSurgery
Association*
2960 Green St.
P.O. Box 5186
Harrisburg, PA 17110
717-260-9808; Fax: 717-260-9809
http://www.irsa.org
irsa@irsa.org

*Intracranial Hypertension
Research Foundation*
6517 Buena Vista Dr.
Vancouver, WA 98661
360-693-4473; Fax: 360-694-7062
http://www.IHRFoundation.org
contact@ihrfoundation.org

*Intractable Childhood
Epilepsy Alliance*
http://www.ice-epilepsy.org
info@ice-epilepsy.org

*John Douglas French
Alzheimer's Foundation*
11620 Wilshire Blvd.
Ste. 270
Los Angeles, CA 90025
http://www.jdfaf.org
jdfaf@earthlink.net

*Johns Hopkins University
School of Medicine*
Department of Psychiatry and
Behavioral Sciences
Meyer 4-113, Chairman's Office
600 North Wolfe St.
Baltimore, MD 21287-7413
410-955-5212
http://www.hopkinsmedicine.
org/Psychiatry/specialty_areas/
neuropsychiatry/

Lee Allison Company
1820 W. Webster Ave., #301
Chicago, IL 60614-2927
888-434-8437; Fax: 773-276-7184
http://www.leeallison.com/
info@leeallison.com

Les Turner ALS Foundation
5550 W. Touhy Ave.
Ste. 302
Skokie, IL 60077-3254
888-679-3311; Fax: 847-679-9109
http://www.lesturnerals.org
info@lesturnerals.org

*Lewy Body Dementia
Association*
912 Killian Hill Rd., S.W.
Lilburn, GA 30047
800-539-9767; Fax: 480-422-5434
http://www.lbda.org

LGS Foundation
192 Lexington Ave.
Ste. 212
New York, NY 10016
718-374-3800
http://lgsfoundation.org/index.
html
info@lgsfoundation.org

March of Dimes
1275 Mamaroneck Ave.
White Plains, NY 10605
888-663-4637
http://www.marchofdimes.com
askus@marchofdimes.com

Massachusetts General Hospital
Frontotemporal Disorders Unit
Boston, MA
1-617-726-5571
http://www.ftd-boston.org

Mayo Clinic
Department of Neurology
http://www.mayoclinic.org

Meningitis Foundation of America, Inc.
P.O. Box 1818
El Mirage, AZ 85335
480-270-2652
http://www.musa.org

Michael J. Fox Foundation for Parkinson's Research
Grand Central Stn.
P.O. Box 4777
New York, NY 10163-4777
800-708-7644
http://www.michaeljfox.org

Migraine Research Foundation
300 East 75th St.
Ste. 3K
New York, NY 10021
212-249-5402; Fax: 212-249-5405
http://www.
migraineresearchfoundation.org
contactmrf@
migraineresearchfoundation.org

Multiple Sclerosis Association of America
706 Haddonfield Rd.
Cherry Hill, NJ 08002
800-532-7667; Fax: 856-661-9797
http://www.msassociation.org
msaa@mymsaa.org

Multiple Sclerosis Foundation
6520 North Andrews Ave.
Ft. Lauderdale, FL 33309-2130
888-MSFOCUS (673-6287); Fax:
954-351-0630
http://www.msfocus.org
support@msfocus.org

Muscular Dystrophy Association
National Office - 222 S.
Riverside Plaza
Ste. 1500
Chicago, IL 60606
800-572-1717; Fax: 520-529-5300
http://www.mda.org
mda@mdausa.org

Myelin Repair Foundation
18809 Cox Ave.
Ste. 190
Saratoga, CA 95070
408-871-2410
http://www.myelinrepair.org/
info@myelinrepair.org

Narcolepsy Network, Inc.
129 Ripple Ln.
North Kingstown, RI 02852
888-292-6522; Fax: 401-633-6567
http://www.narcolepsynetwork.
org
narnet@narcolepsynetwork.org

*Nathan's Battle Foundation
[For Batten Disease
Research]*
459 South State Rd. 135
Greenwood, IN 46142
317-888-7396; Fax: 317-888-0504
http://www.nathansbattle.com
pmilto@indy.net

*National Academy of Elder
Law Attorneys, Inc.*
1577 Spring Hill Rd., Ste. 220
Vienna, VA 22182
703-942-5711; Fax: 703-563-9504
http://www.naela.org

*National Ataxia Foundation
(NAF)*
2600 Fernbrook Ln.
Ste. 119
Minneapolis, MN 55447
763-553-0020; Fax: 763-553-0167
http://www.ataxia.org
naf@ataxia.org

*National Cancer Institute
(NCI)*
NCI Public Inquiries Office
9609 Medical Center Dr.
Bethesda, MD 20892-9760
800-422-6237
http://www.cancer.gov

*National Council on Patient
Information and Education*
200-A Monroe St.
Ste. 212
Rockville, MD 20850-4448
301-340-3940; Fax: 301-340-3944
http://www.talkaboutrx.org
ncpie@ncpie.info

*National Diabetes
Information Clearinghouse
(NDIC)*
1 Information Way
Bethesda, MD 20892-3560
800-860-8747; Fax:
703–738–4929
http://www.diabetes.niddk.nih.
gov
ndic@info.niddk.nih.gov

National Eye Institute (NEI)
National Institutes of Health,
DHHS
31 Center Dr., Rm. 6A32 MSC
2510
Bethesda, MD 20892-2510
301-496-5248
http://www.nei.nih.gov
2020@nei.nih.gov

National Headache Foundation
820 N. Orleans
Ste. 411
Chicago, IL 60610-3131
http://www.headaches.org
info@headaches.org

National Heart, Lung, and Blood Institute (NHLBI)
NHLBI Health Information
Center
P.O. Box 30105
Bethesda, MD 20824-0105
301-592-8573
http://www.nhlbi.nih.gov
nhlbiinfo@nhlbi.nih.gov

National Hospice and Palliative Care Organization
1731 King St.
Alexandria, VA 22314
800-658-8898; Fax: 703-837-1233
http://www.nhpco.org
E-mail: consumers@nhpco.org

National Hydrocephalus Foundation
12413 Centralia Rd.
Lakewood, CA 90715-1653
888-857-3434
http://nhfonline.org
info@nhfonline.org

National Institute of Child Health and Human Development (NICHD)
National Institutes of Health,
DHHS
31 Center Dr.,
Bldg. 31, Rm. 2A32
Bethesda, MD 20892-2425
800-370-2943; Fax: 866-760-5947
http://www.nichd.nih.gov

National Institute of Mental Health (NIMH)
Science Writing, Press, and
Dissemination Branch
6001 Executive Blvd.
Rm. 6200, MSC 9663
Bethesda, MD 20892-9663
866-615-6464; Fax: 301-443-4279
http://www.nimh.nih.gov
nimhinfo@nih.gov

National Institute of Neurological DisoRd.ers and Stroke
P.O. Box 5801
Bethesda, MD 20894
800-352-9424
http://www.ninds.nih.gov

National Institute on Aging (NIA)
Bldg. 31, Rm. 5C27
31 Center Dr., MSC 2292
Bethesda, MD 20892-2292
800-222-2225
http://www.nia.nih.gov
niaic@nia.nih.gov

National Institute on Disability and Rehabilitation Research (NIDRR)
U.S. Department of Education
Office of Special Education and
Rehabilitative Services
400 Maryland Ave., S.W.
Washington, DC 20202-7100
202-245-7459
http://www.ed.gov/about/offices/
list/osers/nidrr

National Kidney & Urologic Diseases Information Clearinghouse (NKUDIC)
3 Information Way
Bethesda, MD 20892-3580
800-891-5390
http://www.niddk.nih.gov
nkudic@info.niddk.nih.gov

National Library of Medicine (NLM)
8600 Rockville Pike, Bldg. 38,
Rm. 2S10
Bethesda, MD 20894
888-346-3656; Fax: 301-402-1384
http://www.nlm.nih.gov

National Meningitis Association, Inc.
P.O. Box 60143
Ft. Myers, FL 33906
866-366-3662; Fax: 877-703-6096
http://www.nmaus.org

National Multiple Sclerosis Society
733 Third Ave., 3rd. Fl.
New York, NY 10017
800-344-4867; Fax: 212-986-7981
http://www.nationalmssociety.
org
info@msnyc.org

National NeuroAIDS Tissue Consortium
401 N. Washington St.
Ste. 700
Rockville, MD 20850
866-668-2272; Fax: 301-576-4597
https://nntc.org/
nntc@emmes.com

National Organization for Rare Disorders (NORD.)
55 Kenosia Ave.
Danbury, CT 06810
800-999-NORD. (6673); Fax:
203-798-2291
http://www.rarediseases.org
orphan@rarediseases.org

National Parkinson Foundation, Inc.
200 SE 1st St.
Ste. 800
Miami, FL 33131
1-800-473-4636
http://www.parkinson.org
contact@parkinson.org

National Prevention Information Network
https://npin.cdc.gov/NPIN
info@cdc.gov

National Rehabilitation Information Center (NARIC)
8201 Corporate Dr.
Ste. 600
Landover, MD 20785
800-346-2742; Fax: 301-459-4263
http://www.naric.com
naricinfo@heitechservices.com

National Shingles Foundation [For Research on Varicella Zoster]
603 W. 115 St.
371
New York, NY 10025
212-222-3390; Fax: 212-222-8627
http://www.vzvfoundation.org
Shingles@ShinglesFoundation.org

National Sleep Foundation
1010 N. Glebe Rd.
Ste. 310
Arlington, VA 22201
703-243-1697
http://www.sleepfoundation.org
nsf@sleepfoundation.org

National Stroke Association
9707 East Easter Ln.
Ste. B
Centennial, CO 80112
800-787-6537; Fax: 303-649-1328
http://www.stroke.org
info@stroke.org

Neurologic AIDS Research Consortium
Department of Neurology
Washington School of Medicine
Campus Box 8111
660 S. Euclid Ave.
St. Louis, MO 63110
Fax: 314-747-8177
http://neuro.wustl.edu/
patientcare/clinicalservices/narc/

Neuropathy Association
110 W. 40th St.
Ste. 1804
New York, NY 10018
212-692-0662; Fax: 212-692-0668
http://www.neuropathy.org
info@neuropathy.org

NIAID Office of Communications and Government Relations
5601 Fishers Ln., MSC 9806
Bethesda, MD 20892-9806
866-284-4107; Fax: 301-402-3573
http://www.niaid.nih.gov
ocpostoffice@niaid.nih.gov

Northwestern University Feinberg School of Medicine
Cognitive Neurology and
Alzheimer's Disease Center
320 E Superior, Searle 11
Chicago, IL 60611
312-908-9339; Fax: 312-908-8789
http://www.brain.northW.e.rn.edu
CNADC-Admin@northW.e.rn.edu

Office of Rare Diseases Research
National Center for Advancing Translational Sciences (NCATS)
National Institutes of Health,
6701 Democracy Blvd
Ste. 1001, Bethesda, MD 20892
301-402-4336,
http://rarediseases.info.nih.gov
info@ncats.nih.gov

Office of Special Education & Rehabilitative Services
U.S. Department of Education
400 Maryland Ave., SW
Washington, DC 20202-7100
202-245-7468
http://www.ed.gov/about/offices/list/osers

Paralyzed Veterans of America (PVA)
801 18th St., NW
Washington, DC 20006-3517
800-232-1782; Fax: 800-795-4327
http://www.pva.org
info@pva.org

Parkinson's Disease Foundation
1359 Broadway, Ste. 1509
New York, NY 10018
800-457-6676; Fax: 212-923-4778
http://www.pdf.org
info@pdf.org

Pathways
150 N. Michigan Ave.
Chicago, IL 60601
800-955- 2445; Fax:
312-893-6621
http://www.pathways.org
friends@pathways.org

Patient Recruitment and Public Liaison Office Clinical Center National Institutes of Health
10 Cloister Ct., Bldg. 61
Bethesda, MD 20892
800-411-1222; Fax: 866-411-1010
http://clinicalcenter.nih.gov/
prpl@mail.cc.nih.gov

Pedal-with-Pete Foundation [for Research on Cerebral Palsy]
P.O. Box 1233
Worthington, OH 43085
614-527-0202
http://www.pedal-with-pete.org
pwp@pedal-with-pete.org

Pediatric Brain Foundation
2925 E. Battlefield Rd. Ste. 225B
Springfield, MO 65804
310-889.8611
http://www.
pediatricbrainfoundation.org/
info@pediatricbrainfoundation.
org

Pediatric Hydrocephalus Foundation, Inc.
66 Caroline St.
2nd Fl. Woodbridge, NJ 07095
732-634-1283; Fax: 847-589-1250
http://www.hydrocephaluskids.
org
info@hydrocephaluskids.org

PPA Support Group
www.groups.yahoo.com/group/
PPA-support

Prize4Life
P.O. Box 5755
Berkeley, CA 94705
617-545-4882
http://www.prize4life.org
contact@prize4life.org

Project ALS
801 Riverside Dr.
Ste. 6G
New York, NY 10032
855-900-2257; Fax: 646-559-9290
http://www.projectals.org
info@projectals.org

Radiological Society of North America
820 Jorie Blvd.
Oak Brook, IL 60523-2251
800-381-6660; Fax: 630-571-7837
http://www.rsna.org

RE Children's Project
79 Christie Hill Rd.
Darien, CT 06820
http://www.rechildrens.org
swohlberg@rechildrens.com

Restless Legs Syndrome Foundation
3006 Bee Caves Rd.
Ste. D206
Austin, Texas 78746
512-366-9109; Fax: 507-287-6312
http://www.rls.org
info@rls.org

Spina Bifida Association
1600 Wilson Blvd.
Ste. 800
Arlington, VA 22209
202-944-3285; Fax: 202-944-3295
http://www.
spinabifidaassociation.org
sbaa@sbaa.org

The Charlie Foundation for Ketogenic Therapies
515 Ocean Ave.
Ste. 602N
Santa Monica, CA 90402
310-393-2347
http://www.charliefoundation.
org

United Cerebral Palsy (UCP)
1825 K St NW
Ste. 600
Washington, DC 20006
800-872-5827
http://www.ucp.org
info@ucp.org

United Leukodystrophy Foundation
224 North Second St.
Ste. 2
DeKalb, IL 60115
800-728-5483; Fax: 815-748-0844
http://www.ulf.org
office@ulf.org

University of California, Los Angeles
Frontotemporal Dementia &
Neurobehavior Clinic
300 UCLA Medical Plaza
Ste. B200
Los Angeles, CA 90095
310-794-1195; Fax: 310-794-7491
http://www.ftd.ucla.edu/clinic

University of California, San Francisco
Memory and Aging Center
Sandler Neurosciences Center
675 Nelson Rising Ln.
Ste. 190
San Francisco, CA
1-415-476-0670
http://www.memory.ucsf.edu/ftd
webmaSte.r@memory.ucsf.edu

University of Pennsylvania Health System
Penn Frontotemporal
Degeneration Center
3 W. Gates
3400 Spruce St.
Philadelphia, PA 19104
215-349-5863; Fax: 215-349-8464
http://ftd.med.upenn.edu

Wake Up Narcolepsy
P.O. Box 60293
Worcester, MA 01606
978-751-3693
http://www.wakeupnarcolepsy.
org
info@wakeupnarcolepsy.org

Well Spouse Association
63 W. Main St.
Ste. H
Freehold, NJ 07728
800-838-0879; Fax: 732-577-8644
http://www.wellspouse.org
info@wellspouse.org

World Health Organization
Ave. Appia 20
1211 Geneva 27
Switzerland
(+ 41 22)791 2111; Fax: (+ 41 22)791 3111
http://www.who.int,
info@who.int

YoungStroke, Inc.
P.O. Box 692
Conway, SC 29528
843-655-2835
http://www.youngstroke.org
info@youngstroke.org

Index

Index

Page numbers followed by 'n' indicate a footnote. Page numbers in *italics* indicate a table or illustration.